The Perfect
Gene Diet

The Perfect Gene Diet

Use Your Body's Own Apo E Gene
and an Integrative-Medicine Approach
to Treat High Cholesterol, Weight Problems,
Heart Disease, Alzheimer's . . . and More

Pamela McDonald, N.P.

HAY HOUSE, INC.
Carlsbad, California • New York City
London • Sydney • Johannesburg
Vancouver • Hong Kong • New Delhi

Published and distributed in the United States by: Hay House, Inc.: www.hayhouse.com • *Published and distributed in Australia by:* Hay House Australia Pty. Ltd.: www.hayhouse .com.au • *Published and distributed in the United Kingdom by:* Hay House UK, Ltd.: www .hayhouse.co.uk • *Published and distributed in the Republic of South Africa by:* Hay House SA (Pty), Ltd.: www.hayhouse.co.za • *Distributed in Canada by:* Raincoast: www.raincoast.com • *Published in India by:* Hay House Publishers India: www.hayhouse.co.in

Originally published in 2007 by Penscott Management Corporation under the title *The Apo E Gene Diet.* "The Apo E Gene Diet" is a trademark of Penscott Management Corporation. "Apo E Gene Diet," patent pending.

Design: The Vivere Design Team

Library of Congress Control Number: 2010920949

ISBN: 978-1-4019-2848-3
Digital ISBN: 978-1-4019-2937-4

13 12 11 10   4 3 2 1
1st edition, October 2010

Printed in the United States of America

For
Granddad,
Richard,
Victoria,
Alison,
and Paige.

Just use love

Contents

Foreword by Dr. Wayne W. Dyer xiii

WHY I WROTE THIS BOOK xv
The Role of Nutrition and Integrative Medicine xix
How Can This Book Help You Now? xxi

INTRODUCTION
How to Use This Book 1

CHAPTER ONE
Backpack or Bedpan, Health Is a Choice 3
Diet and Gene Interactions Shape the Potential for Health or Disease . . . 5
Genetic Risk and Family History 5

CHAPTER TWO
An Introduction to the Apo E Gene 7
What Exactly Do We Mean by Genes? 9
What Is the Apo E Gene? 10
2.1 Percentage of Apo E Genotypes in the General Population. 10
What Does Apo E Mean? 11
Making Connections: Genotype, Gene-Supportive
   Environment, and State of Health 11
Inflammation: A Poor Match Between Environment and Genotype . . 12
You Are What You Eat 13

CHAPTER THREE
**The Connection Between a Gene-Supportive Environment
and the Apo E Gene** 15
Cardiovascular Disease and the Apo E Gene 16
Not All Cholesterol Is Bad 17
Looking Deeper into the Cholesterol Pots: LDL and HDL 18
First, the Bad News: LDL Cholesterol, Large and Small 19
Artery Wall Disease Progression 20
LDL Pattern B: Why Is It Dangerous? 21
The Good News: HDL2b 22
Two Healing Worlds 23
3.1 Optimal Cholesterol Screening Panel Results 27
Your Cholesterol Level and the Apo E Gene 27
The Interconnections among Environmental Factors 28
Alzheimer's Disease and the Apo E Gene. 29
Future Directions—A Useful Genetic Test to Help Guide Your Diet . . 30
Genetic Risk and Family History 31
A Patient's Story: Sam 32
How Different Genotypes Use Fuel Differently 34
3.2 Food-Type Preferences of Apo E Genotypes 34
Caloric Requirements and Your Optimal Health 35
3.3 Sample Meal Schedule 36
3.4 Incorrect Fuel Delivery 37
3.5 Correct Fuel Delivery 37
Multilevel Stress 38
A Patient's Story: Dr. Amanda 41
3.6 Apo E Gene-Supportive Environment (GSE) 43

CHAPTER FOUR
Setting the Stage for the Apo E Gene and Diet 45
General Recommendations for Implementing a
   Diet Based on the Apo E Gene 47
General Recommendations for Optimal Health 48

CHAPTER FIVE
Apo E Gene Testing and Advanced Cholesterol Testing 51
Apo E Gene Testing and You 52
Advanced Cholesterol Testing 54
Dietary Options Without Testing 55
A Patient's Story: Dora 56
Protecting Your Medical Records 58
How to Get Tested 58

CHAPTER SIX
Now That You Know Your Apo E Genotype 59
My Story: Pam 60
How to Choose a Medical Provider 63
Selecting a Medical Practitioner 64
Integrative-Medicine Resources 65
Learning Who You Are—Self-Exploration 65
A Patient's Story: Rebecca 66
Integrative-Medicine Questionnaire 67

CHAPTER SEVEN
Making the Changes You Want to Make 73
Stages of Change 74
Connecting with a Support Person 77
At a Glance—Principles and Behaviors to Always Consider 81

CHAPTER EIGHT
Food: The Foundation 83
Carbohydrates 83
Carbohydrates, Glycemic Index, and Glycemic Load 84
A Patient's Story: Alexis 85
Fat 86
Protein 87
Major Food Categories: What They Do, and How 88
How Food Becomes Fuel 89
Popular Diets Are Harmful to Your Health 90
A Patient's Story: Scott 91
Popular Diet Review 94

CHAPTER NINE
Good Food, Bad Food 97
Mega-Fake Food World 98
Toxins and Processed Foods 100
So What Can We Do? 102
A "Normal" Day's Diet 103
Decaffeinated Coffee May Increase Disease Risk 104
Toxins, Genotype, and Toxin-Clearing Abilities 106

CHAPTER TEN
Fat City 109
Fats, Inflammation, and the Immune System 110
The Good: Fats That Decrease Inflammation in the Body 113
The Bad: Saturated Fats 115
The Ugly: Trans Fats 116
How to Avoid Trans Fat 118
Garbage In = Garbage Out (GIGO) 119
How Much Protein Do We Need? 119
Milk Protein 120

CHAPTER ELEVEN
Individual Medical and Nutritional Recommendations
Based on Apo E Genotype 123
Recommendations for the Apo E 2/2 Genotype 124
Recommendations for the Apo E 2/3 Genotype 124
Recommendations for the Apo E 3/3 Genotype 125
Recommendations for the Apo E 4/2 Genotype 126
Recommendations for the Apo E 4/3 Genotype 127
Recommendations for the Apo E 4/4 Genotype 128
Diet, Hygiene, and Dental Health 129

CHAPTER TWELVE
Movement and Exercise 131
A Patient's Story: Lilian 132
Health Benefits of Exercise. 133
Elements of a Safe and Healthy Exercise Program 135
Exercise Warning Signs 136
Evaluating Your Overall Health 137
Guidelines for Beginning an Exercise Program 140
Exercise Zone Scale and Exercise Effort Level 143
12.1 Percentage of Nutrients Used by Genotype
    for each Recommended Exercise Plan 144
Garbage In = Garbage Out—Again. 145
What a Complete Exercise Program Should Contain 146
Flexibility Training Prescription 147
Stretching Exercises 148
Strength Exercises 151
Progressive Exercise Schedule 156
A Patient's Story: James 161
Pedometer Program Log. 166
Daily Food Log 167

CHAPTER THIRTEEN
Healthy Foods and Other Nutrients. 169
Water 169
Apo E Gene Top 15 Healthy Foods. 171
Garlic: Our Aromatic Friend 171
The Mysterious Mushroom. 172
Tea Therapy 174
Take a Tea Break. 175
Ginger 176
Ginger Beer Recipe. 176
Dark Chocolate 177
Soy—An Excellent Food, with Cautions 177
A Patient's Story: Jeff 178
Smart Foods 181
13.1 Key Types of Phytochemicals and Phytonutrients 182

Alcohol—Good or Bad? 182
Sodium in the Diet. 184
Micronutrients 186
Choosing Dietary Supplements or Vitamins 187

CHAPTER FOURTEEN
Shopping and Dining Tips for Health 189
Restaurants 191
Mindful Dining: Setting a Table Fit for a King and Queen 194
Learning from Our Past 194

CHAPTER FIFTEEN
The Harmony of Mind, Emotions, Body, and Spirit 199
Evidence of the Mind/Emotion/Body Connection 201
Levels of Awareness 202
Where Are *You* in This Model? 207
How Does This All Fit into a Diet Based on the Apo E Gene? 207
Learning Who You Are and What You Want 208

CHAPTER SIXTEEN
Tools for Change 217
Expressive Arts Therapy 217
Mindful Breathing 218
Meditation 219
Meditation/Visualization Chakra Chart 223
Guided Imagery 224
Gratitude 225
A Day with God (Whoever/Whatever "God" Is to You) 226

CHAPTER SEVENTEEN
Planning and Supporting Your Nutritional Change 231
The Sense of Taste and Nutritional Change 231
A Patient's Story: Janet 232
Personal Nutritional Change Process 234
17.1 Sample Nutritional Change Plan Form 234
17.2 Nutritional Change Plan Form 235
Supporting Nutritional Changes 236
Making Nutritional Change 237

CHAPTER EIGHTEEN
Steps to Determining Your Diet Based on the Apo E Gene 243
The Apo E Gene-Supportive Environment—Evaluation Levels 244
A Diet Plan That's Right for You, Based on Your Apo E Gene 245
Step 1: Determine the Calories Required for Daily Activities 245
Step 2: Determine Your Body Composition—
    The Bathroom Scale and Beyond 246
Bio-Impedance—Body-Composition Test 248
Exercise: Finding Your Ideal Body Composition 248
18.1 Lean Mass Recommendation for Males and Females 249

18.2 Body Mass Index (BMI) 250
Step 3: Identify the Perfect Gene Diet Nutritional
   Recommendations for Your Genotype 252
Apo E Menu Suggestion Plans for Each Genotype
   and Different Caloric Levels. 255
Food Exchange List 256

CHAPTER NINETEEN
Sample Meal Plans by Genotype and Calorie Allowance 261
Important Points to Remember 262
Suggested Diets: Apo E 4/4 264
Suggested Diets: Apo E 4/3 275
Suggested Diets: Apo E 4/2 286
Suggested Diets: Apo E 3/3 298
Suggested Diets: Apo E 2/3 310
Suggested Diets: Apo E 2/2 322

CHAPTER TWENTY
Recipes for the Apo E Gene 333
Apo E Gene Breakfasts 338
History of Scottish Oatmeal 339
Apo E Gene Soups 349
Apo E Gene Entrées 355
Apo E Gene Vegetarian Entrées 360
Apo E Gene Pacific Rim Sauces and Salsa 366
Apo E Gene Salads and Salad Dressings 372
Apo E Gene Side Dishes. 377
Food for Thought 382
Happy Families and a Cornish Tradition—Pasties 383
The Magic Ingredient for Cornish Pasties 387
Apo E Gene Desserts 389
Consider Black Currants. 390
Apo E Gene Teas 397
Apo E Gene Waters and Iced Tea/Lemonades 401
Apo E Gene Herbs for Cooking and Health 403

APPENDIX A
Optimal Nutrition for Babies and Young Children 405
Breast Milk and the Apo E Gene. 407
Recommendations of the American Academy of Pediatrics 407
Nutritional Value of Breast Milk. 408
Nutritional Concerns about Formula 408
Physical and Psychological Benefits to Baby and Mother 409
Infant Nutrition and the Apo E Gene 411
Nutritional Recommendations by Age and Genotype 411
Introducing Solid Foods 411
Nutrient Recommendations for Apo E Genotypes 414

APPENDIX B
Apo E Gene Additional Calorie Levels. 417
Apo E 2/2: 1,200–3,600-Calorie Serving Sizes 418
Apo E 2/3: 1,200–3,600-Calorie Serving Sizes 418
Apo E 3/3: 1,200–3,600-Calorie Serving Sizes 419
Apo E 4/2: 1,200–3,600-Calorie Serving Sizes 419
Apo E 4/3 and 4/4: 1,200–3,600-Calorie Serving Sizes 420

APPENDIX C
Autism Diagnoses, Nutrition, and Windows of Opportunity 421

APPENDIX D
Apo E Gene Research 427

APPENDIX E
Anonymous Apo E and Advanced Cholesterol Testing 431
Select the Testing Kit You Want 431
Apo E Gene Seminars. 432
Apo E Gene Testing Companies 432

Acknowledgments 433

About the Author. 436

Foreword

by Dr. Wayne W. Dyer

The book you now hold in your hands can and will not only change your life for the better, but if you read and apply it seriously, it will very likely save you from an unnecessarily early demise. This is quite a claim, and the reason I can speak from such an authoritative position is because that is precisely what it has done for me.

I have heard it said that a coincidence is nothing more than God hiding behind a cloud and smiling. Well, the day that Pam McDonald came into my life, God was not only smiling behind that cloud, but I'm certain that he was winking and clapping for having arranged such a fortuitous meeting.

Pam and one of her colleagues had come to Maui to meet with me and share some of the enormous successes they'd had in treating patients with serious disease via the new integrative-medical science, in combination with the teachings I've been speaking about publicly for the past 35 or so years. They didn't know exactly where I lived, so they both followed their intuitive knowing and simply waited in the grassy area near the beach in west Maui where I live part-time. On the day we met, I had just returned from a visit to a medical team and had been informed that I was living with a medical condition called Chronic Lymphocyte Leukemia (CLL). Someone or something smiling from behind the cloud urged me to go outside and take a walk on a path that I had never taken before at a time when I had never exercised before. As I walked—my mind in a quandary as I attempted to grasp what I'd just heard a few hours before—I was approached by Pam and her colleague Kim. They asked if I could take a few moments to share the excitement they felt concerning their work and how my own life's work had been so instrumental to them in applied integrative medicine.

My mind at that moment was not open to talking to anyone about anything, since I was somewhat in shock about what I had just learned. All I really wanted to do is go for a long walk alone and meditate and ask for Divine guidance as to what my next step should be. As I have said so often, in times of need, God can come to you in a myriad of disguises, so have a mind that is open to everything and attached to nothing.

After talking politely for a few moments, I simply blurted out what I'd just learned about the leukemia diagnosis, and Pam said to me without hesitation, "I thought I came here to share our findings in integrative medicine and the Apo E Gene diet, but obviously I was sent here to help you heal your own body." Since that day, Pam McDonald, the author of this life-changing—no, life-saving, book—has been my constant integrative-medicine practitioner, and has personally guided me to a whole new level of mind/body health.

This book is loaded to the gills with specific information that will indeed transform your life in so many ways. Basically, the book is well written and professionally researched in order to be of assistance to anyone embarking on a healing path. If this were not true, I would not be writing this Foreword and endorsing this material enthusiastically.

What the book doesn't do, however, is tell you about the spiritual consciousness embedded in the author, who painstakingly researched and wrote this amazing material. Pam McDonald lives and breathes what she writes about. She immediately arranged to have my blood tested and discovered that I was a 3/3 on the Apo E gene scale. She designed a specific diet for me, taking into account the fact that the test revealed I had one of the highest cholesterol traits predictive of aggressive heart disease she had ever seen—even thought my routine-screening cholesterol test showed me to be in the normal range. She further noted that based upon my genetic coding, the medications I was taking were completely wrong for my genetic trait.

Pam took it upon herself to prescribe the correct treatment, along with dietary recommendations that would serve to reduce my cellular inflammation and put me back on to a regimen of well-being in harmony with my own genetic blueprint. As a 3/3, the worst thing I could do was go on a low-fat diet. Indeed, I learned that my body could not process and break down certain foods that I had been eating for a lifetime. It was Pam who arranged to have my blood properly processed. And she was also the one who called me every day to ensure that I understood which foods I had to avoid and which ones I needed to make the major focus of my new eating regimen.

It was Pam who arranged on her own time and at her own expense to meet with me in San Diego to reinforce the essential connections between the kinds of food I was eating and my ability to live out my life from a place of well-being, balanced with my own genetic traits. It is still Pam who sends me messages and updates on a regular basis to remind me to stay on the path of the Perfect Gene Diet, which, by the way, is simple and easy and in no way a sacrifice or a hardship. It is the love and higher consciousness in these remarkable women who researched and wrote this book that I want to acquaint you with here in these moments before you immerse yourself in this information.

This is not a book with a radical new diet for you to experiment with as you lose those extra pounds. Rather, it is an approach that, with a simple test, will evaluate your individual genetic map and then provide you with the correct do's and don'ts—nutritionally, physically, and spiritually—to keep you balanced with respect to the DNA model that was handed to you at birth.

Pam McDonald is not just an integrative-medicine practitioner, but she embodies the idea that when people with serious chronic conditions such as heart disease , Alzheimer's, leukemia, diabetes, and so on become aware, they need not stay stuck in the progressive deterioration that accompanies these chronic illnesses. Their symptoms can and will begin to disappear, and they'll start to look and feel better.

Since I have been on the Perfect Gene Diet, I have managed to improve my white blood count; take off 18 excess pounds without even feeling like I'm dieting; enhance my lung capacity; increase my energy; and, more important, simply feel better each and every day. And Pam McDonald has gone from being a stranger who had used my materials in concert with her work and who wanted to share it with me, to being the single most significant person—medical or otherwise—who has helped me get and stay on a dietary regimen perfectly compatible with what God had in mind when he brought this body of mine into this physical world from the infinite, formless world of Spirit.

I personally took this book to my publisher and made the case to Hay House to bring this message to the masses. This has been publisher Louise Hay's mission for as long as I known her, and when I told Hay House of my strong feelings about this, along with the integrity and commitment of its author to making this shift toward an integrative-medicine approach, my publisher jumped on board and elected to bring it to you. I am so proud to write these few supportive words in the opening pages of this monumental work, and I endorse the Perfect Gene Diet wholeheartedly. I also endorse the author, and I especially want to thank God for urging me to go out into the world on that day of my own diagnosis and meet the women who brought a sense of sanity back to my eating regimen, which allowed me to continue to help others as a result of the help that has been delivered to me.

Why I Wrote This Book

"Let food be thy medicine and medicine be thy food."
— Hippocrates

During my 28 years as a medical professional working in Great Britain and the United States, I have witnessed illness and disease at all stages. I have seen everything from simple coughs and colds to the most deadly cancers. Unfortunately for most of us, disease shows up when least expected and can create life-shattering consequences. Disease brings with it many painful problems, yet few are more devastating than the emotional distress and panic that people experience when diagnosed with a life-threatening illness. Observing firsthand the response people have to these diagnoses has been the worst side of my job. For each patient who feels panic, I feel and internalize the panic myself. (In fact, I believe almost all patient-oriented practitioners do the same.) My immediate response is to help them deal with their initial pain. However, my long-term goal is to help prevent disease from occurring in the first place, and I consciously undertake this task one patient at a time.

For instance, some of my patients can count themselves among the millions of obese Americans—not only adults, but now even children as young as toddlers. All of them face unpleasant health futures with heart disease, hypertension, and diabetes poised to walk in the door opened by extra weight. I tell my overweight patients that, despite all the "popular" information available today about diets, each individual's approach to weight loss must be a personalized endeavor, and I work with them to create individual weight-loss programs based on their own variation of the Apo E gene. Often, I begin by discussing with them the reasons why obesity has reached epidemic proportions in the United States.

I believe the main reason is our move away from whole, natural foods to highly processed food products. We have also left behind healthy home-cooked meals in favor of fast food and restaurant meals, affording us little control over the content of what we eat. The food in many restaurants, fast-food establishments, schools, and even hospitals is highly processed and often preserved in ways that are harmful to the body. Furthermore, we tend to eat too fast, with little emphasis on mindful eating, which would strengthen our mind-body-spirit connection and enhance our enjoyment of life. Then, as we gain weight, we jump into the latest in-vogue diet, trying to find a quick way out of the unhealthy eating patterns we have been following for years. All of this only encourages obesity, chronic inflammation of the body, and the development of chronic illness.

As a culture, we need to realize that the most favorable diet for the human body requires understanding the connection between each person's genetic makeup and its response to the nutritional environment that is provided by our diet—specifically the differences in how each individual's body responds when exposed to the three major food groups: carbohydrates, fats, and protein. Among my patients who want to lose weight, confusion is the number one problem. Many people today don't know what to eat to be healthy, partly because the medical community doesn't give clear messages about nutrition. This is, sadly, understandable because doctors themselves receive no meaningful training in nutrition.

Thankfully, this is changing. Over the past few decades the medical field has been jolted into noticing how powerfully nutrition can affect a person's health. We can thank Dr. Robert Atkins for *Dr. Atkins' Diet Revolution;* Dr. Robert Superko for *Before the Heart Attacks;* Dr. Arthur Agatston for *The South Beach Diet;* and Dr. Dean Ornish for *Stress, Diet and Your Heart.* Without question, these diets produced some interesting information about how different eating patterns can be a powerful tool and affect a person's health in both the short and long term—in both positive and negative ways. These diets gained not only the attention of the lay public, but also of the medical community. In particular, the Atkins diet shifted so many people's weight in such a significant way (although perhaps not the best way—more on this later) that the medical community couldn't help but notice. For the first time, the medical community in general began to consider that maybe diet really *does* make a difference in a person's health, and we should pay attention to nutrition as a useful tool, not only in battling obesity, but also in disease prevention.

However, all these diets, no matter how good or bad, are recommended for the general population as "one diet fits all" plans. Fortunately, medical science has recently concluded that diets are an individual matter, with no particular popular diet working well for everyone. We now have enough information to shift from mass diet recommendations to the safer science of nutritional medicine, delivered by licensed medical professionals who have the scientific training, the knowledge of the human body, and the understanding of how the human body functions in tandem with the mind and spirit to efficiently utilize food as medicine. If this tool of nutrition is well implemented, patient well-being will be taken to a new level. As a health-care professional, I am not convinced that the local gym or the commercial diet center provides the safest environment for diet and exercise. In those environments, many patients are receiving misinformation and potentially harming themselves. I believe that the medical professionals most qualified to offer the best guidance about diet and exercise are the properly trained M.D.'s, nurse practitioners, osteopaths, physician's assistants, registered dietitians, and exercise physiologists. By properly trained, I mean skilled in nutrition science, exercise physiology, and the mind/body/emotions connection— all working together to bring about healing, wellness, and optimal health.

It is time that the medical establishment came together to recognize that nutritional medicine is one of the most important supports for the health of the entire nation. With the epidemic of obesity well under way, we can make monumental changes by focusing on the correct nutrition and disease-prevention strategies for *each individual patient*. In my heart and as a scientist, I know the epidemic of obesity, heart disease, stroke, cancer, and all the other chronic illnesses can be greatly slowed or even stopped. However, as a medical community and as a country, we need to act now and begin working together. This means not only focusing on educating our physicians and other medical professionals about disease prevention, but also enlisting the entire medical community, plus the food industry, our educational institutions, and our local and national food businesses, in a concerted effort to help prevent a human health disaster—and maybe an economic disaster as well. This type of collective undertaking can create a health outcome where everybody wins.

Truly, this is a monumental task, but we can start by educating ourselves about appropriate care and therapies to help prevent disease. One of the most cost-effective therapies is teaching people how to make appropriate nutritional choices, since good nutrition can have the most positive effect on a person's health. In fact, it is the number one integrative-medicine tool used today.

In addition, we should strongly consider utilizing integrative, healing-oriented medicine as a practical method simply because it takes into account the whole person—body, mind, spirit, and physical environment, including all aspects of a person's lifestyle. This kind of medicine focuses strongly on the patient-provider relationship and makes use of the best therapies, both conventional and alternative, for each individual patient at their particular time of need.

Today we live in a world where the medical delivery system is too overtaxed to meet many of the real needs of patients, and where the patient is dealing with new stressors, from ubiquitous junk food to the popular, but frequently unhealthy diets advertised through high-powered media channels. We need new guidelines to be able to move forward in a beneficial, meaningful way to help both the patient and the system make the transition to a supportive environment, especially nutritionally.

During my integrative medicine training I was taught the following powerful principles that can help guide us during this time of transition:

- Focus on and utilize the principles of a patient-focused health-care system.

- Ensure that patient and practitioner are partners in the healing process.

- Take into consideration all factors influencing health, wellness, and disease, including body, mind, spirit, and physical environment.

- Facilitate the body's innate healing process by the appropriate use of both conventional and alternative methods.

- Use effective natural and less invasive interventions whenever possible.

- Neither reject conventional medicine nor accept alternative therapies uncritically.

Good medicine is based on good science; it is inquiry-driven and open to new paradigms. Alongside treatment, the broader concepts of health promotion and the prevention of illness are paramount. Practitioners of integrative medicine should exemplify its principles and commit themselves to self-exploration and self-development.

Stay Focused on Your Goals

Before you read any further, I would like you to keep in mind one simple but essential idea: *First dream about a life that will make you completely happy—create your life in your mind, stay focused on that life which is yours—then write it down on paper. And every day refine your life in words by writing it out on paper for that particular day.* There is a simple reason for this: Our subconscious mind will always lead us to take action on what we focus on. If you wish to have good health, then you must focus on *having* good health, not on being sick, or even on not being sick. With the latter, your energy is still on what you don't want, not what you want.

If you want to lose weight and become more physically fit, then you need to focus on being healthy and physically fit, rather than on not being overweight and ill. Being overweight is a *symptom,* not the *problem.*

Clear your mind and focus on what you want. *Write it down.* Refuse to let *anything* get in the way of what you want. This may be as straightforward a task as losing weight, or something more complex, such as improving your whole health to prevent or reverse a chronic illness such as arthritis, stroke, high blood pressure, diabetes, heart disease, etc. At the same time, expand your focus to include your body, mind, spirit, and physical environment.

The Role of Nutrition and Integrative Medicine

Curbing the escalating rates of chronic illness—from obesity to heart disease, stroke, and cancer—is possible when we recognize the role of nutrition in health and healing, and focus on what is right for each individual patient. We can start by educating ourselves on how to make appropriate nutritional and lifestyle choices to prevent disease. But we need to act now. Good nutrition has a powerful effect on a person's health, and is the number one integrative-medicine tool.

We must begin to educate physicians, nurse-practitioners, and physician's assistants about the role of nutrition in disease prevention; and also focus on bringing the food industry, educational institutions, and media together to serve the health needs of our nation's population. I believe this is both possible and necessary if we are to prevent a human health disaster—and quite possibly an economic disaster from the widespread decrease of job productivity and spiraling treatment costs, as these unwell people get sicker. Such a collaborative effort can create a win-win outcome for the health status of human beings and the economy.

A major force in forwarding this change will be the training of more integrative medicine practitioners. We will look at the principles and practice of integrative medicine in more depth in a later chapter. For now, it is helpful to understand a basic distinction between allopathic and integrative medicine. Allopathic medicine, using drugs and surgery, is our current norm for treating disease. It is an excellent model for treating many acute symptoms and diseases, but it has limited value in treating chronic illnesses or bringing about healing.

Integrative medicine has a much wider foundation and has been called the medicine of the future, a future that is already here in a number of areas of the country. Integrative-medicine providers are fully trained in conventional allopathic medicine and then undergo additional training in integrative medicine.

At my clinic in Danville, California, we practice integrative medicine. This means that, as well as utilizing medication and surgery, we incorporate diet, exercise, botanical herbs, mind-body medicine, massage therapy, craniosacral therapy, stress reduction, prayer, meditation, and/or guided imagery in our treatment plans. These are all very effective therapies that gently shift the energy of the body and support its own internal healing processes.

We have found that to prevent the major diseases such as obesity, diabetes, cardiovascular disease, autoimmune disease, and cancer, we must look closely at each person's specific individual genetic instructions or recipe. Utilizing this recipe as a guide to helping people shape their environment is proving to be a very powerful tool for prevention. I call this creating a gene-supportive environment, or GSE.

Many people think they know what to do to be healthy, yet cannot seem to take the requisite actions and accomplish their goals. Why? Have you ever wondered why you have not been able to stay with a low-fat diet along with a typical gym's standard high-intensity exercise program ("no pain, no gain")? It could be that your body does not have the genetic makeup to be able to tolerate a very low-fat, low-carbohydrate, or even high-protein diet. Similarly, your body may not tolerate a high-intensity exercise program because it may not be able to tolerate that kind of exercise. Just as individuals have different nutritional needs, they have differing predispositions to being supported by a particular style of movement.

As already noted, research (see Appendix D) suggests that when a person follows the nutritional guidelines for their genotype, they have a far greater chance of attaining optimal health and avoiding chronic disease. I am very excited by these discoveries and know that we are only seeing the tip of the iceberg. It is in part my excitement at the prospects these discoveries hold for our health that has prompted me to write this book. I want to see this research more widely available to both laypeople and professionals, to seed both more research and greater application of what we already know.

I believe that mature adults must be responsible for, and take care of, their own physical and mental health. Daily health-promoting practices are vital for maintaining good health of the body, mind, emotions, and spirit. Part of this prevention practice is medical screening. With today's advanced technological tools, medical practitioners can detect many medical problems and treat them before they become life-threatening.

How Can This Book Help You Now?

My immediate intention with this book is to share information that can support you in both achieving optimal levels of health and well-being, and in minimizing the likelihood of your developing the debilitating diseases that are normative within our culture today. More specifically, this book can guide you to better health. It can give you important information about the correct diet, exercise, and other gene-supportive environment issues relevant for your Apo E genotype. While there are general guidelines for all the genotypes, I will address the pros and cons of having your Apo E genes analyzed, so that if you decide to be tested and learn your genotype, you can then create a more gene-supportive environment for yourself. What you will be advised to do may be as straightforward a task as losing weight or something more complex such as changing many factors in your life to prevent chronic illness. I know this method can work for you because it has worked for hundreds at my clinic.

I was asked by many of my colleagues and friends to include some of my experiences while writing this book. As a trained practitioner in allopathic medicine, alternative medicine, and integrative medicine, I believed that this required me to commit myself to self-exploration and self-development before embarking on the writing of what you hold in your hands. So I am including a small part of my own personal journey. In summary, my hope is that this information will help you in making a happier and healthier life for you.

My promise is to bring the very best information on the Apo E gene and its effects on health to my readers and the patients in my clinics. As we learn more about the specifics of each type's gene-supportive environment, I will update this information via my website: **www.ThePerfectGeneDiet.com**.

Introduction

This book is not a book about diets in the usual sense of the word. I debated using the word "diet" in the title for months. Colleagues encouraged me to use it to reach an audience that might not otherwise pick up the book, but it is most definitely not a "diet book." Now that it's in your hands, please expand your thinking about the word "diet." *I define "diet" as recommendations for individual nutritional, exercise, and other lifestyle factors that lead to disease prevention and a healthy life. This is a perfect integrative-medicine solution.*

How to Use This Book

The information in this book can help you make your health even better than it already is.

When you begin reading, you may first want to flip through the entire book to any part that attracts your attention. Then, as you begin to move more systematically through the book from the beginning to the end, you will see the full picture of how your Apo E gene and the internal environment you create in your body with food, exercise, and stress contribute to your health and to the prevention or creation of certain illnesses, particularly heart disease and Alzheimer's disease.

There is a detailed explanation of the Apo E gene, what it does in the body, and the different genotypes or variations of this gene. In addition, there is a discussion of how to get gene-tested and the necessary precautions to take before deciding to take such a test. Since this book is based on the principles of integrative medicine, which is based on mind, body, emotions, and spirit, I provide details about it, as well as how to find a medical practitioner and further support to guide you in implementing the information in this book.

You will find nutritional information on the Big Three—carbohydrates, fats, and proteins—along with a list of beneficial foods and practical advice on exercise—all related to each Apo E genotype.

I have included tools you can use to explore who you are, to understand more about where you have come from, and where you and your health could be headed. You will find information, along with further resources, about how to make positive changes in your life and improve your health based on your Apo E genotype.

Next, there is a lengthy list of nutritional recommendations, based on Apo E genotypes and calorie allowances, followed by some delicious recipes. Finally, several appendices will offer additional information.

Many of my patients have used these same procedures, tools, and nutritional guidelines, and found them to be helpful and healthy. I wish the same results for you.

Chapter One

BACKPACK OR BEDPAN, HEALTH IS A CHOICE

I believe that we almost always have a choice between health and chronic illness. We can choose to be healthy and be out backpacking, or we can choose to be sick, possibly living out our days in an institution using a bedpan, our independence lost as a result of chronic illness.

Keep in mind that chronic illness does not just "show up" one day to cause problems. Some diseases take decades to develop, and many of them develop silently, often with few or no symptoms. Understanding this, and knowing that you do have a choice of taking action—or not—to safeguard your health, is the first step in preventing many chronic diseases from gaining a foothold. It's much better to live your life in a way that will prevent disease, rather than learning that you have developed an illness after it's too late to reverse the accumulated damage.

To do this, we need to become more focused on both our wellness and disease prevention—to look a little deeper than we have in the past, asking questions that will change our lives by enhancing our health and wellness. I hope the information contained in this book will do just that.

Diabetes, insulin resistance, glucose intolerance, and heart disease can be well established without giving any major warning signs. Sometimes the first knowledge of such a condition arrives with a full-blown heart attack or stroke. Being overweight or obese is one of the most obvious signs that one or more of these diseases is present (although even thin people can be over-fat). Keep in mind—being overweight is not only about your body image. Being overweight is a symptom of a serious underlying problem, *not the problem itself.* Many of us think we know what to do to be healthy, yet cannot seem to accomplish this goal. Why? Have you ever wondered why you have not been able to stay with a low-fat diet along with a rigorous exercise program? It could be that your body does not have the genetic makeup to be able to tolerate a very low-fat, or a low-carbohydrate, or even a high-protein diet.

Remember, we have choices where our health is concerned, and we need to connect our lifestyle with its direct health outcomes. Some of these choices depend on our own individual genetic makeup, tests for which I will be describing in this book.

I am committed to helping you become the healthiest you can be and also being a role model for my patients. Personally, when I reach 75, I want to be outside backpacking, hiking, biking, or skiing with my children and grandchildren, not spending my days institutionalized, needing help getting to the bathroom.

Historically, health recommendations focus on what is right for the general public (such as: "Eat a low fat diet"), not for the individual. Therefore, when you read the information in this book and ask, "Should I get these tests?" make your decision with the assistance of a medical practitioner who is skilled in these areas rather than following guidelines believed to be good for the health of the general population. You do not want your health to be evaluated on the "average scale," because what you will end up with is the "average" heart attack.

As you will learn in this book, you will likely cause a chronic illness for yourself if you consistently create the wrong body chemistry through the wrong diet and wrong exercise regimen for whichever of the six different Apo E genotypes you happen to be. That's why general diet recommendations such as "Eat a low-fat diet" or "Eat a low-carbohydrate diet" are not right for everyone. For some Apo E genotypes, a low-fat diet can actually create heart disease. So, a logical solution is to learn about the Apo E gene and how it matches your diet and lifestyle.

Diet and Gene Interactions Shape the Potential for Health or Disease

With our new understanding of the human genome and the arrival of DNA testing, it is possible to recognize interactions between what we eat and how our genes function, and how these interactions may contribute to disease. Diet can change how different genes will express themselves and how they will adapt to different environments. Coupled with the existence of polymorphism, or the presence of several different "blueprints" of genes in different individuals, environment then plays a specific role in either reducing or increasing the risk of certain diseases. One example of this phenomenon is the variations of the Apo E gene, a major subject of this book.

We now have the technological capability to look at our genetic type in order to determine the likelihood of our developing a chronic disease. If we know our genotype, we can make fundamental decisions for preventing the development of a particular chronic disease. While we don't yet understand the purpose of all of the genetic information in our bodies, we know enough to apply how certain gene traits interact with particular dietary regimens. This will improve our health today, rather than waiting decades until a disease announces itself with a health crisis.

I will highlight some common tests that may help prevent certain chronic illnesses. While by no means a complete list, they are important examples that have been used successfully for disease prevention. It is extremely important to remember that the passageways to illness vary from person to person, based on each person's combination of genes and the dietary factors that influence them.

When it comes to our personal daily chemistry requirements—mainly our food—we are unique individuals in every way, and each of us has specific individual dietary needs. Research clearly shows that the same food can be either a nutritional medicine or a toxic irritant, depending on your particular genotype. So to help remember that everything you eat influences what goes on in your cells, I've created the expression "From Your Plate to Your Cells.™"

Genetic Risk and Family History

The unique body that is "you" is a combination of genes passed down from your ancestors. A look back at your family's medical history can offer clues to inherited disease patterns as well as steps that will prevent them.

In this context, "inherited" means much more than just the physical, genetic components of your body. It includes the entire scope of your family's culture—beliefs, customs, practices, social behavior, and attitudes. It is helpful to be aware of how strongly you accept the elements of your family's culture, as well as what other beliefs, customs, behaviors, etc., you have picked up on your own. All of these elements influence your journey through life and will affect your body, mind, spirit, emotions, and internal and external environments.

You probably know at least a little about your family's medical history, and even this can be helpful. Perhaps you know that your maternal grandfather was a hardworking farmer and lived to be 97, even though he ate all the "wrong things," at least according to what we believe today. So you assume he had "good genes."

That could be true, but it also could be true that while he had a genetic predisposition to heart disease, his lifestyle of hard physical labor for many years kept their expression in check. He may even have had the worst possible genetic traits for developing heart disease—a positive LDL Pattern B trait, Lp(a), and an Apo E 4/3 (which you will learn about later in this book)—but still remained healthy thanks to his lifestyle.

So, have you inherited his gene—one that could predispose you to heart disease if you eat the wrong diet? Many of us have these genes and don't know we have them, but if we have a gene unsupportive environment (GUE) we can develop a silent disease. What has changed is our food environment, and as long as we have a terrible nutritional environment in this country, we are at risk for turning on these silent diseases.

We must consider that the environment we live in today is completely different from that of just two generations ago, with much less physical activity and far fewer whole, healthy foods readily available. If you share Grandpa's genetic traits relating to heart disease, but live today's high-stress, nutritionally manipulated, and chemically exposed lifestyle, you probably will not be so lucky.

For now, know that many people have unrecognized hereditary cholesterol factors that can increase their risk of heart attack, even at an early age. Eighty percent of heart disease is said to be genetic, so genetic testing is crucial to knowing your own health status. Just as important is knowing that a family history of heart disease is the most powerful element you and your medical practitioner can use in determining how to reduce your risk.

There is no way to know for sure without genetic testing.

Chapter Two

AN INTRODUCTION
TO THE APO E GENE

"All we know is still infinitely less than all that remains unknown."
— William Harvey

"You're one fit guy, Rick," Dr. Humphrey told my husband. "You have the cholesterol results of a 19-year-old."

After his annual physical exam with all the standard and necessary blood tests, including a screening cholesterol panel, this was welcome news. But Rick, age 47, wondered, "Am I truly free of disease?" He wanted more definitive proof, real peace of mind about his health. He wondered if the screening cholesterol test told him all he needed to know.

Rick had good reason to question the test results. When he was 12, he watched his father's transformation from a healthy, active man to being bedridden with a heart condition and diabetes. The heart disease meant he could no longer be physically active, which led to his gaining a great deal of weight around his midsection. This in turn led his body to express type 2 diabetes, which, in a vicious circle, worsened his heart disease. To make matters much worse, he was also battling colon cancer.

Rick's sadness and grief over his father had never left him. After watching his father's health degenerate over a matter of months, one of Rick's most vivid, and terrifying, childhood memories was witnessing his father have a heart attack.

It motivated Rick to keep himself as healthy as possible; he didn't want his children to watch him die young or to suffer these same health problems. For years, he had followed a low-fat diet and a strenuous exercise regimen, believing the experts who said this was the best way to keep his heart in good shape.

Still, he had his doubts. So even with excellent results from his cholesterol screening, he asked what other tests he could take. Dr. Humphrey didn't believe any further testing was necessary, but in the face of Rick's determination, he recommended a heart scan. I decided to join him.

A few weeks later, Rick and I went for EBT heart scans near our home in Walnut Creek, California. Mine showed no evidence of heart disease. When Rick's scan was complete, he hopped off the table, eager to see his results. We were stunned. His scan revealed coronary plaque—the beginnings of heart disease. Rick was silent on the ride home, and when we arrived, he disappeared. I found him sitting on the edge of our bed and crying, terrified about the condition of his heart. "Am I going to die?" he asked. In reply, I promised I would do everything possible to solve this mystery. It's true that arterial inflammation can be stopped and reversed, but 50 percent of people who have heart attacks also have normal cholesterol levels and no other apparent reason for their heart attack.

When Dr. Humphrey heard Rick's results, he was also surprised. How could someone apparently as fit and healthy as Rick—someone who had religiously followed the recommended guidelines for maintaining a healthy heart—have coronary heart disease?

For three weeks I scoured the scientific literature to find the answer to that question. What I discovered about genetic heart-disease risk factors and the Apo E genotype, not only changed Rick's health for the better, but also broadened my work with heart disease and led to improved outcomes for many of my patients.

In brief, Rick was eating the wrong foods for his Apo E genotype. His low-fat diet did not provide enough long-term fuel in the form of fats, which, combined with his strenuous exercise routine, placed harmful levels of stress on his body's systems. He was eating the wrong kind of protein for his genotype—too much animal protein and not enough plant protein, which turned on a genetic pattern related to LDL cholesterol production that increased his arterial plaque production by 50 percent. Furthermore, the small amount of fat he was eating came mostly from meat containing saturated fat, which increases arterial inflammation. And finally, to top it off, his high intake of carbohydrate foods elevated his insulin level, which also has been shown to encourage arterial plaque.

Rick began eating correctly for his genotype: non-inflammatory fats in the form of olive oil and nuts, soybeans and avocados; fewer high-glucose carbohydrates; and more plant protein, including beans, soy nuts, and lentils. His LDL cholesterol normalized, his percentage of body fat decreased, and his insulin resistance—a precursor to type 2 diabetes—resolved. He also cut back on exercise.

Rick was actually killing himself by following the guidelines touted in recent decades as being the best, and perhaps only, way to prevent heart disease. To be fair, genetic testing was not available when the guidelines were developed; however, in light of what we are now learning about the Apo E genotypes, simply evaluating total cholesterol in terms of LDL and HDL is not enough. It is also important to evaluate 13 other kinds of total cholesterol. Finally, to complete the picture, it is necessary to determine a person's Apo E genotype, which will reveal the correct diet and exercise regimen that will truly maintain heart health and also help prevent serious illness such as vascular diseases and Alzheimer's disease.

Since the completion of the Human Genome Project in 2003, scientists have found many genes that are involved in a variety of disease states. It is becoming common to hear media reports about new research that clearly shows how many of our diseases have genetic components. Genetic research will doubtless continue to make new discoveries in this area, supporting more disease prevention through practical applications of this information. It is possible that in the near future, the Apo E gene will be linked to a lot more disease states than are currently proven.

What Exactly Do We Mean by Genes?

When you want to build a house, you have an architect draw blueprints. Your builder then looks at the blueprints to know exactly what to build. The same process occurs with the body—only our genes are the blueprints for our body. *And,* unlike a house, the body is being rebuilt every second of every day.

Besides the builder and the blueprint, another major factor in house building is the quality of the materials used. When built with poor-quality materials, buildings deteriorate rapidly. When built with high-quality materials, structures such as St. Paul's Cathedral in London can stand for hundreds of years. Your body follows the same process—if you use high-quality materials, it will last much longer. *This book is about choosing the right materials to go with your specific blueprint.*

What Is the Apo E Gene?

The human body has 23 pairs of chromosomes. Each chromosome is made up of many genes. We will look mainly at a particular gene on chromosome 19—the Apo E gene (Apo is short for apolipoprotein—see box, page 11), which was discovered in the early 1970s. We single out this gene because certain variants of the specific pair of Apo E genes you inherited from your mother and father influence your predisposition to certain illnesses.

There are three Apo E gene variations, or *genotypes,* that occur naturally in humans: Apo E 2, Apo E 3, and Apo E 4.

Since genes come in matching pairs—we each have two copies of every gene—one from each parent, there are six possible combinations of pairs. If you received an Apo E 2 from each parent, the shorthand description would be E 2/2. The other five combinations are E 2/3, E 3/3, E 4/2, E 4/3, and E 4/4.

As you can see from the table below, the most common gene, Apo E 3/3, is found in approximately 64 percent of the population. It is considered the "neutral" Apo E genotype.

2.1 Percentage of Apo E Genotypes in the General Population		
Apo E 2	2/2	1%
	2/3	10%
Apo E 3	3/3	64%
Apo E 4	4/2	2%
	4/3	18%
	4/4	5%

Combinations that include either the Apo E 2 or Apo E 4 are considered "alternative" expressions of the more common Apo E 3 pairing; and they process foods differently from the way in which an Apo E 3's will.

For optimal health, you need to match your particular genotype with the most gene-supportive environment (GSE) you can create. You do that through what you eat, how you exercise, and how you respond to stress, which is largely determined by how you think.

What Does Apo E Mean?

Our body has evolved a very complex biochemical method of moving fats around inside it. Why all this complexity?

You already know that oil and water don't mix. That's what our body (water-based) is up against when it must absorb and use fats (oil-based). Our blood is a water-based solution for transporting nutrients and oxygen to the cells. Any fats that need to travel in it wouldn't dissolve; they would just clump up and clog the system.

To get around this inconvenience, our body has created a wonderful method of packaging the fats and oils in molecular "suitcases" that keep the fats from coming in contact with the water of our blood.

That's where this strange word "Apo" with an "E" attached to it comes in. Apo is short for *apolipoprotein*.[1] It has the letter "E" because it's one of a whole series of apolipoproteins –A, B, C, D, etc. The Apo E *gene* gets its name from the fact that it's the part of the blueprint in charge of synthesizing apolipoprotein E, an important component of cholesterol metabolism.

In a larger sense, the Apo E gene is involved in the energy system of the body—and energy is key to every system in the body. Apo E can be found in many places: blood, spleen, liver, intestine, brain, kidney, and other peripheral parts.

Making Connections: Genotype, Gene-Supportive Environment, and State of Health

The Apo E gene can *provide good health* if the body is given the correct foods and other gene-supportive environment (GSE) factors for its Apo E type. On the other hand, the Apo E gene can *impair good health* if the body is given the wrong foods and other gene-unsupportive environmental (GUE) situations.

---

1   Derivation of apolipoprotein: Apo•lipo•protein. Apo = separated from or derived from; lipo = fat; proteins are made of amino acids and essential to all cellular structures. The apolipoproteins are the protein components of lipoproteins that remain after the lipids to which the proteins are bound have been removed.

The Apo E gene is the key to making the right match. Here's where knowing your Apo E genotype can help determine the environment that will best support you in developing and maintaining a safe, optimal level of cholesterol in your system.

Before we go any further, let me clarify what I mean by "environment." Everything that surrounds or goes into your body or mind is an element in your environment and subsequently impacts your health. This means your thoughts become as much a part of you as the food you eat. So while your food intake is an important element in your environment, you are much more than just the food you eat.

Your environment, so defined, largely determines your health. More specifically, it consists of:

- what you eat
- the way you move and exercise your body
- the quality of your mental and emotional experiences (including how you deal with stress and emotional energy)
- the strength and quality of your intention for what you want
- what you think others want from you
- the physical environment that surrounds you—is it pleasing or stressful?
- your spiritual beliefs

With today's affordable technology for analyzing people's genotype, we can easily learn a person's Apo E genetic recipe. While we have a lot to learn about what each of the thousands of genes we have in every cell actually does, we can make excellent use of the ones that we do understand—like the Apo E gene—to make recommendations for the ideal gene-supportive environment for any individual.

Inflammation: A Poor Match Between Environment and Genotype

Chronic diseases such as diabetes, obesity, gouty arthritis, hypertension, cardiovascular disease, multiple sclerosis, chronic kidney disease, Alzheimer's disease, Parkinson's disease, and cancer all have in common the long-term presence of low-grade cellular inflammation that is largely the result of *a poor match between environment and genetic makeup—the gene-unsupportive environment* (GUE) that I described above. I will describe the mechanisms of inflammation in detail in a later chapter, but for now, it's important to know that when a normal, healthy cell is exposed to an inflammatory environment over a long period of time, the cell becomes aplastic (unable to replicate properly). How this *dis-ease state* manifests in your body can range from high cholesterol levels, cardiovascular disease, and vascular dementia, to cancer, Alzheimer's disease, Parkinson's disease, and more. In most cases these degenerative killer diseases are the result of imbalances of the body's ability to regulate its processes that are usually present for 30 or more years before they are noticed. Some can even begin before birth, in a toxic womb environment.

Put simply, the wrong environment for a particular Apo E genotype can push the body to produce high levels of cellular inflammation as it attempts to fight the effects of its environment. This can result in chronic illnesses, including cancer.

Remember, it's about the gene and the environment the gene is exposed to. The body knows what to do when it has an occasional or brief imbalance. But when it becomes chronically overwhelmed and unbalanced from consistent exposure to an unsuitable environment, it cannot function as it should. Such an imbalance between genotype and environment will likely lead to chronic illness.

This means that while you may, over many years, be eating a "health-conscious" diet like the popular low-fat diets and never develop a disease, another person may follow the very same diet and develop a serious illness. Could this be, in part at least, because the so-called healthy diet advocated by the media may not be right for everyone?

We are unique individuals in every way, even when it comes to our personal daily dietary requirements. Knowing this, food can be used as nutritional medicine if we eat the appropriate foods in the correct amounts. This is why I developed a diet based on the Apo E gene. My experience has shown me again and again that **one diet does not fit all.**

You Are What You Eat

The foundation of an individual diet recommendation, and your optimal gene-supportive environment, is a nutritional plan that focuses on eating the optimal percentages from The Big Three food categories—carbohydrates, fats, and proteins. There is a unique optimal combination of these that creates the ideal diet for each of the six Apo E genotypes. Creating this optimal balance in your diet is a prerequisite of good health.

Why? The Apo E gene has been shown to be the number one factor affecting how your body uses The Big Three, and this influences the likelihood and severity of your developing some diseases. It is very important to eat the right balance of The Big Three.

We have all heard the saying "You are what you eat." Now, more than ever, research shows this to be true. The food you eat today becomes the cellular makeup of your tissues tomorrow—food that goes into your body becomes your body. Eating the right diet for your Apo E genotype is one of the best investments you can make in your health. A healthy diet can be delicious and health-promoting, supplying the nutrition your body needs, based on your current health and Apo E genotype.

✿

Chapter Three

THE CONNECTION BETWEEN A GENE-SUPPORTIVE ENVIRONMENT AND THE APO E GENE

All Apo E genotypes require a specific fat combination for optimal cell health. In other words, your Apo E genotype determines the optimal type and amount of dietary fat needed to ensure the correct percentages of "fuel" for your body to function properly. A diet based on your Apo E gene provides the recommended amounts and types of fats for optimal cell health for each genotype. A mismatch between genotype and fat intake creates a gene-unsupportive environment. The Apo E 4s have the greatest difficulty clearing fats from their bodies, especially the more complex inflammatory fats, and must significantly limit saturated and trans fats. However, everyone, no matter what their Apo E genotype, should minimize inflammatory fats.

It is important to realize that the presence of Apo E 4 does not cause cardiovascular disease and other conditions like Alzheimer's disease. Nor does it necessarily mean that the person will develop such diseases. What is important is matching your diet—and lifestyle—to the needs of your genes. Since each Apo E genotype has an individual set of dietary recommendations linked to it, knowing your type can prevent diseases that are common to your genotype. I will later discuss diet, exercise, and lifestyle for each Apo E genotype.

You can't change your genes, but you can change how they perform by creating a gene-supportive environment (GSE) for them to function in. But first, let's look at what can happen in a gene-*un*supportive environment (GUE), using some of the research that establishes a clear connection between the Apo E gene and cardiovascular disease as well as other chronic illnesses such as Alzheimer's disease. Please keep in mind that *statistics never relate to the individual person because no situation or circumstance is ever quite the same for any two individuals.*

Cardiovascular Disease and the Apo E Gene

Cardiovascular disease accounts for the number one and number three causes of death (heart attack and stroke) in the United States. Combined, these account for 40 percent of all deaths. Cardiovascular disease is a progressive, deteriorating, inflammatory disease leading first to damage of cells, major organs, and eventually whole body systems. It is a gradual process that can begin in childhood—as young as 5. Upon reaching a certain age, usually around 40 to 50 but sometimes younger, the risk of heart attack jumps dramatically. Following a heart attack, many people fail to make a full recovery, with approximately 40 percent dying within a year. Within six years, nearly half of those surviving have become disabled.

The work performed by the heart is demanding and never-ending. Your heart is only the size of two fists, but the energy produced by this tireless little machine over a 50-year period could move a battleship. It beats thousands of times a day, pumping hundreds of gallons of blood. Never stopping day or night, your heart works twice as hard as the largest muscles in your body. A damaged heart almost inevitably means a damaged life.

The heart requires a constant supply of blood to provide it with oxygen and the necessary nutrients, via three main coronary arteries. If a blockage occurs in one of these arteries, the heart becomes deprived of oxygen, resulting in the death of some of its cells—a heart attack.

Cardiovascular disease is a disease of inflammation, but the impact of inflammation is not limited to the arteries. Inflammatory disease can occur anywhere in the body, down to the deepest crevices between cells, sparing nothing and generating a complex chain reaction.

Consuming the wrong fuel for your body's genetic makeup causes the body to create the wrong internal environment. This causes a reaction that harms the major fluid delivery system of the body—the arteries—and leads to the deterioration of entire body systems because these "rivers" of the body have become a toxic waste dump and are spewing toxins and inflammatory by-products everywhere.

Inflammation results when the body is unable to keep up in the process of healing itself by clearing these bad fats from the bloodstream. Overexposure to the wrong dietary fats raises LDL and lowers the HDL—see the illustration on page 20.

Specialized immune cells, clotting substances, and proteins, along with seven kinds of "bad" lipoproteins (LDLs), then form a "scab" (arterial plaque) in an attempt to protect the inner lining of the arteries to heal the arteries. (See box on page 18: "Looking Deeper into the Cholesterol Pots: LDL and HDL").

Not All Cholesterol Is Bad

Arterial plaque is similar to the plaque that forms in your mouth if you don't floss, but plaque on your teeth won't kill you. Inside your "plumbing," it's a different matter. Everyone "knows" that too much cholesterol is bad for us—but it's not quite that simple. First, we need to learn more about two components of cholesterol that few people understand—low-density lipoproteins (LDL), the "bad" type of cholesterol, and high-density lipoproteins (HDL), the "good" cholesterol.

While the cholesterol inside LDL lipoproteins is called the bad cholesterol, it is not the *cholesterol* that is bad; it is instead *how* and *where* cholesterol is being transported, and in what amounts, over time, it is being deposited into the artery wall.

Besides the "bad" cholesterol (LDL) wreaking havoc by inflaming your arteries, the problem is compounded if your genetic makeup doesn't provide you with enough of the "good" cholesterol (HDL)—your body's arterial self-cleaning ability will not be adequate for the job. This means more rapid plaque buildup, with arteries clogging even faster. While many other factors are involved in the development of arterial plaques, it is the Apo E gene that determines your levels of HDL and LDL.

Again, we find that knowing your Apo E genotype is crucial in determining how your body will respond to its environment, and particularly, what food components are helpful and which are toxic for your genotype.

Looking Deeper into the Cholesterol Pots: LDL and HDL

To understand the impact of cholesterol on your health, we need to look more closely at the components of cholesterol.

The Specifics

The usual blood tests, called a cholesterol panel, done during routine checkups, are for the main categories of cholesterol and fat. They are:

- total cholesterol
- total LDL (bad cholesterol)
- total HDL (good cholesterol)
- triglycerides (fatty acids)

But testing for just these basic groups reveals only so much. In fact, the testing most commonly done does not even measure the LDL directly but calculates it from a formula based on the other three values. Furthermore, research shows that 80 percent of patients who developed coronary artery disease have the same total cholesterol level as those who did not develop the disease. To learn what's *really* going on in our arteries, we must look more deeply at several of the 12 different subtypes of cholesterol particles contained in the two major cholesterol groups—LDL and HDL. I often refer to these major categories of cholesterol as "pots." To see inside these pots requires more sophisticated testing than the typical cholesterol panel. Fortunately, these tests are now available and affordable so that what we find inside these pots can tell us a lot more about the health of our arteries.

There are seven kinds of cholesterol particles in the LDL pot, but only three of these concern us here. There are five kinds in the HDL pot, only one of which is important to us here. The composition of the 12 kinds of cholesterol particles in these two pots is determined first by what type of Apo E genes you have, and more important— because you can change it—the gene-supportive environment you create for your arteries by what you eat, what kind of exercise you get, and how you think.

First, the Bad News: LDL Cholesterol, Large and Small

How does an artery become damaged? Understanding how our body's vascular plumbing system—especially the arteries—becomes damaged by imbalances in the cholesterol it creates is critical to understanding what causes chronic heart disease.

LDL's job is to carry cholesterol and fatty acids from the liver, where it is synthesized, to the cells where it is used by your body in a variety of ways. This sounds reasonable, so how does LDL get such a bad rap?

Well, first you need to know that LDL cholesterol comes in seven sizes, called type I, IIa, IIb, IIIa, IIIb, IVa, and IVb (the larger the number, the smaller the size). LDL's bad rap comes from three of these. The first is IVb, the smallest of the stew. If you have elevated levels of IVb, you have a much greater risk of developing artery damage. But that's not all—having more than 15–20 percent of the IIIa and IIIb types also puts your arteries at risk.

So why are these three smaller ones bad for you? They are so small that they can easily slip in between the cells that line the insides of your arteries. In fact, they are twice as likely as the larger types of LDL to do this. When they do this slippery thing, they cause the arteries to become inflamed in reaction to the invasion, and that's not good.

One way to think of these culprits is as little metal chips with spikes on them that, once they get inside the artery's lining, make a multitude of cuts that cause inflammation, which then needs to be healed by your immune system. The smaller the chip, the more places it can cause damage. When the inflammation reaches a certain level, your immune system's attempt to repair the artery's wall becomes overwhelmed. Plaques of hardened calcium and cholesterol then form in your arteries in a misguided attempt to seal the damage off.

Here's where the Apo E genotypes come in. They determine what happens to the different types of fats, proteins, and carbohydrates that you eat. For example, if you have the Apo E 4 gene—the 4/4, 4/2, or 4/3—and eat a lot of fat, the likelihood of inflammation in your arteries is higher. To a lesser extent, arterial inflammation occurs with the Apo E 2 gene—either the 2/2 or the 2/3 combination.

For arterial health, each genotype has both an ideal kind, and combination of, fats, proteins, and carbohydrates—and hence, heart health—so knowing the right balance for your particular genotype is crucial.

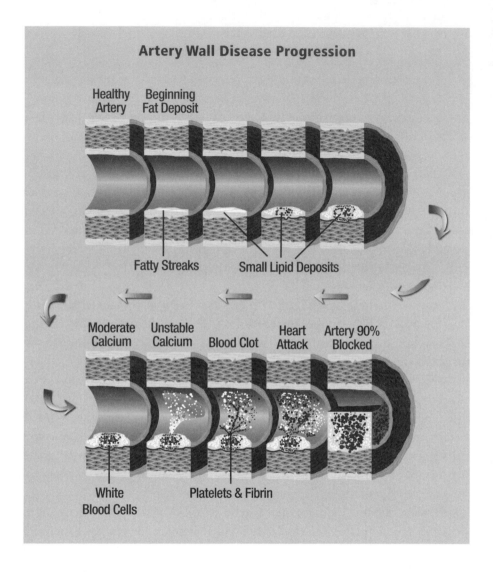

LDL Pattern B: Why Is It Dangerous?

LDL Apo E gene-unsupportive environment (GUE)
• Small dense LDL Pattern B
• High insulin

LDL Apo E gene-supportive environment (GSE)
• Large LDL Pattern A

Oxidation

Rapid LDL Entry into artery walls

Poor Artery Flexibility

Individuals have different environments for expressing their genotype, meaning how the genetic data appears in their body or tissue structure—think blue eyes, a long nose, or a certain LDL particle size. While eye color and nose length don't change, your LDL particle size *can change*, depending on the type of diet and other gene-supportive environmental factors. What matters is how this gene's requirements for optimal functioning are being met. Approximately one in four people has the LDL Pattern B genetic risk factor for too much small, dense, bad cholesterol. Even though this disorder is associated with three times the risk of heart attack, the standard cholesterol test will not find this condition, common as it is.

In the case of the LDL Pattern B trait, eating the wrong diet for a person's Apo E genotype "turns on" the Pattern B type gene, giving the body a genetic instruction resulting in the production of smaller LDL particles in the liver. If the gene is not present, it cannot be turned on. Approximately 50 percent of men and 30 percent of premenopausal women with heart disease have the Pattern B trait.

What does "turning on" a particular gene mean? The expression "turning a gene on" may conjure up an image of a little man standing by the DNA double helix in a plumber's suit holding a wrench and waiting to be called upon to turn a gene on or off. However, what actually happens is that if the body contains a gene that prefers a certain mix of nutrients in its diet but cannot find it, the body becomes unbalanced. This compromised state then encourages the body to try to find its own balance.

The Good News: HDL2b

While the various components of the LDL pot carry cholesterol out to your cells, HDL carries the surplus back to the liver where it is recycled. In this way, HDL provides our body with a natural artery-cleaning service. You simply cannot have too much of this good type of cholesterol, and later we will see how your diet and exercise program can cause even more HDL to be produced.

In my experience, the Apo E 2 and the Apo E 3 genotypes tend to have higher levels of HDL, especially HDL2b.

So how does HDL2b relate to artery disease? If you have too much bad LDL and not enough good HDL, especially HDL2b, your body can't clean its arteries properly, and the cholesterol accumulates and causes them to narrow—and thus begins cardiovascular disease.

HDL2b works for the body's vascular system in at least two ways. It lowers blood "thickness"—a tendency to clot inappropriately—and it is a powerful antioxidant that stops molecular damage to the vascular system.

Having levels of HDL2b greater than 20 percent for men and 30 percent for women contributes to optimal artery health. To achieve these levels, I advise patients to first be tested for HDL2b because despite high HDL levels, I often see very low HDL2b levels. Unless your HDL2b levels are normal or above, your ability to clean your arteries is hindered.

It's important to know that not all advanced cholesterol-testing methods are the same—some can be off by as much as 40 percent—leading to the wrong treatment plan.[1] Once you know your true levels, you can make any necessary dietary and lifestyle changes.

---

1   Comparison of traditional and alternative laboratory methods. Determination of lipid measurement Lp (a) and LDL phenotype. Presented by H. Robert Superko, M.D., at American Heart Association 42nd Annual Conference on Cardiovascular Disease Epidemiology and Prevention. Honolulu, HI, April 23–26, 2002.

Two Healing Worlds

In 2006 I went to Phoenix to meet Wayne Dyer and hear his latest message. I wanted to bring his latest thinking and wisdom back to my patients, since I had been recommending that they read or listen to his message for several years.

I found that when using Wayne's work and mine together, patients got better faster. Not in a Band-Aiding way like with our traditional allopathic model's 15-minute visit that ends with a prescription for the latest $10 pill, but in a human, mindful way, whereby a patient could be supported in discovering and embracing a clear path that will prevent, stop, or reverse frightening diseases.

After hearing a most amazing lecture, I was able to ask Wayne for some professional advice about how I could perfect my speaking abilities because I was giving a talk in a month at Dr. Andrew Weil's annual "State of the Science" nutrition conference for medical professionals in San Diego. My audience was well educated in the science of nutrition— physicians, dietitians, research scientists, nurses, exercise physiologists, etc.—so I felt very anxious about this talk and wanted to gain advice from the best so I could give the best possible talk on preventing and healing heart disease.

Wayne's ability to deliver a message is very special. I resonate strongly with his style—clearly coming from his heart and soul. My question for Wayne was, "How do you do the lectures you do and be so great— what gives you the confidence to be so amazingly good?"

Wayne, being Wayne, replied with a question "Do you know your message well?" I replied, "Yes."

"Then it is easy. Speak from your heart. Be you, and you have nothing to worry about because that is your message. If you can do that, you will give the best lecture and people will love it."

I immediately knew that he was 100% correct and thanked him.

In June of 2009, my dear friend and colleague, Kim Evans, asked if

I would go to Maui with her. She wanted us to share with Wayne the stories of our patients' successes so that he could see how integrative medicine, genetics, and his work had changed so many of our patients' lives. I immediately agreed.

When patients are sitting face-to-face with a medical provider who gives them a serious diagnosis of heart disease, cancer, dementia, Alzheimer's disease, or diabetes, they need to be given a path that leads to a healing solution, not just for the physical body, but for the mental, emotional, and spiritual bodies as well. They need to be given hope and support and examples of how they can make changes—a feeling that they can change their lives and their physical bodies. They can focus on what they want in their lives, and look forward to a future of health.

I knew that Wayne's message had given many of Kim's and my patients hope and health. The success of this coming together of two worlds—the physical importance of matching environment with genetic makeup, and the power of the mind's intention—which Kim and I practice daily with patients, is no accident. It encourages people to focus on what they want, not on what they don't want.

This may be very simple to say and hear, but once a person is able to understand this concept as it is told in a Wayne Dyer sort of way, it has the power to shift the most horrific disease states.

The day Kim and I were to meet with Wayne was a very special day. Our intention was written out and focused with love. Our mission was to deepen the experience of healing and miracles that had been going on for so many years in our practices.

We were staying at the Westin Hotel in Maui, and we had Wayne's address but were not sure where his home was relative to the hotel, so we decided to find it ahead of time. After walking the entire beach in the wrong direction and not finding his home, we walked back to a grassy area on the other side of the Westin, where Kim suggested we just sit on the grass and see if some additional information would come to us. Kim is extremely intuitive and follows her intuition all the time—she is usually right. In less than 6 or 7 minutes, Wayne came walking down the path, and we said hello. We were talking for maybe 10 minutes when he shared with us the diagnosis of leukemia he had been given that morning. He had not even had time to tell his family.

Immediately Kim and I felt that our mission was much bigger and much more important than just sharing our successes. We both felt that an integrative-medicine approach for Wayne's situation would be helpful, as well as the Perfect Gene Diet work. A few hours later, after talking further, we felt as if we had a spiritual agreement to be a part of his healing and to show up on the very day he was diagnosed with this serious illness, and be there for him in whatever capacity we could best serve. One thing he said that day was: "I feel a lot of love coming from both of you [our written intention from that morning]." He even said, "I feel as if you have come here to help save my life." We had no idea how big this intention would prove to be. It surprised us both—but it was perfect.

Over the next few months, Wayne learned that his genetic profile explained why he had heart disease. He had the genetic Lp(a) cholesterol trait with one of the highest Lp(a) levels[2] I had ever seen. This can cause some of the most aggressive types of heart disease and stroke in men. In addition, the medication that Wayne was taking would not treat this particular type of elevated cholesterol—his medications were completely wrong for his genetic Lp(a).

In addition, the combination of two medications he had been taking had recently been implicated as worsening heart disease, as well as having the potential to cause cancer. I then prescribed the correct treatment, as well as a gene-supportive environment with dietary recommendations that would help reduce his cellular inflammation.

---

2   Lp(a) is not routinely tested with the cholesterol screening panel that is usually ordered by your primary-care doctor or your cardiologist.

While many people take years to change old patterns, Wayne did it immediately. As soon as he learned what he had to do, he was ready to go to work—he came out of the house where he was staying in San Diego with an avocado in his hand and told me (I was in San Diego, too), "Look, Pam, I am changing already." He had gone into the house to find an avocado just as I shared a study on how avocado can reduce cholesterol with plant stenol.

Over the next few months I helped Wayne shift his eating patterns. He immediately felt better and began to shift his body composition. Other things had been shifting, too. The bigger message of nutrition had not only crept into his life through me, but was also coming from other authors who were touching Wayne's life and providing him with more information from every angle. Nutrition as a healing tool was now a reality for him as he saw firsthand how it could be used. Intuitively, he knew this and was using nutrition in a very effective way—especially now that it mattered more than ever before. He was also learning how an individual nutritional plan, based on a person's individual genetics, was very important to someone's health, in contrast to the one-diet-fits-all method.

When I first talked to Wayne in Maui, I instinctively felt that it was not the right time to give him my book. My goal was to help with whatever he needed, and then, if my book would help bring more knowledge to him, I would be guided to give it to him. It was months after I first began to help Wayne with his heart disease mystery, that I knew it was now okay to give him the book, as it would bring him additional information and guidance.

Wayne loved the book and felt that it would be an excellent resource to help not only him, but many people in the coming years. He is extremely supportive of how we've integrated his ideas into our work. I greatly appreciate his commitment to help get this message out to the world.

3.1 Optimal Cholesterol Screening Panel Results

	Situation	Optimal Level
Total cholesterol	You do not have heart disease	less than 200 mg/dl
	You have heart disease	less than 150 mg/dl
Total LDL	You do not have heart disease	less than 100 mg/dl
	You have heart disease	less than 70 mg/dl
Total HDL	Men	greater than 50 mg/dl
	Women	greater than 60 mg/dl
Total triglycerides	All situations	less than 150 mg/dl
HDL2b	Men	greater than 20 mg/dl
	Women	greater than 30 mg/dl
LDL small particle size		
IIIa + b	All situations	less than 15 mg/dl
IVb	All situations	less than 5 mg/dl
Lp(a)	All situations	less than 30 mg/dl
Blood glucose	Normal range	65 to 99 mg/dl
		Note: 100 to 125 means you are glucose-impaired. Greater than 125 mg/dl means you are diabetic.

Your Cholesterol Level and the Apo E Gene

Maintaining a healthy level of cholesterol is essential to your cardiovascular system. Although researchers are not completely certain about the exact level of cholesterol for optimal health, it appears to be below 70 mg/dl (that's milligrams per deciliter—there are almost 30,000 milligrams in an ounce, and a deciliter is 1/10 of a liter, or about 3.3 fluid ounces—not very much!).

Of the three kinds of Apo E genes, the 4s (especially that 5 percent of the population who have two of the Apo E 4 genes) are the most sensitive to high-fat diets and need more carbohydrates than the other types, or their cholesterol will be higher.

The Apo E 2s are the reverse, having the best ability to handle fats but an inability to process elevated levels of carbohydrate without increasing their triglyceride and cholesterol levels. This genotype is able to tolerate non-processed low glycemic load carbohydrates well, producing a slow rise in blood glucose and insulin levels (for example, whole grains, legumes, whole fruits, and vegetables—see Chapter 11, page 123) but cannot handle refined, processed carbohydrates without producing rapid increases in triglycerides, and blood glucose and insulin levels.

If you have cholesterol triglycerides, and blood glucose and insulin problems, it's important to know which Apo E genes you have. You can then adopt the dietary recommendations that can prevent this disease from being expressed.

The Interconnections among Environmental Factors

Your arterial health depends not only on your genotype but on many environmental factors—from your body composition, diet, and exercise program, to the psychological factors of the way you think, how you manage stress, how you view the world, and how you think the world views you. These factors are not independent of each other but *highly interconnected*. For example, the way you think influences the chemistry in your brain, which, in turn, changes your body's food needs. This is an aspect of that ever-present, but often ignored, mind-body connection I will describe in more detail below.

A diet based on your Apo E gene takes into account not only your diet and exercise program, but also how your stress levels are influencing your LDL and HDL levels because excessive stress affects how your body performs. If you are in a constant state of stress, your body is constantly in the fight-flight-or-freeze response, producing ever more cholesterol in anticipation of this pattern continuing. Knowing what genes you have gives you the power to intelligently create a gene-supportive environment through what you eat, how you exercise, and how you think.

Alzheimer's Disease and the Apo E Gene

Cognitive decline in old age has been seen throughout history. However, it was not until the early part of the 20th century that a collection of brain-cell abnormalities was specifically identified by a German physician, Alois Alzheimer, for whom the disease was named.

Nearly a century later, a high risk for Alzheimer's disease was associated with the Apo E 4 gene. Immediately following this discovery, ethical dilemmas associated with genetic testing led to the conclusion that medical records should be kept private in order to protect the rights of patients. Guidelines for genetic testing for Alzheimer's disease determined that individuals should not be tested without their primary medical providers' support and guidance. In 1997, President Clinton proposed a law that would make it a crime for employers or insurance companies to discriminate on the grounds of genetic-testing data they obtained. While his proposal did not become law, half the states in the USA have adopted this policy.

Not all people with Apo E 4 develop Alzheimer's disease, especially those who have created a gene-supportive environment. But without a gene-supportive environment, 90 percent of the 4/4 combination and 49 percent of the 4/3 and 4/2 variants develop the disease. This is a relatively exclusive Apo E club since it is estimated that only 5 percent of the population has the Apo E 4/4. The percentage of the population with the Apo E 4/3 and 4/2 genotypes totals 20 percent.

Conversely, not all people with Alzheimer's disease have the Apo E 4 genotype. What I do know from my clinical practice is that Apo E 4s who eat a high-fat diet have a very high cholesterol level. My patients with two copies (Apo E 4/4) consistently have total cholesterol levels in the 300s and 400s, with LDL in the 200s and 300s. Extremely high levels of LDL (bad) cholesterol cause high levels of inflammation in the blood vessels, including those in the brain. Therefore, a connection between Alzheimer's disease and one's diet is not surprising.

Research is proving that medication is not the answer for treating or preventing Alzheimer's. What works is a multilayered approach of gentle behavioral strategies, based on a gene-supportive environment (GSE). These help prevent and reverse the dysfunction associated with Alzheimer's—specifically preventing the oxidative damage that leads to cell degeneration, loss of synapses, and amyloid accumulation—all culminating in cognitive decline.

Since medication is not proving to be a real solution, what can we do, and where are we to go from here? Looking at our genetics, and seeing how our body is set up for the clearance of fat and cholesterol, is an important step. Especially as the Apo E gene is the most important gene we know of in 95 percent of all

Alzheimer's cases. In the meantime, we can make day-to-day changes to stop incremental dysfunction in the brain.

First, eat a diet that matches your Apo E genotype, avoiding the inflammatory foods that your genetic type is less able to clear. Avoid toxic chemicals such as preservatives, dyes, synthetic hormones, pesticides, heavy metals, herbicides, etc. Include a rich supply of antioxidants for cell protection, and exercise as a healing regenerative tool for regrowing brain cells.

How does the regrowing of the brain work, you ask? A protein produced in the brain called Brain-Derived Neurotrophic Factor (BDNF) triggers the process of growing back damaged brain cells. With exercise, BDNF is produced in high levels—essentially a growth factor for the brain (or a brain fertilizer) that helps grow back neurons.

Exercise increases BDNF specifically in areas of the brain where we see Alzheimer's disease develop. Exercise is critical for the health of the human brain, especially in cases of Alzheimer's.

As with all chronic diseases, Alzheimer's results from the interaction of genetic, environmental, and lifestyle factors over many years, causing changes in brain structure and function. While it is a complex disease with no single, clear-cut cause, for those with a 4/4 genotype, carefully creating your nutritional environment will likely postpone or prevent the development of Alzheimer's disease.

In summary, of the many theories about this disease—from toxic factors like aluminum or zinc or smoking being the causative agent—having an Apo E 4 gene (or two) seems to have the strongest connection—resulting in elevated insulin, cholesterol, and fats, with a corresponding cellular inflammatory process in the brain.

Future Directions—
A Useful Genetic Test to Help Guide Your Diet

In my clinical practice I am often able to discern trends in diseases. From these examples, I hope that you can see that the Apo E gene is a powerful component of our total genetic blueprint—a major factor in our overall state of health. For this reason, I believe this gene will be the focus of much future research in the areas where it interacts with our specific environment—our diet, exercise, thought patterns, and any medications we're taking, as well as its connection with heart disease, cancer, and many other chronic diseases, especially those involving the immune system.

In my opinion, not enough attention is being paid to the nutritional connection of these diseases with the Apo E gene. With more attention paid to that connection and with the right nutritional adjustments, reducing the risk of chronic disease is possible, and the risk of cardiovascular disease and Alzheimer's disease in particular can be lowered.

Furthermore, I think the risk for Apo E 4 genotypes extends beyond just Alzheimer's disease and heart disease. Given that my clinical experience has shown that patients with certain genotypes have certain disease clusters or associated illnesses, the development of many chronic illnesses may turn out to stem from imbalances within each Apo E genotype and how the person's environment supports (or doesn't) their specific genotype.

Genetic Risk and Family History

Looking back at your family's history can provide ideas of what diseases have occurred in your family. That gives you an idea of what you might have inherited and what might be needed to prevent a recurrence of untimely death. Remember that not only do you inherit the physical components of your body, but also the entire scope of your family's culture—through exposure to their beliefs, attitudes, customs, practices, and social behavior.

In addition to what has been imprinted by your family, the wider culture you live in also creates much of your belief structure. It's important to understand this, since it is your beliefs that shape your mind, body, emotions, spirit, and soul and show up in the environment you create around you. All of these factors will influence your journey through life.

Even a casual examination of your family's medical history can be helpful, but uncovering it can be difficult because with families scattered all over the world, as many are today, their health information is scattered with them. My patients often give a description like, "Grandpa lived until he was 97 years old. He was a farmer, and he lived in all that fresh air. But he ate all the wrong things. He must have had good genes to live that long." Perhaps he did indeed have good genes, but the question that begs to be asked is: Was his environment gene-supportive? He could have had so-called bad genes, but perhaps his genes had not "turned on" or been expressed negatively to adversely affect his health.

A farm diet, despite being high in animal fats, was usually replete with pure, whole foods—produce from the garden, eggs from free-range chickens, regular eating patterns without skipped meals, and a higher quality of life with a positive attitude of creating and producing—a sound foundation and mission.

All that plus a high amount of physical exercise could have promoted perfect health for Grandpa. The question then becomes: What have his descendants inherited? Is there a risk of genetic heart disease or not?

Many people have unrecognized hereditary cholesterol factors that can increase their risk of disease. Therefore, an accurate family history—or at least as accurate as you can gather—can help you decide whether or not to consider a more advanced cholesterol test. Selective testing can then assist your medical provider in evaluating the true risk of vascular disease.

The social milieu and working environment our family of origin likely experienced is not the same as the more sedentary lifestyles most of us live today. Even if Grandpa had a positive LDL Pattern B trait, Lp(a), and even an abnormal Apo E 4/3, eating whole foods and staying extremely active for his entire life might have kept these traits from "turning on," so that he lived a long and healthy life. However, with today's high-stress, nutritionally manipulated, chemically exposed, less-active lifestyle, he might not have been so lucky.

Remember, we know that a large percentage of heart disease is genetic, so getting genetic testing is important. A family history of *any* chronic disease, however, is the most powerful message you can get for the importance of a risk-reduction program targeting that disease.

A Patient's Story: Sam

Having been in the medical field for about 30 years, I can safely say I've seen my share of interesting situations. One I've encountered frequently is patients with the "doc in a box" mentality, where they demand a test immediately just because they want it right then, without even understanding what the test is all about or what the results might mean to their lives.

Many people have come to our office, insurance card in hand, demanding to have "this new Apo E test." They say a friend who's had the test referred them, and then they hold out their arm to have blood drawn, and "Oh, by the way, you can just call me with the results." But we don't operate this way.

One day a man named Sam walked into our office, handed his

insurance card to Barbara, our office manager, and said he was ready for his blood test.

Barbara looked at the schedule and didn't see his name listed. Neither did she recognize him.

"I don't seem to have you on the schedule," she said. "Are you sure you're in the right place?"

"Isn't this Pam McDonald's office?"

"Yes."

"Then I'm here for that Alzheimer's disease test."

Barbara asked if he meant the Apo E gene test. He agreed that was the one.

"Have you seen Pam before?" she asked. "Are you her patient?"

"No. I've never met her," Sam said. "I was just looking at getting that test today. I understand you don't have to fast for it. I have good insurance, and they'll pay for it. And if they don't, you can bill me."

Barbara knew that Sam had no idea what the Apo E test was all about and asked why he was interested.

"I've got Alzheimer's disease in my family," Sam replied, "and I want to get tested to know if I'm going to get it."

When Barbara recommended that he make an appointment for a consultation to learn more about Apo E gene testing, he became agitated. "I want this test done today," he insisted as he pulled out his credit card and placed it on the counter. "I have a lot of money. I can pay for the test."

I came around the corner at that moment and saw the distress on Barbara's face. She asked Sam to take a seat and filled me in on the situation.

I invited him into my office and asked him to sit down so I could tell him more about the gene test and the Apo E gene. Still upset, he wasn't inclined to listen, but I asked him to give me about 20 minutes of his time to provide some critical information, and then I would answer all his questions. Ten minutes later, he returned his credit card to his wallet in very slow motion. He began to relax and sat back in his chair. When I had finished talking, his face showed surprise at what he had learned.

"Wow," he said. "I had no idea this test was so powerful and important. Thank you."

Sam did return later for Apo E gene testing, along with other tests so that we could see the larger picture of his health. He chose not to know his Apo E gene type, saying as long as I knew it and could prescribe the right nutrition, exercise, and stress-reduction plan for him, that was just fine. He knew that if he ever changed his mind and wanted to know the test results, all he had to do was ask.

Sam began following the appropriate plan for his Apo E genotype and now says his health has never been better.

How Different Genotypes Use Fuel Differently

The digestive system basically consists of various organs that function to break down food into components the body can use. The goal is to transform healthy, whole food into small, nutritionally loaded, fuel packages that can be placed in the cells. Now we must ask how fuel use relates to the Apo E gene.

Each Apo E genotype has a preference for the different types of fuel provided by the different foods that can be eaten—from the short-term carbohydrates that burn quickly, to the long-term fats that burn slowly—summarized in the following table.

3.2 Food-Type Preferences of Apo E Genotypes	
Apo E 2/2	Prefers more long-term fuel
Apo E 2/3	Prefers more long-term fuel
Apo E 3/3	Prefers a balance of long- and short-term fuel
Apo E 4/2	Prefers a balance of long- and short-term fuel
Apo E 4/3	Prefers more short-term fuel
Apo E 4/4	Prefers more short-term fuel

The Apo E 4 combinations cannot effectively use fat in high amounts. Apo E 4 genotypes need to rely on moderate glycemic load, and carbohydrates such as vegetables and fruit, high in antioxidants and fiber.

The Apo E 3 genotypes have neutral or normal ability to use cholesterol, fat, and glucose as fuel. A balanced combination of moderate fat and carbohydrate intake is required for this genotype, avoiding all high glycemic load carbohydrates. In my practice, I often see trends related to genotypes, such as more insulin resistance and type 2 diabetes with the Apo E 3/3 genotype than any other. I am not sure what the reason is, but one interesting consideration is that Apo E 3/3 people cannot tolerate a low-fat diet or imbalance in the Big Three—they require 25 percent of their calories to come from healthy fats.

The Apo E 2 genotype tends to utilize fat as the preferred source of fuel, rather than carbohydrates. This genotype should avoid all high glycemic load carbohydrates in preference to moderate glycemic load carbohydrates.

You need to take into consideration the quality, quantity, and usability of any fat, protein, or carbohydrate based on your genotype. This next diagram (on page 37) shows blood glucose levels with both incorrect and correct eating habits.

Caloric Requirements and Your Optimal Health

In today's complex and fast-paced technological world, many people are willing to open a bottle of pills or try almost any kind of treatment that promises fast weight loss, including extreme diets with no science behind them. More and more people are becoming overweight and adopting a sedentary lifestyle. But we don't *have* to give up good health in today's world. We can live a healthier life if we become mindful of creating a gene-supportive environment and choose with care our food and our physical activities, as well as use some time-tested preventive and treatment methods based on an integrative medical approach.

The first thing to determine is how much fuel your body actually needs to maintain optimal daily functioning. In order to accomplish this, we must understand what a calorie is and how this may affect our fuel requirements.

Your body needs energy every second of every day. Every single bodily function, from thinking a thought to the complex operation of growing a body, requires fuel to energize it. Energy is measured in calories, with one calorie being the amount of energy required to increase the temperature of one gram of water by one degree Celsius. The calories that measure the energy in foods are in reality kilocalories (1,000 calories = 1 kilocalorie—sometimes capitalized to show the difference or referred to as kcal). The calories of the fuel we burn comes from carbohydrates, protein, and fat—what I like to call The Big Three—and is delivered via the intestines throughout the day. For some people, a fourth fuel is alcohol, but at the expense of getting no other nutrients, just empty calories. Caloric needs are individual, and everyone has a set calorie requirement per day to function well. Here are the fuel ratings for The Big Three, plus alcohol:

- 1 gram of carbohydrate provides 4 calories.
- 1 gram of protein provides 4 calories.
- 1 gram of fat provides 9 calories.
- 1 gram of alcohol provides 7 calories.

In addition to the proper amount of calories, it is important to divide calories among foods that are effective and beneficial to your body. It is very easy to overfeed your body by eating more than is necessary. For maximum benefit, your caloric intake should be spread throughout the day in smaller meals. Most of us are in the habit of having three meals a day, at set times, but there is no conclusive evidence to support any benefits from this pattern. In fact, many of my patients don't even eat breakfast, so starting with lunch, they have a concentrated feeding schedule over about 6 to 8 hours, leaving the other 16 to 18 hours with no food fueling the body.

We can learn a lot about how our bodies *should* be fed by seeing how long it takes to digest a normal portion of carbohydrates, proteins, and fats. In terms of quantity, we need to look at the size of the stomach. Should we be eating smaller meals, more frequently? The answer is yes. Frequent meals with smaller amounts are better suited to fulfill our fuel needs.

So how to split 2,000 calories over a 15-hour period? With properly sized meals, the ideal spacing between them is about three hours. This means six meals, which will maximize the body's balance of blood glucose and other nutrients. Here is a sample meal schedule, but be aware that individual caloric requirements will vary.

3.3 Sample Meal Schedule		
7 A.M.	Breakfast	400 calories
10 A.M.	Morning snack	200 calories
1 P.M.	Lunch	500 calories
4 P.M.	Afternoon snack	200 calories
7 P.M.	Dinner	500 calories
10 P.M.	Evening snack	200 calories

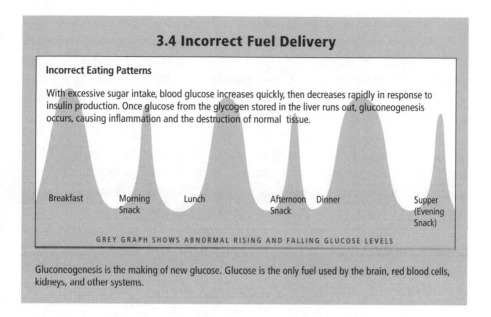

3.4 Incorrect Fuel Delivery

Incorrect Eating Patterns

With excessive sugar intake, blood glucose increases quickly, then decreases rapidly in response to insulin production. Once glucose from the glycogen stored in the liver runs out, gluconeogenesis occurs, causing inflammation and the destruction of normal tissue.

Breakfast   Morning   Lunch   Afternoon   Dinner   Supper
                    Snack   Snack   (Evening
                                                                                                                          Snack)

GREY GRAPH SHOWS ABNORMAL RISING AND FALLING GLUCOSE LEVELS

Gluconeogenesis is the making of new glucose. Glucose is the only fuel used by the brain, red blood cells, kidneys, and other systems.

3.5 Correct Fuel Delivery

Correct Eating Patterns

Normal blood glucose levels maintained with balanced short- and long-term fuel intake. No gluconeogenesis.

Breakfast   Morning   Lunch   Afternoon   Dinner   Supper
                    Snack   Snack   (Evening Snack)

GREY GRAPH SHOWS NORMAL RISING AND FALLING GLUCOSE LEVELS

This is an ideal eating schedule, and the only difference in its applicability between one person and the next is the caloric amount and when they sleep. For example, a very physically active person will have a higher caloric need than someone sitting behind a desk all day. The following represents a way to determine your own required daily intake of calories.

The first step is to calculate your daily caloric requirement. (We will look in detail at just how you can do that in Chapter 18.)

The second step is to start to learn the caloric content of your typical meals. Read the labels on food products so you know their caloric content. Serving size is important. Learn to recognize what a healthy serving—for you—of different foods looks like. Many people will be surprised to learn that a nutritionally balanced serving of carbohydrate, fat, and protein is far different than what we are used to eating. Serving sizes are included in the individual diet section (see pages 264–332).

In the beginning, using a timer can remind you to eat a meal or snack at appropriate times of the day (many cell phones have countdown timers). Many people find that their stomach works like clockwork after a very short time. I usually eat breakfast at 6:00–6:30 A.M. and by 9:30 or 10 A.M. I am ready for my snack. I can tell the time by my stomach—I am not one to miss a meal.

The next important step is to eat the correct foods so your calorie intake is just right for you—not for your friend, your husband, or your wife—*you*. While making dietary changes, you must regularly double-check your diet with your body composition to be sure that you are neither gaining nor losing an excessive amount of lean or fat mass too quickly. Once you reach the ideal weight, your body composition should be checked at least twice a year. Make food enjoyable by trying new recipes with new spices and whole food ingredients.

Multilevel Stress

Stress can be caused by mental, emotional, or physical strain. Stress comes in many different forms, some are related to emotional negativity, others to major life events such as getting married, a death, or job change. Stress can sometimes be tolerated, and sometimes not. What is stressful for one person may not be stressful to another. For example, some people consider a wedding to be a calm, beautiful, positive event. For most of the people involved, however, a wedding is a high-stress event. No matter what causes the stress, it requires and produces a host of chemicals and hormones within the body, the emotions, and the mind. Our physical body and nervous system, when stressed, require a large and continuous flow of fuel (glucose) in our bloodstream. When we do not eat correctly and keep our bodies fit and healthy, we are less able to tolerate stressful events.

Feeling stressed all day long is hard enough on a body, but skipping meals only causes it more stress. Not taking time to eat and rest properly causes the body to attempt to feed itself internally, causing stress on the cells. Typically, a busy person who does not eat may feel fatigued and take a caffeine drink to correct this feeling. But the caffeine stimulates the nervous system, which in turn requires more fuel or blood glucose, so it becomes a Catch-22, creating ever-more stress. Fundamentally, this is the internal cell stress we do not see. But if it goes on for an extended period of time, we begin to see chronic illness creeping into the body. The body shows very few signs that chronic illness, silent at first, is developing.

Let's look in more detail at a day in the life of a highly stressed person:

6 A.M. Wakes up. Skips breakfast. The body now has to make its own fuel because, during prolonged fasting like this, the body needs energy and will break down muscle to get it. Gluconeogenesis, or the breaking down of body tissue to feed itself, is set in motion. The by-products of gluconeogenesis are urea and ammonia, which create inflammation in the body—so an inflammatory process is now activated.

7 A.M. Drives to work. With a stressful drive, cortisol production increases. More fuel is required. More fuel required means gluconeogenesis continues, with still no food intake.

8 A.M. Gets to work. Drinks a cup—or two—of coffee. Coffee is a stimulant. Still no food, work stresses are beginning to build, cortisol is produced in still higher amounts. Gluconeogenesis continues—further inflammation.

11 A.M. or noon. The body begins to feel highly compromised. Keep in mind that the last time this person ate was probably dinnertime, around 7 P.M. the night before. It is now 11 A.M. We are looking at 16 hours without eating. The body can become very fatigued very quickly.

This person's day is an abnormal, self-imposed, multilevel, internal stress event. Yet this type of eating behavior is common among my patients. Why? Because people believe that if they don't eat, they will not gain weight. This cycle can be changed, but first it must be identified as an unhealthy behavior.

The symptoms of stress can vary from butterflies in the stomach to life-threatening, pure panic events. These, in turn, can elevate blood pressure and create heartbeat irregularity. Many people spend their lives with their nervous systems turned on high, and when coupled with poor fuel intake, this translates into more stress chemistry. This high-stress setting requires a lot of fuel in the way of glucose. It is as if the body has the gas pedal pushed to the floor and the engine is revving at top speed, but the wheels are not moving. When the nervous system goes into overload due to stress, we can begin to manifest physical symptoms, and extended stress with no relief can lead to chronic illness and depression.

The body doesn't have any way to counteract or use this level of stress—physically a fight-or-flight reaction—unless it runs or fights. The natural physical preparation of a fight-or-flight reaction is to increase fuel in the blood, increase oxygen and blood to the brain and large muscles, decrease fuel to the gut, and improve lung function to take in more oxygen. These are all basic reactions to be able to either fight or run.

If you are sitting in a meeting and are given some stressful information, and stress in the past has trained your body to prepare for either fight or flight, then your body becomes over-stressed with no outlet. This can harm you on many levels, physical and psychological. How this harm manifests is unique to each person.

You can control or change your reaction to a stressor. It just takes practice and patience. What does your body need at this point? It needs to shift out of this fight-or-flight reaction state into a calmer, restful state, so that you can logically think about the situation you are experiencing. An excellent way to calm the autonomic nervous system is by breathing deeply and slowly. Using the breath to help lower an elevated stress reaction is very effective (see page 218). Our breath is a connector between our conscious mind and our sympathetic and parasympathetic nervous systems, those automatic unconscious systems that function without our having to think about them.

As important as many other heart disease risk factors are, knowing your family history, your genotype, and how to intervene in multilevel stress events is of utmost importance in ensuring you'll end up with a backpack rather than a bedpan.

In the following chapter, we will look in more detail at what I believe to be our best path to developing and sustaining a healthy body, mind, emotions, and spirit—the perfect integrative-medicine solution.

A Patient's Story: Dr. Amanda

Amanda, 49, is a cardiologist who came to me for both personal and professional reasons. She wanted to learn more about her own health, and also gain knowledge she could share with her patients.

She had some real concerns about her own health. Her cholesterol levels had been high in the past, she had recently been diagnosed with elevated glucose levels—a warning sign for future diabetes—and her family had a history of cardiovascular disease and stroke. And, she added with a laugh as I took her medical history, "Can you do something about these terrible hot flashes and night sweats?" Then, in a more serious tone, "I'm sick and tired of feeling so terrible because of them."

As a cardiology specialist, Amanda was a busy professional. She also had a family—two children and a husband—who depended on her at home. She struggled with balancing all aspects of her life, including her own health. Typically, she got up at 7 A.M. to get herself ready for work and the kids for school, feeding them a quick breakfast of toast or cereal and then simply grabbing a glass of juice and a cup of coffee for herself before rushing out the door to drop off the kids at school then get to her office or the hospital. She usually didn't eat before 10 or 11 A.M., unless she grabbed a snack bar from the box she kept in her desk.

Her blood tests revealed that her total cholesterol was 243, her LDL was 164, and her blood glucose was 108—all high. She also had an elevated Lp(a), which is an element of cholesterol not tested in the standard cholesterol panel. Lp(a) at high levels has a tendency to increase the risk of heart attack and stroke, and Amanda's was twice the safe level. Her Apo E genotype was 3/3 (not able to tolerate a low-fat diet or long periods of fasting), and her body composition was 34 percent body fat.

She also kept a diet log for a week, which showed her diet was low in fat—something she believed necessary to keep her weight down—and that she frequently skipped meals.

These results motivated Amanda to make some changes in her life. First of all, she underwent a full cardiovascular screening to see if she had developed any disease. Fortunately, her results were negative. We worked together to set some goals. For the first week, she focused on her daily schedule so she would have time to eat right and exercise. Since this would take the cooperation of her family, she called a meeting to explain what she needed to do and why she wanted to do it. Her family easily agreed to help out.

With her new, healthier schedule, Amanda got up earlier so she could have time to eat a healthy breakfast based on her Apo E 3/3 requirements and walk for exercise every day. Throughout the day, she began to eat her meals and snacks on a regular basis. She also changed her schedule at work so she could have a break in the morning and afternoon to relax and eat a nutritious snack and have a soothing cup of green tea. Amanda treated herself to fresh flowers on her desk and bought a beautiful new teacup so she could enjoy her breaks even more.

Six weeks after beginning her new way of living, Amanda's total cholesterol had dropped to 187, her LDL was 84, her Lp(a) had dropped by a third, and her fasting blood glucose was a normal 89. While she still had night sweats, her daytime hot flashes had decreased. She had lost three pounds and 3 percent of her body fat while increasing her lean muscle mass.

Amanda saw very clearly how her old eating habits and stressful schedule were harming her health—and how the changes she made were reversing that trend. Not only was she sold on the diet plan based on the Apo E gene for herself, she began using the new information in her own cardiology practice.

3.6 Apo E Gene-Supportive Environment (GSE)					
	Apo E 2		**Apo E 3**	**Apo E 4**		
Genotype	2/2	2/3	3/3	4/2	4/3	4/4
Incidence Of Gene Expression	1%	10%	60%	2%	20–22%	5–7%
Genetic Base Pairs 112 and 158	TGC/ TGC (Cys/Cys) TGC/ TGC (Cys/Cys)	TGC/ TGC (Cys/Cys) TGC/ CGC (Cys/Arg)	TGC/ CGC (Cys/Arg) TGC/ CGC (Cys/Arg)	CGC/ CGC (Arg/Arg) TGC/ TGC (Cys/Cys)	CGC/ CGC (Arg/Arg) TGC/ CGC (Cys/Arg)	CGC/ CGC (Arg/Arg) CGC/ CGC (Arg/Arg)
Toxic Clearance	Very High Clearance	Moderately High Clearance	Moderate Clearance	Moderate Clearance	Poor Clearance	Very Poor Clearance
Gene-Supportive Environment (GSE) Diet	Very High Fat No Processed Carbo-hydrate	High Fat No Processed Carbo-hydrate	Moderate Fat	Moderate Fat Strict Limitations	Low Fat Strict Limitations	Vegetarian Strict Fat Limitations
Alcohol	Benefit with normal triglycerides has been shown to increase HDL		Increases LDL	Strong recommendation to avoid All Alcohol Increases LDL and decreases HDL		
High-Fiber Diet, Whole Soy Food, Plant Sterols & Stanols	Optimal servings of these foods reduce LDL cholesterol in all genotypes					
Omega-3 Supplement	Decreases triglycerides, small dense LDL and increases HDL		Decreases triglycerides, small dense LDL and increases HDL	Decreases triglycerides, small dense LDL. Increases LDL and decreases HDL		
Exercise maintains a Gene-Supportive Environment (GSE)*	55% Aerobic 45% Anaerobic	55% Aerobic 45% Anaerobic	50% Aerobic 50% Anaerobic	50% Aerobic 50% Anaerobic	75% Aerobic 25% Anaerobic	75% Aerobic 25% Anaerobic

*Do not exercise unless you have eaten.

Each Apo E gene requires an optimal gene-supportive environment (GSE). Chart 3.6 on page 43 outlines these differences.

Chapter Four

SETTING THE STAGE FOR THE APO E GENE AND DIET

"Cure sometimes, heal often, support always."
— Hippocrates

As an integrative-medicine nurse-practitioner, I am dedicated to disease prevention. I have developed an integrative-medicine diet and disease-prevention program by drawing on the knowledge and experience I have gained through my formal medical education, my clinical practice, and my integrative-medicine fellowship, as well as my life experience. I began using this program with patients in 2002, and as of this writing have seen several hundred patients (The Heart Health Watchers program, Danville, California).

As noted earlier, this diet is not a diet in the usual sense of the word. I use the word "diet" to mean *a series of specific recommendations for individual nutritional and other environmental factors that lead to disease prevention and a healthy life,* based on your individual Apo E genotype. This personalized plan for your genotype—your gene-supportive environment—will guide you in choosing the optimal:

- fat content, with the correct types of fats
- carbohydrate content, with the correct types of carbohydrates
- protein content, with the correct types of proteins

- caloric content, for your needs
- amount and kind of exercise
- balance of stress and relaxation in your life
- quality of mental and emotional environment
- type of energy and intentions you allow into your life (the spiritual component)
- physical environment (esthetics and other factors in the physical space around you)

The elements of this program draw strongly on the principles of integrative medicine. According to the University of Arizona's Program in Integrative Medicine, which is internationally recognized as the leading program in integrative medical education, integrative medicine is a healing-oriented type of medicine that takes into account the whole person (body, mind, and spirit), including all aspects of his or her lifestyle. It emphasizes the therapeutic relationship and makes use of any appropriate therapies, both conventional and alternative. The principles of integrative medicine[1] are:

- Patient and practitioner are partners in the healing process.
- All factors that influence health, wellness, and disease are taken into consideration, including mind, spirit, and community, as well as the body.
- Both conventional and alternative methods are used appropriately to facilitate the body's innate healing response.
- Effective natural, and less invasive, interventions are used whenever possible.
- Integrative medicine neither rejects conventional medicine nor uncritically accepts alternative therapies.
- Good medicine is based in good science. It is inquiry driven and open to new paradigms.
- Alongside the concept of treatment, the broader concepts of health promotion and the prevention of illness are considered paramount.
- Practitioners of integrative medicine exemplify its principles and commit themselves to self-exploration and self-development.

---

1   Based on the program in Integrative Medicine, University of Arizona, School of Medicine.

My experience in supporting patients in implementing the changes required by a diet based on the Apo E gene has led me to develop a number of general recommendations that apply to all, regardless of their particular genotype.

General Recommendations for Implementing a Diet Based on the Apo E Gene

These general recommendations will help you be successful in making changes in your current lifestyle:

- Use the principles of integrative medicine that:
  - take into account the whole person—body, mind, emotions, spirit, environment, and lifestyle
  - emphasize a supportive, caring, therapeutic relationship
  - make use of all appropriate therapies, both conventional and alternative, and
  - use culturally appropriate, natural, effective, minimally invasive interventions whenever possible

- Find a practitioner who is:
  - trained in integrative medicine, since nutrition and exercise are two very powerful tools of integrative medicine
  - committed to a healthy lifestyle, self-exploration, and self-development

- You will then be guided and supported in:
  - stimulating your body's innate healing with foods that match its genetic instructions
  - utilizing all three food categories (fats, proteins, and carbohydrates) in an optimal balance for your genotype (unless a medical condition prevents this)
  - focusing on foods that do not cause inflammation and are easily assimilated, metabolized, and cleared by your body
  - counting *all* calories (if weight is an issue)
  - choosing natural, whole (that is, unprocessed) foods whenever possible
  - utilizing routine blood chemistries and physical evaluations to make adjustments as treatment progresses

 ◆ implementing the exercise program that is best for your
   individual Apo E genotype
 ◆ adopting practices for managing life stressors (includes use of proven
   gentle techniques such as stress reduction, breathing exercises, prayer,
   or meditation)
 ◆ choosing and using appropriate natural supplements
 ◆ creating a pleasing, esthetic physical space around you

While an understanding of the whole picture, starting with the Apo E
genotype, is necessary to make appropriate recommendations for an *individual*,
the more general recommendations below apply to all types.

General Recommendations for Optimal Health

Improving Your Nutritional Intake

It has been my experience that the correct nutritional intake is one of the most
important factors for good health. The physiological environment you create as
a result of the foods you eat, combined with your Apo E genotype, are crucial
factors in preventing disease and maintaining your cellular balance. These
components are all part of creating the right internal environment:

 • Choose organic, whole foods—when possible.
 • Eat plenty of fruits and vegetables.
 • Eat balanced amounts and types of proteins, carbohydrates, and fats.
 • Eat mindfully and slowly.
 • Choose appropriate food portions.
 • Cut back on excessive caffeine and alcohol.
 • Avoid GMO, chemically treated, and processed food.
 • Stop eating on the run.
 • Eat foods that taste delicious and feed your soul as well as your body.

Regular Physical Activity

Regular physical activity is as important as good eating habits. The following
routines are a few examples of beneficial activities that contribute to optimal
health. Whether it's one of these, a combination, or other activities, you'll get the
greatest benefit if you do them regularly.

- aerobic (cardiovascular) exercise
- anaerobic (strengthening) exercises
- flexibility exercises
- daily walks

Greater Self-Awareness

As you make your lifestyle changes, you can enhance the process by some form of self-expression that helps you to stay in touch with how you are feeling as you go along. Be sure to choose a form of self-expression that you enjoy and can do regularly. These are a few examples:

- painting, sculpting, or other art practice
- music
- journaling or writing

Relaxation or Stress-Reduction Practices

These examples are just a few techniques my patients have used successfully. Try one that appeals to you:

- meditation, contemplation, or prayer
- mindfulness practice
- a balance between work and play

Spiritual Practices

While the following examples may be unfamiliar, try them on for size. This is no different from trying new foods. If you don't like the flavor of the activity, then find something else:

- inward disciplines (meditation, prayer, study)
- outward disciplines (simplicity, solitude, submission, service)
- incorporate disciplines (confession, guidance, worship, celebration)
- remember the things for which you are grateful

Other Recommendations

The following suggestions are general recommendations for overall health and well-being:

- Improve your sleep patterns.
- Start a new class (for instance, educational or development class, yoga, tai chi).

- Practice preventive oral hygiene (flossing, regular dental checkups).
- Stay connected with friends and family.
- Be optimistic.
- Be caring and kind.

Unhealthy Practices or Behaviors to Eliminate

Practicing the positive behaviors above will likely make it easier to eliminate unhealthy behaviors. Take some quiet time to think about particular behaviors that are in your best interest to change. The following are examples of behaviors to eliminate:

- poor nutrition
- poor exercise and movement habits
- drug/alcohol abuse
- speeding
- tobacco use
- negative thinking

Chapter Five

APO E GENE TESTING AND ADVANCED CHOLESTEROL TESTING

"How very little can be done under the spirit of fear."
— Florence Nightingale

While our medical system has not yet fully embraced genomic information, nor applied it effectively to clinical medicine, the facts are that it is now possible to use genetic testing to help prevent some of the serious chronic illnesses that are appearing in near-epidemic proportions. A number of high-quality testing programs can give effective assessment and treatment options. One example is the subject of this chapter: advanced cholesterol testing coupled with Apo E testing. Just because you do not currently exhibit any signs of disease, this does not mean you will not develop them. Now is the best time for prevention. A high blood cholesterol level, as well as other risk factors, can lead to serious problems in the future, so finding out your total cholesterol, HDL, LDL, and triglyceride levels—the basic cholesterol panel—is an important first step in determining your risk for heart disease and Alzheimer's disease.

In addition to these routine blood tests, two advanced kinds of testing are valuable, and these are the subject of this chapter. One test is for the Apo E gene, while the other is an advanced cholesterol test. The Apo E gene is the number one gene affecting cholesterol. Besides the genetic testing, it's useful to consult with your practitioner to determine if you want to do the advanced cholesterol testing to learn your cholesterol subfractions—those components in the "pots" discussed previously.

However, there are important issues to be considered before deciding to have these tests, which must be done with the support of a health-care provider who may not even be familiar with them. In this chapter, my intention is to help you decide if either test is appropriate for you.

If you decide to do either or both tests, you can send for a kit (see Appendix E) that will make it easy for your provider to order the tests for you, since they can only be ordered by a licensed professional. They are simple blood tests that can be drawn at a local lab and then sent off to a special lab for analysis. About a week later your provider should have the results. In the meantime, you can study Chapter 6. This will help prepare you for possible changes that the tests may indicate are advisable for you to make in creating your optimal gene-supportive environment.

Apo E Gene Testing and You

A large percentage of heart disease is known to be genetic. So, as experience with patients has also shown me, even more important than looking beyond total cholesterol levels is testing for the number one gene that affects cholesterol and heart disease—the Apo E gene.

Most people are not sure how they feel about genetic testing or what to do with the results if they have been tested. Because it is such a new technology, most people have never discussed a genetic test with a medical provider, let alone had one performed. Yet if you have had a baby born into your family in the past few years, chances are the baby has had a genetic test for phenylketonuria (PKU). The routine genetic testing of newborns can identify genetic disorders that must be treated early in life, and is the most widespread use of genetic testing. All 50 states have passed laws requiring that newborns be tested for PKU because if it is not identified and treated very early with dietary restrictions, it causes mental retardation.

While the medical industry is in its infancy with respect to genetic testing and handling its results, we know enough to say that proper genetic testing can provide you with some important information that can help you determine how to best protect or improve your health. This does not mean that everyone should be gene tested. There are some involved, complicated medical and ethical issues associated with gene testing. I won't get into the debate about genetic testing from a philosophical standpoint, but rather share with you certain conditions under which you may—or may not—want to consider genetic testing. Your decision about whether or not to take the Apo E genotype test should be made with the help of a practitioner, ideally the one who will then order the test for you if you decide in favor. The guidelines below can help you and your practitioner make the right decision for you.

Drawbacks of Testing

The decision to get tested for the Apo E gene is not easy, and one of the main reasons is because your health-insurance company and your employer could find out that you have an above-average risk of developing Alzheimer's disease or cardiovascular disease. Besides their knowing, you might rather not know that unless you make major changes to how you live your life, you have a 90 percent chance of developing Alzheimer's disease. If you are considering the test because your family has a history of Alzheimer's disease, or you have very high cholesterol, you should talk with a medical provider who has experience performing these tests and can help keep your test results confidential.

The Apo E test, along with an advanced cholesterol test, can give you clear nutritional direction and guidance. The question then becomes whether *you* need an Apo E gene test, or just advanced cholesterol testing. Personally, I think it depends on what you want, need, and are willing to do. I do not recommend that testing be done just to find your risk of contracting Alzheimer's disease. Rather, the decision to be tested should be based on your desire to obtain the information necessary for proper nutritional guidance and assistance in preventing chronic illness.

Reasons for Doing Apo E Genetic Testing

Indications and warning signs that may be a reason for genetic testing are a familial or personal history of:

- severe cardiovascular disease
- Alzheimer's disease
- Parkinson's disease
- severe neurological disease
- gout
- alcoholism
- high triglycerides and/or LDL
- insulin resistance or diabetes
- substance abuse
- morbid obesity
- depression/anxiety disorder or other mood disorders

- confirmation of a high cholesterol disorder potentially being affected by the Apo E gene
- confirmation of a diagnosis of late-onset Alzheimer's disease in a symptomatic adult or to reduce risk with dietary prescription
- assistance with treatment of multiple sclerosis by dietary prescription
- assistance with treatment of Parkinson disease by dietary prescription

At the same time, if you have one of the following chronic illnesses or conditions and you are not getting better with your current care plan, you may want to consider getting an Apo E test to help improve your dietary patterns.

Here are just a few conditions that I have seen find exceptional success with dietary change related to an Apo E genotype:

- acne
- gout
- depression
- chronic pain
- high cholesterol
- hypertension
- multiple sclerosis
- anxiety
- fibromyalgia
- insomnia
- glucose intolerance
- arthritis
- diabetes
- alcoholism
- ADD and ADHD
- cardiovascular disease
- Parkinson's disease
- severe perimenopausal symptoms
- chronic obesity
- insulin resistance
- menopausal symptoms

I strongly recommend that you find a medical provider who has been trained in the advancing field of genetic heart disease and in integrative nutritional medicine to support you. More information on medical providers can be found at: **www.ThePerfectGeneDiet.com**.

Advanced Cholesterol Testing

You may want to consider getting advanced cholesterol testing if you:

- eat an inflammatory diet
- are an Apo E 4 genotype who eats an inflammatory diet
- have high levels of LDL (bad) cholesterol (not resolving)
- have low levels of HDL (good) cholesterol (not resolving)
- are unable to tolerate cholesterol medications

• experience high levels of stress

If the majority of the situations above apply to you, you *might* be at high risk of developing chronic illness, heart disease, or Alzheimer's disease.

By contrast, you will have a low risk of developing a chronic illness if you:

• are an Apo E 4 with a normal LDL (bad) cholesterol
• are an Apo E 4 with a high HDL (good) cholesterol
• have a balanced lifestyle
• eat a diet low in inflammatory foods
• pursue a well-established aerobic exercise program
• have healthy relationships
• are happy and involved in life with little or no stress
• are creating and living a life you love

Answering yes to the majority of these indicates you probably wouldn't benefit from advanced cholesterol testing.

On the other hand, if you don't know your Apo E genotype and you switch to a low-fat diet, and your small, dense LDL level then worsens, it may well be due to eating the wrong diet. Genetic testing might show that you are an Apo E 3/3 that can't tolerate a low-fat diet. Or that you are an Apo E 2/3 or 2/2 that needs to eat a much higher-fat diet.

Dietary Options Without Testing

In the absence of knowing your specific Apo E genotype, dietary improvements can be accomplished by *trial and error*—seeing what different diets do to your cholesterol levels. This requires monitoring your diet and body composition extremely carefully. I have tried this trial-and-error approach many times with patients and can tell you, it is not easy—it requires accurate, detailed diet documentation; a strict exercise log; multiple testings; and office visits. It is time-consuming, and patients soon get fed up with the rigid process. The frustration rate is very high, but if you are willing to monitor your diet, perform the exercise, commit to the testing, stick with the logging journal for your diet and body composition, and are patient, it will work. Rarely in this trial-and-error plan do you or your health provider ever find your Apo E genotype. You follow a general "What's good for one, is good for all" nutritional plan, and a "general" exercise plan, and watch to see what your cholesterol does.

A Patient's Story: Dora

For 16 years, Dora had been working with her primary-care doctor to solve her cholesterol mystery. Despite trying many different medications, reading all the books about lowering cholesterol and following their advice, and even trying some of the popular diets, Dora was never able to bring her cholesterol level below about 400—*double* the recommended maximum level for good heart health. When this lovely 75-year-old woman came to see me, she was not following any particular cholesterol-lowering program because she was stymied, as was her primary-care doctor, about what approach to try next. Nevertheless, she was still determined to reduce her cholesterol levels.

She had good reason. As she told me while relating her medical history, nearly every immediate family member suffered from severe heart disease, and many had already died. Clearly, she faced multiple risk factors for heart disease, and perhaps even Alzheimer's disease, since certain Apo E genotypes carry a higher risk for both. People with the Apo E 4/4, in particular, are more prone to Alzheimer's disease, although Dora said none of her family members had exhibited symptoms. I saw no hint of cognitive impairment in Dora, whose delightful sense of humor never failed to cheer me. Very no-nonsense and polite, she was also bright, aware, alert, and happy. She is also one of the most determined people I know. While her children were young, she worked nights as a telephone switchboard operator to support them, coming home in time to get them off to school and then sleeping during the day while they were gone. It was this same brand of perseverance that motivated her to solve the perplexing mystery of her cholesterol levels.

Once I explained that advanced cholesterol testing and an Apo E test could give her very detailed information, Dora eagerly agreed to have the tests done. The results showed extremely high total cholesterol and high LDL—not unexpected—as well as Apo E 4/4, passed to her from both of her parents.

Her test results of January 4, 2005, blew the top off the charts with a total cholesterol level of 489 and an LDL level of 381—both extremely high. Her HDL was 67, in the high range.

Now we had a very specific genetic road map, which we could use to structure her particular diet and exercise program. Since Dora had never been able to physically tolerate either drugs or botanical supplements typically used to lower cholesterol, we decided on a no-medicine approach using only diet and exercise in line with her Apo E 4/4. These top two integrative-medicine tools would be a true test of the right program for her genotype.

I recommended a diet for Dora that would reduce all her cholesterol levels. She was to make the changes slowly so her body could adjust. First of all, it was important for her to avoid skipping meals, with breakfast, lunch, dinner, and three healthy snacks spaced three hours apart. She was to eat 1,600 to 1,800 calories a day, divided this way: 25 percent protein from plant sources and fish (very little red meat, limited to only once every 24 to 48 hours), 55 percent carbohydrates from low-glycemic foods such as whole grains, and 20 percent fat in monounsaturated and polyunsaturated forms. In addition, Dora was to begin walking on a treadmill every day, beginning with 10-minute sessions and slowly increasing the time.

A month later, Dora's total cholesterol was 243, her total LDL was 160, and her HDL was 57. At the time of her third test, on March 11, 2005, her results had improved even further: total cholesterol of 214, total LDL of 142, and total HDL of 65. The final result: one very happy patient with exceptional results. A summary of her progress is as follows:

January 4

Total cholesterol:	489 mg/dL *(Optimal: below 200. High: over 240.)*
LDL cholesterol:	381 mg/dL *(Optimal: below 100. Very high: over 190.)*
HDL cholesterol:	67 mg/dL *(Low: 40. High: 60.)*

After a month of Apo E 4/4 genotype diet and exercise protocol with no medications:

February 8

Total cholesterol:	243 mg/dL
LDL cholesterol:	160 mg/dL
HDL cholesterol:	57 mg/dL

March 11

Total cholesterol:	214 mg/dL
LDL cholesterol:	142 mg/dL
HDL cholesterol:	65 mg/dL

Five years later, Dora still comes to see me occasionally, and she's holding her own.

Protecting Your Medical Records

As I mentioned earlier, in 1997 President Clinton proposed a law making it a crime for employers or insurance companies to discriminate on the grounds of any genetic testing data they obtained, but only half of the states in the United States adopted this policy. In any case, it's essential to protect patients' medical records to prevent discrimination as a result of such testing data.

With our current public policy, genetic testing can be a double-edged sword, helping to save lives and improve the quality of life for some, but causing financial loss for others, such as when a person's job, medical coverage, or both are lost based on genetic testing. Therefore, until we get our genetic medical record protection policies in place, I recommend that patients pay for the Apo E gene test privately to keep the results confidential.

Another option is to use an identification number rather than your name. I have set up a foundation, described in Appendix E, for anonymous Apo E gene and advanced cholesterol testing that will help protect patients and their medical records.

How to Get Tested

If you have decided to have genetic or advanced cholesterol testing, see Appendix E for information on ordering a kit that you can take to a practitioner to order for you.

Chapter Six

NOW THAT YOU KNOW YOUR APO E GENOTYPE

After getting your Apo E gene test results, you may have to devise a clear plan with respect to your current health and what you want to accomplish for your future health. Therefore, you must carefully consider your options.

Option 1
You might have been curious to find out your Apo E genotype, but you do not want to change your current behavior. Now that you know your genotype, you may choose to do nothing and simply continue living your life in the same way, allowing your behaviors and environment to determine your health outcome. For example, you now know you are an Apo E 4/4, but you choose to just wait and see if any health complications arise, taking your chances in the nutritionally manipulated environment of conventional foods. With this option, you now have a better understanding of the risk involved, but that's all, so I would not recommend taking the test.

Option 2
Having been tested, you may now know that you have a higher-risk type of Apo E gene but believe that certain medications will help reduce your risk of chronic illness even though you are not able or willing to make significant lifestyle

changes. Medication is a powerful tool, but not the only answer. You need the right medications. This means that finding a provider trained in the advanced field of lipid science and metabolic disease is very important when choosing to take the medical-treatment route. When choosing this option, make sure you find a good medical provider who is up-to-date on the latest treatment options and supports your request to reduce your risk of chronic illness over your lifetime, not just in the short term.

Option 3
If the test showed that you have a higher risk genotype and you're willing to follow a lifelong prevention program that includes all possible options, you can draw on allopathic medicine and alternative methods to reduce your risk of chronic illness—the path of integrative medicine. The full disease prevention program you will develop with your medical provider may engage you in the most comprehensive process you have ever undertaken, yet it could yield some of the best possible long-term positive health benefits.

Now that you have decided to take the path of integrative medicine and optimize your health and well-being, you need to be sure that you have a medical provider who will support you in your endeavors to enhance your health.

My Story: Pam

As an integrative-medicine practitioner, I never want to recommend a treatment or perform any procedure on a patient unless I have either first thoroughly researched it or experienced it myself. So, soon after I began testing and working with the Apo E gene material, I had myself tested for two reasons: One, so I could better understand what my patients would go through; and two, when a family member's results came back and we discovered she had an abnormal Apo E genotype, I wanted to see if I also had an abnormal variant.

While I was curious to know my own Apo E genotype, did I want to know if I had an abnormal variant, especially 4/4? Given that I knew the possible outcomes of having such a variant—none of them good without intervention—I wasn't sure if I could face that knowledge. But then, I figured, not knowing and not intervening with the correct diet, if necessary, was worse.

I went to see my physician, who is also a friend and colleague, and explained why I wanted to have this gene test. He agreed with me and signed the order to have my blood drawn. I took it to my dear friend Betty, a medical assistant and phlebotomist, so she could take the necessary sample. I put my arm down so she could reach the vein at the crook of my elbow, but just as she moved the needle toward my arm, I jerked it back.

"Not so fast," I said. "Betty, do I really want to do this?"

Understanding my reason for hesitating, she asked, "Do you want to talk to the doctor again?"

"No." But I didn't put my arm back down on the table, either.

Betty sat down and looked me in the eyes. "Think about why you're doing this. You just told me that you want to have yourself tested so you can experience what your patients will experience, yes?"

I had to agree with her. "You're right. I need to know how this feels. Go ahead."

I surrendered my arm, and Betty drew the vial of blood.

A few weeks later, I walked into the building where my doctor has his office. He was walking down the hall toward me.

"Hi, Pam. Did you see your results? You're Apo E 4," he called down the hall and continued into his office.

I stopped in my tracks, feeling as if all the blood in my body had suddenly gushed from my body. Shaking and speechless, I just stood there. I couldn't believe the results—and I couldn't believe my doctor would deliver them in such a public, insensitive way. Finally, I walked into his office and sat down in the chair across from him.

"Are you all right?" he asked.

"Wow. Do I have one 4 or two?" I knew that an Apo E 4/4 is the worst variant; a 4/3 would at least be a little better.

"You're a 4/3. What does that mean?" he said. No wonder he had been so breezy about delivering the results in the hallway. Not familiar with the Apo E gene, he didn't know what they meant.

So I explained my own gene test results to my doctor. While the 3 is a good transporter of fats and cholesterol, I told him, the 4 is the one that doesn't work so well and, with the wrong nutrition, can cause serious health problems.

Seeing that I was shaken, he then summarized all the current disease-preventing practices I already perform on a daily basis—exercise, good diet, stress reduction, mind-body-spiritual practices, etc.

"Think about it, Pam. You are a healthy person," he said. "You have extremely low cholesterol, your subfraction cholesterol is completely normal, and you have a negative heart scan, so your diet is clearly the right one for you. You've created the right environment for your genotype without even knowing it. And with these results, we know you're living the life journey you created, and your purpose is much bigger than you knew."

He was right. I was healthy, and now knew how to stay that way. I was actually very lucky, since I was one of the people who could actually tolerate a low-fat, higher-carbohydrate diet because of my specific Apo E gene combination. I decided to remember his words and continue living my life as I had been.

This was an important lesson for me. I had received Apo E test results in the worst possible way. However, I believe that this happened exactly the way I was supposed to experience it—I now knew how not to deliver painful or frightening results to patients who chose to have the Apo E gene test. I became even more protective toward my patients, and careful about how I explain the test and the results. Yes, my experience was perfect.

How to Choose a Medical Provider

Selecting the best possible medical provider can be a daunting process even under the best of circumstances, since the health-care provider–patient relationship involves something we all value most—our health. Use care when choosing a medical provider so that the outcome provides a fulfilling relationship.

The best time to choose a health-care provider is before you need one. It's best not to wait until you or a loved one is faced with an illness or emergency. Know that not all medical providers are created equal, or have the appropriate training. You will usually make the best choices after some research. Write down your requirements for a health-care provider and order each according to its importance to you. Then proceed to research the possibilities using the information sources available.

It is helpful to remember the distinction between allopathic and integrative medicine. Allopathic medicine is the model our current medical system uses for treating disease. It derives its name from "allele," which means "opposite," and seeks to find drugs or procedures that will reverse the symptoms. It tends to ignore, or at least not directly address, the underlying problem the symptoms are pointing to.

Integrative medicine has been called the future of medicine. It is relatively new on the scene, and there are not very many practitioners as yet. However, I suggest you locate a physician or nurse-practitioner trained in integrative medicine if at all possible.

While some medical providers have a philosophy that fits your belief system, others may not. It is vitally important that you inquire about a practitioner's training and background. Many medical providers say they can care for your total health; however, when you question the extent of their specific training, you may see some important deficiencies in their ability to appropriately evaluate and treat your whole health picture.

For example, the therapy provided by a professional chiropractor can be valuable when used with a primary-care provider—such as an M.D., D.O. (doctor of osteopathy), N.P. (nurse-practitioner), or P.A. (physician's assistant)—but not in place of them. I also work with some exceptional chiropractors who provide excellent care within the boundaries of their training. However, some patients are under the impression that chiropractors are medical doctors because of the word "doctor" in their degree—D.C. (doctor of chiropractic)—but chiropractors are alternative-medicine providers who aren't necessarily trained to deal with all medical conditions.

The world of alternative medicine is wide and varied. Some practices of alternative medicine are safe, some are very questionable, and some are outright dangerous. Most people do not have the background to discriminate between safe and unsafe practices of alternative-medicine practitioners. It is wise to get guidance from a primary-care provider trained in integrative medicine before attempting to utilize any nontraditional therapy or practice. Integrative-medicine practitioners have been educated in many fields of medicine, not just traditional allopathic medicine. They can help you identify the differences between safe, and some of the potentially harmful, medical treatments that are sometimes used despite concerns about their efficacy and safety.

Selecting a Medical Practitioner

The following guidelines will help you select a medical practitioner who is appropriate for you:

- Consider your personal likes and dislikes of any potential providers.
- Consider their education, training, and competence.
- Consider choosing an M.D., N.P., D.O., or P.A. for your main advisor.
- Consider a provider known for caring about his or her patients.
- Consider a provider who takes the time to listen to you and your concerns.
- Choose a medical provider who is able to explain information clearly and at your level of understanding.
- Choose a medical provider who will anticipate potential long-term health problems.
- Choose a provider who practices not only disease management but also disease prevention.
- Choose a medical provider who personally practices what he or she teaches.

Additional factors that might affect your choice of a medical provider include:

- your health-insurance plan
- the location of the medical provider's office
- the location of the hospital where the provider treats patients
- the age and gender of the medical provider—some women prefer women and some men choose to see only male providers
- cultural considerations, such as language and belief systems— someone with the same faith or religious beliefs, such as someone who offers prayer and spiritual guidance as an option

Integrative-Medicine Resources

The following Websites are examples of good programs; they can also direct you to trained integrative-medicine practitioners:

Duke Center for Integrative Medicine:
www.dukehealth.org/Services/IntegrativeMedicine

Andrew Weil, M.D.:
www.DrWeil.com

Scripps Center for Integrative Medicine:
www.scrippshealth.org

University of San Francisco, Osher Center for Integrative Medicine:
www.osher.ucsf.edu

University of Arizona Program in Integrative Medicine:
www.integrativemedicine.arizona.edu

Your main medical provider is a key player with respect to providing you with important information, guidance, and support. Knowing who you are and what you want is also key. Once you have found a medical provider, the following section will help guide you with regard to your next steps.

Learning Who You Are—Self-Exploration

As we mature, we develop a sense of who we are, what we want, and why we want it. Some of us may be more aware of this than others. Regardless of where you are in this process, the following questionnaire will help you think more deeply about who you are, where you have been, how the world influences you, and what you want out of your life.

Integrative medicine puts a lot of emphasis on the value of the patient-provider relationship. As well as deepening your understanding of who you are at this point in your life, this questionnaire will allow your medical provider to learn more about you. This will be helpful when, together, you develop your care plan.

A Patient's Story: Rebecca

Rebecca was 26 when she first came to see me. She was chronically ill, with severe, chronic pain in her feet and ankles. This wasn't surprising since she weighed 254 pounds, with a little more than half her weight, or 51.5 percent, being body fat. For many years, Rebecca had tried most of the popular diet plans—Atkins, Jenny Craig, Weight Watchers— and she had even worked with two local weight-loss providers in her struggle to lose weight and keep it off. None of them had worked. In fact, she had continued to gain weight, even though she had followed each plan religiously. Finally, she came to see me, determined once and for all to lose weight, lose her pain, and be healthy.

As always with new patients, I took a detailed medical history. Rebecca's family had a strong history of heart disease; and she suffered severe headaches, chronic pain, terrible acne, kidney stones, and chronic constipation. Her gallbladder had been removed as a result of gallbladder disease. Not surprisingly, she also suffered from deep depression. Her modest job created high levels of stress for her.

I also gave Rebecca the Integrative-Medicine Questionnaire, which contains questions that help both my patients and me to understand their past, their beliefs, and what they really want out of life (see page 67 for this questionnaire). I also gave her a physical exam, and she had an Apo E gene test. She was an Apo E 4/3. Now it all made sense why she had never been able to lose weight—and even gained pounds—on the popular alternative low-carb, low-calorie, and high-protein diets that seemed to produce such good results for other people. Relieved and happy to know the reason, she was more than ready to test the nutritional plan that was best for her genotype. More than once, she asked me why no one had ever told her about this process before.

She studied the Big Three food groups—carbohydrates, protein, and fat—and how they applied to her Apo E 4/3. Very slowly, Rebecca began making dietary changes according to her genotype. At her next visit, her weight had increased by two pounds, but that did not deter her. The next time, she weighed 246 pounds—she had lost 10—and by six months, her weight was 223 and her body fat was 46 percent. In addition, her cholesterol improved, her acne had completely disappeared, as had her constipation and chronic pain.

Six months after that, or one year after her first visit, she had slimmed down to 197 pounds and 41 percent body fat. She had lost 59 pounds, of which 42 pounds were fat.

Today, Rebecca continues following her prescribed Perfect Diet and exercise and stress-reduction plan. She is happier and healthier than at any time in her life, feeling like a beautiful woman who has gained control of her health.

"I've changed my life for good," she says, "and I won't ever look back."

Integrative-Medicine Questionnaire

Review this section in a quiet, comfortable, relaxing place. Do not rush through the questions—think carefully, and be open and honest with yourself. You may want to use a separate pad of paper or a journal in which to write your answers.

Growing Up

- Where were you born?
- Close your eyes, relax for a few minutes, and think back to some of your first memories.
- Describe who you were as a child (happy, sad, joyful, carefree, afraid).
- Describe who you were as a teenager (happy, anxious, nervous, carefree, relaxed, isolated, connected).
- Can you identify any major experiences or life lessons from those early years?
- Other than being born in a certain place because your parents lived there, can you find or imagine any "higher purpose" or spiritual reason why you were born into that physical place?
- Describe who you are now.
- How would you describe yourself to another person?

- Imagine how someone who knows you very well would describe you.

- Imagine how someone who knows you casually would describe you.

- Write down some key experiences from your life and how they have shaped you and made you the person you are today; include:

  - any and all significant relationships

  - any significant events connected to an educational experience or career

  - how these affect the way you are viewed in, or you view, the world

Who and What Is Most Important to You Today?

Rate each of the areas below on a scale of 1 to 5 (where 5 is of highest importance), and jot down any thoughts this question brings up:

_____Health (mind, emotions, body, spirit, environment)

_____Partner (husband, wife)

_____Family (children, grandchildren)

_____Family of origin (grandparents, mother, father, brother, sister, children, aunts, uncles)

_____Self-developed/created family

_____Career (Is your work fulfilling the part you think you were meant to be playing in the world?)

_____Friends (lifelong, deep friends to casual acquaintances)

Having identified who and what is most important to you, write your response to the following questions:

- What does family represent to you?
- What do friendships represent to you?
- What do work associates represent to you?
- Are there any other key people in your life?
- Who can you trust and go to in times of stress?
- Are these trusted ones family, friends, life teachers, helpers, counselors, advisors, or tutors?
- Do you communicate openly with these people?
- Do you convey your wishes and desires from your true heart?

- Is it easy or difficult for you to communicate openly with others?
- Are you satisfied with the work you are currently doing?
- Have you ever asked yourself what is your purpose on this earth, and does your current work fit with your purpose or heart's desire? The following questions can guide you in determining this:
  - Do you feel as if your work flows from your heart or is it restrictive, unsafe, controlled, or limited in nature?
  - At the end of the day, has the time and effort you have spent with people at work left you with positive or negative feelings?
  - What kind of work relationships do you want to have with others?
  - What kind of work relationship do you want to have with yourself?
- How do you want to think—negatively or positively?
- How does having your heart's desires change your current life?

Overall Health

Keep in mind that not everyone functions in an optimal way when a low-stress lifestyle is followed. Some individuals actually function better under higher stress situations than lower stress situations.

- Are you aware of whether you best function in lower or higher stress situations?
- When stress is excessive, do you focus on excuses or finding blame in others?
- Do you see life situations as opportunities or problems?
- Most of the time do you consider yourself to be healthy or sick?
- Do you think a lot about your health? If so, what aspects do you think are the most important?
- If you think a lot about illness, what are the specifics of the illness you are preoccupied with? Is it a chronic illness or a brief or occasional illness?
- Is your health-care provider a licensed primary-care provider trained in allopathic medicine?
- Is your provider one who fits your needs and can evaluate your entire health, not just a small, specialized piece of it?
- How do you describe your relationship with your current health-care practitioner?
- Do you feel restricted in your communication (perhaps due to fear of being rejected if you make a request)?

- Do you feel like you have enough energy every day, or are you fatigued much of the time?

- Do you sleep well?

- Do you get enough sleep?

- Do you have a preset bedtime?

- Do you have a sleep routine that works for you?

- Do you take any supplements or medicines to help you fall asleep?

- Do you use any other sleep aids, such as alcohol or drugs?

- If you do, is this a chronic habit or infrequent practice?

- Do these supplements or medications fit with your belief system?

- Do you wake up within a few hours of going to sleep?

- Do you wake up most nights to go to the bathroom, or for another reason?

- Do you wake up on your own when it is time for you to get up, or use another method such as an alarm?

- How do you feel when you awaken: happy, sad, depressed, fresh, energized?

Nutrition

- Are you aware of the type and quality of food going into your body?

- Have you ever explored the value of the different types of food, such as whole foods versus processed?

- Are you mindful or mindless of the quality and quantity of foods you are consuming?

- Do you have control of the food you consume? Or is someone else responsible for the food you are eating? Family member, caretaker, restaurant, others?

- Do you include supplements and vitamins in your daily life?

- Does your primary-care provider recommend these supplements?

- Are your supplements self-prescribed?

- What do you know about these supplements?

- Have they been prescribed 100 percent for your benefit, or were they prescribed for a provider's financial gain?

- Is your supplement 100 percent pure (at least according to the label)?

- Do you know if your vitamins or supplements are manufactured under the highest-quality conditions?

- Do you know if your supplements interfere with any medication?
- Do you feel 100 percent comfortable with your intake of vitamins and supplements? Are you sure they are the correct ones for you?
- Are you sure that what is on the label of your supplement or vitamin is what is in the bottle or container (vitamins are not FDA regulated)?

Exercise

- Do you move regularly during your day, or are you primarily sedentary?
- What are the levels—low, moderate, high—of your daily activities?
- Do you know what physical activity levels and exercise routines are?
- Do you have a daily exercise routine?
- Do you have a weekly routine?
- Are you limited by sickness or injury?
- Do you like exercise, or are you completely turned off by it?
- Has your experience included friends or family who have exercised or who do not exercise?
- Would you like to learn how to exercise and learn to like exercise?

Relaxation

- Do you know how to relax?
- Do you feel you have any time to relax?
- Do you make time each day to relax?
- Can you define what relaxation is for you?
- When you do relax, do you feel guilty?
- If you do feel guilty, can you identify reasons why?
- Have you ever been given a message that relaxation is a waste of time?

Spirituality and Love

- What is spirituality for you?
- Do you feel connected to a higher purpose/spirit?
- Can you describe what brings meaning into your life?
- When you are in a time of stress, do you look to a source of higher power/God for guidance?
- Have you been loved in the past?

- Do you feel you are loved?
- How is love demonstrated to you and around you?
- Do you love yourself?
- Do you love others?
- Can you express your love?
- When and how do you experience joy?
- When and how do you experience happiness?
- When and how do you experience love?
- When and how do you experience peace?
- How often do you acknowledge and express these feelings and emotions?
- Were you encouraged to ignore or suppress them?
- Can you describe and express love, joy, peace, and happiness?
- Do you actively seek to bring these things into your life; or were you taught and have you been focused on expressing anger, fear, hurt, or unkindness?

As you come to the conclusion of this exercise, take some time to think carefully about the information you have explored here. You can use it to help make changes to improve your health and life. Over the next few days and weeks, I recommend that you write down any thoughts that come out of this exercise that surprise you, as well as strong feelings that come up, be they negative or positive. If you need assistance with what you've discovered, talk with your primary-care provider. He or she can help guide you.

"Wherever you stumble, there you will find your greatest treasure."
— Unknown

Chapter Seven

MAKING THE CHANGES
YOU WANT TO MAKE

Have you ever tried to make a major change in your daily routine and found that it is not as easy as you thought?

For example, have you ever tried to change your eating habits? What about eliminating sweets, candy, or desserts from your diet? If you have tried to do this, you may have failed because this is not an easy change to make. So here are important questions to ask: Do you need to remove these foods from your diet, or can you make them count? Can you make desserts and sweets become part of the important foods you eat?

First, look at your current sweets intake. Is it primarily sodas, candy, and other refined carbohydrates? Then look at the whole foods available to you, and ask yourself if you can make changes where dessert and sweets are concerned so that you are using whole foods instead of processed foods. The answer is yes, you can. A positive behavioral change process like this will enhance not only the quality of your body, but also that of your mind, emotions, spirit or soul, and environment.

Replacing old eating habits with new ones poses a significant challenge for most people. However, if you use the right combination of carbohydrates, fats, and proteins from pure, whole foods at each meal, they become fun foods and no longer pose a behavioral challenge. For example, if you have a cookie made with poor-quality, highly processed ingredients, the cookie will have a negative effect on your body's cells. However, if you make a cookie with high-quality, whole-food ingredients, it will have a positive effect. The cookie has now become a positive food for the body. Once we start eating whole foods on a regular basis, our taste adapts. We no longer crave the unhealthy foods we once ate. In the recipe section (Chapter 20), I have included some fun foods that contain important calories in the form of whole foods.

Viewing food as an essential ingredient in good health is the first step to making changes in your eating behavior. While most people do not connect what they eat with health or disease, making this connection is important. In order to begin changing your behavior, you must first recognize that a change is needed, and then you need to identify how this change will benefit you. Finally, you will have to want to make the change.

Let's look at a method that can support you in this process. Known as the **stages of change,** developed by James Prochaska, Ph.D., and Carlo DiClemente, Ph.D., in the late 1970s, it has become one of the most important approaches to behavioral change in the health field. Here is an outline of each stage, ending with actions you can take to move toward the next level.

Stages of Change[1]

Stage 1: Pre-contemplation
Characterized by the thought, "I don't think I have a problem."

At this level, you are in denial. You see no problem and, therefore, no need to contemplate change. You might say, "There is no problem" or "I don't have to fix what's not broken."

There are no actions you can take at this point since you see no problem or need for change. You may or may not later get a wake-up call and move to the next stage.

Stage 2: Contemplation
Characterized by the thought, "Is change really beneficial?"

You may be saying, "Prove to me that a change is needed."

At this level, you have some knowledge of your disease-promoting behaviors and may be considering making some beneficial changes. You have not yet made a

---

[1]   See *Changing for Good,* by James O. Prochaska, John Norcross, and Carlo DiClemente, HarperCollins, 1994.

pledge because you are still considering the advantages and disadvantages of a major behavior change.

Actions you can take: Consider making a plan for initiating change. Keep it simple. For example, you may love to eat at a fast-food chain three times a week. You should already know that this kind of food, in excess, is not good for achieving and maintaining optimal health. Slowly it may dawn on you that you can't keep this up and expect to remain healthy.

Stage 3: Preparation
Characterized by the thought, "I am going to do this! I'm ready to go for it!"

At this stage, you are ready to get started. You're ready to make a change. You are now developing a concrete plan.

Actions you can take: Develop clear objectives and precise procedures. Plan short-term and long-term goals that are sensible and achievable, along with a clear idea of how to accomplish them, and in what time frame.

Stage 4: Action
Characterized by the thought, "I'm doing it!"

At this level, you have allocated your time and energy to reaching your goal. Even this is a tremendous step forward. In addition, you may develop a strong belief, and the confidence, that what you're doing is good and worthwhile. These feelings will drive you to achieve success—enjoy them.

Actions you can take: Continue to follow up with those assisting you with this change. Their support can be pivotal in linking you to any additional information and resources you may need to maintain and strengthen your convictions that you can make the desired changes. In-person support is best, but you can get good support by phone or Internet if necessary. For example, you might want to eat fast food only twice a week, then drop down to once a week, and also decide that if you eat fast food, you won't "super size" it. Ask your support person to help you stick with these decisions.

Stage 5: Ongoing Maintenance
Characterized by the thought, "It's difficult to think of how I was before."

It may be difficult for you to remember what your behaviors were like before you became dedicated to your good health. When you have sustained the new behaviors for six months to a year, you can consider that you have graduated to ongoing maintenance. When you reach this level, you know the benefits of the behavior change because you can feel and experience it firsthand. At this level, there is only one goal left to focus on: prevention of a setback.

Actions you can take: consider defining some long-term behavior maintenance approaches to prevent reverting to old behaviors. For example, develop a support system, review past journals and logs, keep up with body-composition tests, be proud of your improved health, and focus on how you feel and look now versus how you previously felt and looked.

Stage 6: Relapse or Termination

Characterized by the thoughts "How can I get back on track?" or "Am I done with this now?"

Relapse is common, and being prepared to start over again is important. If you have relapsed, see if you learned something new about yourself and about the process of changing behavior. For instance, ask yourself, "I did it for six days, so what made that work?" Shift your focus from failure to whatever promotes problem solving. Get the support you need to re-engage in the change process. Set realistic goals to prevent becoming discouraged and take positive steps toward that behavior change.

Alternatively, you have conquered the problem and no longer feel the temptation to return to your old, poor behavior. Congratulations! Typically, confidence in success peaks after a year, but temptation may linger for another year or two. Once you no longer feel any temptation at all, you know you have reached your goal and can enjoy your success.

Identifying Your Current Stage

I hope you now have a clearer idea of what it takes to make real and sustainable changes in your life. If you are not ready to make the changes you sense you would need to become a happier and healthier person, then simply do your best to study and follow the information that tells you how to move toward a level where you will be ready to make the next step. It can be very helpful to find a person who will support you in this, and we will look more closely at this in the following pages. Also, ask your medical practitioner for assistance whenever possible. Read health newsletters of reputable institutions like Harvard, Berkeley, Duke, Johns Hopkins, Tufts, and Stanford. You can find some very reliable information on the Internet, too.

Connecting with a Support Person

Changing our behavior long-term requires a strong support system. It is human nature to want to feel connected to others—and to be understood by them. Sometimes, when we are unable to accomplish something by ourselves, we need to involve another person who can help us shift ourselves out of a negative behavior pattern into a positive one. I suggest you identify a support person and schedule a time, daily or weekly, to discuss your progress and the challenges you are facing.

In your session with your support person, the checklist below may help you focus your thoughts and give you both a deeper understanding of where you are and where you want to be.

Support Person "Check-in" Questionnaire

Current Date:_____

Support Person's Name:_____

Medical Provider's Name:_____

Which stage are you in?

Stage 1: Pre-contemplation

____ Stage 2: Contemplation

____ Stage 3: Preparation

____ Stage 4: Action

____ Stage 5: Ongoing Maintenance

____ Stage 6: Relapse or Termination

The six steps in each of the following sections correspond to the Six Stages of Change.

My Mind: Thoughts and Feelings

Step 1: Ask yourself, "Am I, or have I been, focusing my thoughts and feelings primarily on what I want to accomplish, or what I want out of life?"

_____ Yes   _____ No

Step 2: Given your response to the question above, circle a number on the scale below that represents how you are feeling, right now.

Negative   Positive
1   2   3   4   5   6   7   8   9   10

Step 3: Discuss your score and the associated feelings with your support person.

Step 4: After you have shared your feelings with your support person, gently acknowledge, or simply notice, without judgment, the presence of any negative thoughts. Then, withdraw your attention from these and focus on the positive thoughts and feelings associated with what you want to accomplish.

Step 5: Rate your feelings once again by circling the number on the scale below, as it relates to how you are feeling *now*.

Negative   Positive
1   2   3   4   5   6   7   8   9   10

Step 6: At this time, could you benefit from the information or expertise of an additional support person, such as a counselor or medical provider?

If "Yes," I suggest that you do not continue with the following sections until you find an additional support person. If you do not need additional support, continue to the next section.

My Body

Step 1: Ask yourself, "Am I, or have I been, focused primarily on what I want with respect to how I care for my body?"

_____ Yes   _____ No

Step 2: Given your response to Step 1, rate how you are feeling in the present moment by circling a number on the scale below.

Negative   Positive
1   2   3   4   5   6   7   8   9   10

Step 3: Discuss these feelings with your support person. If you know you want to make changes to your weight, body composition (percent body fat and lean mass), body mass index (BMI), body measurements, nutrition, and exercise habits, include how you feel about each of these with your support person.

Step 4: After you have shared your feelings with your support person, gently acknowledge, without judgment, the presence of any negative thoughts. Then, withdraw your attention from these and focus on the positive thoughts and feelings associated with what you want to accomplish.

Step 5: Rate your feelings once again by circling the number as it relates to how you are feeling *now*.

Negative   Positive
1   2   3   4   5   6   7   8   9   10

Step 6: At this time, could you benefit from the expertise of an additional support person?

My Spirit/Soul
Sit quietly and take several deep breaths to calm and focus your energy. When you are ready, move forward to consider the following questions.

Step 1: Ask yourself, "Am I, or have I been, focused primarily on what I want to accomplish, or what I want out of life with respect to my spiritual/soul life?"

_____ Yes   _____ No

Step 2: Having asked this question, how do you feel in this moment? Rate your feelings by circling an actual number on the scale below.

Negative   Positive
1   2   3   4   5   6   7   8   9   10

Step 3: Discuss these feelings with your support person.

Step 4: After you have shared your feelings with your support person, gently acknowledge the presence of any negative thoughts. Then, withdraw your attention from these and focus on the positive thoughts and feelings associated with what you want to accomplish.

Step 5: Rate your feelings once again by circling the number as it relates to how you are feeling *now*.

Negative   Positive
1   2   3   4   5   6   7   8   9   10

Discuss your overall feelings of this session.

Step 6: At this time, could you benefit from the information or expertise of an additional support person, such as a counselor or medical provider?

My Physical Environment

Step 1: Ask yourself, "Am I, or have I been, focused primarily on what I want to create in my physical environment?"

_____ Yes   _____ No

Step 2: Having answered this question, how do you feel in this moment? Rate your feelings by circling an actual number on the scale below.

Negative   Positive
1   2   3   4   5   6   7   8   9   10

Step 3: Discuss these feelings with your support person.

Step 4: After you have shared your feelings with your support person, simply notice, without judgment, the presence of any negative thoughts. Then withdraw your attention from these and focus on the positive thoughts and feelings associated with what you want to accomplish.

Step 5: Rate your feelings once again by circling the number as it relates to how you are feeling *now*.

Negative   Positive
1   2   3   4   5   6   7   8   9   10

Step 6: At this time, could you benefit from the information or expertise of an additional support person, such as a counselor or medical provider?

Congratulations! You now have greater clarity on how you feel and where you are with respect to each of these areas of your life. Now, it is time to write down the goals and tasks to be accomplished in the next few days and/or weeks as they relate to each section. Make your goals both meaningful and achievable. You may want to enlist the help of your support person in doing this! Remember, you can change these as you go along and learn more about what you want and what you can achieve. You may also want to take a look at the chapter "Tools for Change" (Chapter 16).

Discuss how you are feeling now with your support person. Set a date for your next support meeting.

Remember, there is no better time than right now to begin creating the life you want.

At a Glance—Principles and Behaviors to Always Consider

You may want to copy this section and keep it with you at all times.

Keys to Your Perfect Diet

- Educate yourself about nutrition with regard to your own personal health and Apo E genotype.
- Stay open-minded about nutrition—it is an evolving science.
- Find two or three trusted resources to support you in your ongoing nutrition education.
- Drink from a trusted, clean water source. Don't take the water you drink for granted.
- Eat unprocessed—whole food—carbohydrates.
- Eat mostly two types of fats—monounsaturated and unprocessed polyunsaturated fats (omega-3s)—derived from a whole, nonprocessed food source.
- Eat high-quality proteins that contain only nonprocessed monounsaturated and polyunsaturated fats.
- Eat a variety of fruits and vegetables, of all colors, from an organic, non-GMO source.
- Support wholesome local farming, and dine at restaurants that offer healthy menus. Educate yourself regarding local farming and restaurant practices.
- Know what you are putting into your body each day— mindfulness is the key.
- Take only vitamin supplements that apply to your health needs, not what is recommended for the general population.

Choose a high-quality product that is not focused on generating profit. Know the full details behind your personal vitamin (or botanical) regimen. Store them properly (cool, and sometimes refrigerated).

- Know the personal risks and benefits of alcohol as they apply to your health. Do not follow the general population's recommendation.

- Prepare and display your food in a way that is pleasing to you. (Consider china, silver, or crystal over plastic, styrofoam, and paper.)

- Practice stress reduction and align your intention with your goals and desired changes throughout the day.

- Actively and respectfully move your body daily, using stretching, strength, and aerobic exercise.

- Be aware of your surroundings and environment—respect Mother Earth, communicating honestly and with love and kindness.

Chapter Eight

FOOD: THE FOUNDATION

Food is grouped into three main categories: carbohydrates, fats, and proteins—The Big Three. Eating the right balance of these foods for your genotype is a prerequisite for your good health. Understanding what these categories of food are, and how your body uses them, is the first step in choosing the right combinations that meet your body's specific fuel needs.

Carbohydrates

Carbohydrates are the simplest of foods. They provide the body with an immediate source of fuel in the form of sugars and starches that are easily digested and enter the bloodstream as glucose. Glucose is the most basic nutrient that your body needs and uses—the preferred fuel of cells. However, this fuel is short-term; it's quickly metabolized. One gram of carbohydrate yields only four calories of energy.

Carbohydrates, Glycemic Index, and Glycemic Load

Historically, nutritional scientists have tried to devise a method of categorizing carbohydrates to guide wise food choices. Despite public health messages promoting high-carbohydrate, low-fat, low-calorie diet regimens to achieve weight loss, and the public's knowledge of the health hazards associated with being overweight or obese, the prevalence of weight problems in the United States continues to rise. Of particular concern are the increased risks associated with obesity—hypertension, type 2 diabetes, heart disease, and many other chronic disorders. If not controlled, these diseases can pose a significant economic and emotional burden to both those afflicted and to society.

As I've shown elsewhere, of particular concern is the lack of scientific evidence on the safety and efficacy of low- or no-carbohydrate diets on overall health. Because low-carbohydrate diets derive the majority of calories from protein and fat, there is the potential negative impact on cardiovascular health. It is important to have a clear understanding of what carbohydrates really are, and how they are used in the body because I've recommended that people get a minimum of half their calories from carbohydrates—not just any old carbohydrate, but specific ones having a low glycemic load.

What Is This Word "Glycemic"?

Glycemic means "causing glucose in the blood." Before 1981, carbohydrates were seen as two main types, simple and complex, based on the number of sugars in their molecular makeup. The simple carbohydrates are monosaccharides and disaccharides because they have only one or two sugar molecules. The complex carbohydrates are called polysaccharides because they have more sugars in their molecular structure and take longer to be digested.

In 1981 this concept was expanded with the introduction of the *glycemic index* (GI)—a number assigned to each carbohydrate food indicating how much it raises your blood sugar when eaten. The idea caught on and people began to avoid foods with high GIs. In 2002 the GI concept was further refined by taking into account the average serving size, because a high GI food consumed in small quantities has the same effect on blood sugar as larger quantities of a low GI food. This number is called *glycemic load* (GL) and is calculated by multiplying the grams of carbohydrate content in a food times its GI, divided by 100.[1]

What happens when you eat a high GL meal? A quick increase in blood-sugar level causes your pancreas to lower its blood sugar level by producing more insulin. The high insulin level then drops the blood sugar, or glucose level, but at a cost to your body. After a time, the overworked pancreas becomes tired and is unable to produce enough insulin—*insulin resistance*. If your diet continues along the same path, type 2 diabetes will result. If the pancreas is pushed even further, pancreatic cancer may develop.

This is how high GL foods have given carbohydrates a bad name. Low GL foods do not increase the blood glucose as quickly, so less insulin is needed to keep your blood sugar stable. These are the foods we evolved to have as a major part of our diet, and for optimal health, we need to return to.

A Patient's Story: Alexis

Nineteen-year-old Alexis had been diagnosed with abdominal migraines, which are a variant of migraine headaches that cause spontaneous abdominal pain with terrible nausea and vomiting. Not surprisingly, she was suffering anxiety attacks, and she would often sleep more than 12 hours at a stretch from exhaustion. Finally, she was exhibiting signs of anorexia because she rarely felt hungry and also was often afraid to eat because of the severe abdominal pain. Her primary-care doctor had prescribed medications to control the nausea, vomiting, and anxiety, and Alexis frequently required intravenous fluids because of the dehydration caused by vomiting. When she failed to improve, her primary-care doctor recommended that she see me, and her worried parents came with her.

After taking a detailed medical history, I could see that Alexis was healthy and had few other stressors in her life except for the chronic abdominal migraines. Her eating patterns were abnormal and very

---

1 For example, a 100-gram slice of watermelon with a GI of 72 and a carbohydrate content of 5 grams (it contains a lot of water) calculates as 5 x 0.72 = 3.6, so the GL is 3.6. A food with a GI of 100 and a carbohydrate content of 10 grams has a GL of 10 (10 x 1 = 10), while a food with 100 grams of carbohydrate and a GI of just 10 also has a GL of 10 (100 x 0.1 = 10).

unhealthy, mostly fast food when she did eat, partly out of habit but also because of her need to have food quickly, and food that tasted good. Her parents wondered if eating a healthy, nutritious diet would help—I believed that it might—so Alexis agreed to try it. She began eating healthier foods in a regular pattern and felt better for a few weeks, but then the abdominal migraines returned even more severely. So I suggested that she have an Apo E gene test and then refine her nutrition to meet the needs of her genotype.

When her Apo E genotype was revealed to be 4/3, she began eating correctly for that type, which meant more complex carbohydrates on a regular basis. Her health improved dramatically, and the abdominal migraines diminished. She began to sleep much less and her anxiety attacks improved a great deal. I explained the reason for the improvement to Alexis and her parents. Very simply, with her Apo E genotype, her body became extremely stressed when she ate very little and on an irregular basis. Combined with the dehydration, this pattern severely depleted her glycogen stores, which are necessary for providing continual energy to the body, and sent her metabolism into a tailspin. For Alexis, this meant abnormal cell functioning in her intestines, which brought on the abdominal migraines.

Alexis continued her anti-anxiety and migraine medications at previously prescribed levels for a time, and then slowly reduced them under medical supervision.

Fat

Fat is a more complex source of fuel than carbohydrates and is derived from two principal sources—plants and animals. When the body breaks down fat molecules, the end results are compounds called free fatty acids and glycerol. The liver then processes these fats and glycerol into glucose, which can then be used as a fuel source.

Fat, once digested and absorbed, provides a long-term form of fuel in the body because it is a more complex package than carbohydrates and takes longer to break down and use.

The fats in our diet can be classified into four main types: monounsaturated, polyunsaturated, saturated, and trans fat. The monounsaturated and polyunsaturated fats should be consumed in the right proportions for your genotype, or your body can become greatly imbalanced. Again, depending on your genotype, your body can tolerate no saturated fats, or only a limited amount, and we should all avoid trans fats. More on that later.

As we'll see, contrary to popular opinion, we *need* fats in our diet. We need the right kind, though, so choose your saturated fats wisely. I consume mine every other Friday via a small amount of high-quality cheese. I derive great joy from my excellent-quality cheese and consider myself to be a cheese connoisseur, but I must be smart and avoid eating too much. Keep in mind that a single gram of fat yields nine calories of long-term fuel for the body, no matter if it comes from monounsaturated, polyunsaturated, saturated, or trans fat.

Protein

In talking about fats, we need to talk about proteins, too, since all natural unprocessed foods containing protein also contain fats. It seems we cannot open a magazine or turn on the TV without finding some protein drink, bar, powder, supplement, or some other fad idea about protein. Selling protein is a multibillion-dollar business and industry. The fashionable Atkins diet trend gave a tremendous boost to the protein industry, and today billions of dollars are wasted on these processed protein products.

Protein is essential for the development and maintenance of individual cell structure and function, as well as regulating hormonal activity. Coming from both plant and animal sources, it is composed of long chains of amino acids that are linked together and break down into mostly carbon, hydrogen, oxygen, and nitrogen. This last element—nitrogen—is not present in carbohydrates or fats. When the body has to use protein as fuel, rather than as building blocks for cellular repair and maintenance, it produces nitrogen-containing amino acids that are burned and produce a waste product in the liver, urea, which then has to be cleared by the kidneys.

As I said above, protein foods most often contain fat (unless it is processed out). Animal protein contains mostly inflammatory fats, while plant and fish protein contains anti-inflammatory fats. One gram of protein yields only about four calories of energy, so it's not a very good source of energy.

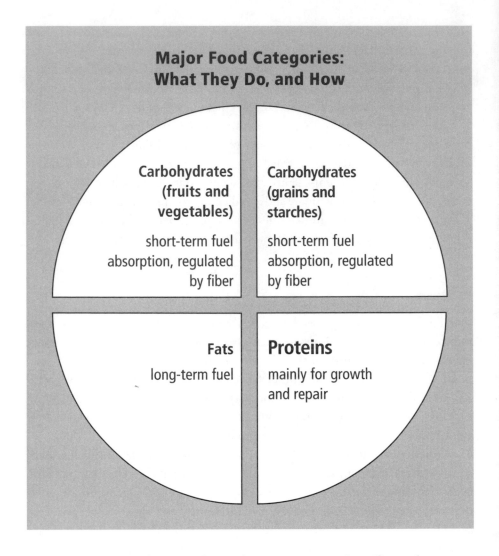

**Major Food Categories:
What They Do, and How**

**Carbohydrates
(fruits and
vegetables)**

short-term fuel
absorption, regulated
by fiber

**Carbohydrates
(grains and
starches)**

short-term fuel
absorption, regulated
by fiber

Fats

long-term fuel

Proteins

mainly for growth
and repair

The interaction between fats and protein is complex. If you do not eat enough carbohydrates, the glucose the body is designed to get from the carbohydrates will have to come instead from breaking down the body's fats and proteins. One of the uses of body fat is to store energy for times of fasting, which allowed our ancestors to weather lean seasons. But when that system is abused by chronic dieting or inappropriate food selections, and your fat stores are mostly used up, you can do a lot of damage to your body. In this situation your internal feeding system can cause rapid protein (muscle) loss and decrease your ability to burn stored fat. You use up your body's muscle mass to generate energy-producing fuel, all because you are not eating the carbohydrates your body needs. In the short term this may not be harmful. However, over a longer term, this can cause excessive, irreversible cellular damage and chronic illness.

The bottom line is that too much protein and small amounts of carbohydrates—as advocated in the Atkins diet—means limited fuel for the brain. A high-protein, restricted-carbohydrate diet puts the body into glucose-deficiency mode, causing major strain to the intestine, liver, and kidneys. The body ends up having to make its own glucose from internal sources to feed the brain and body. High-protein, low-carbohydrate diets are particularly dangerous to an Apo E 4 because the inflammatory fats are more difficult for this genotype to clear from the body, leading to an inflammatory process in the coronary arteries and elsewhere in the body.

How Food Becomes Fuel

First, food is placed into the mouth and begins to be broken down by the teeth and our salivary digestive enzymes. Food then passes down the throat through the esophagus into a baglike holding area called the stomach.

Once in the stomach, food is further broken down with hydrochloric acid, protein-digesting enzymes, and mechanical churning. From the stomach, food is moved into the first part of the small intestine, the duodenum. Here, the liver, gallbladder, and pancreas feed in more chemicals, enzymes, and other substances that play a major role in the breakdown of the stomach contents. Then absorption of the nutrients occurs in the jejunum (middle section of the small intestine) and ileum (last section of the small intestine).

Once most of the nutrients have been absorbed in the small intestine, the remains are passed into the large intestine or colon. Here live trillions of friendly *lactobacilli, acidophilus,* and *E coli* bacteria that are necessary for producing most of our vitamin K and for further breakdown of the unabsorbed food. Also, the colon recovers most of the water and minerals from the digestive juices that are no longer needed. What remains (fiber and a surplus of those friendly bacteria) is first stored in and then passed out of the last part of the colon, the rectum, via the anus.

Your body is now left with a supply of the nutrients absorbed by the intestines, but the ratio of the Big Three needed by the body may not be optimal because one or more of the them were restricted by dietary choices (such as a diet too low in fat). If so, cellular health can become unbalanced, leading to disease.

Popular Diets Are Harmful to Your Health

Most diet books focus on greatly increasing or removing one of The Big Three. Some of the most popular recent trends have been removing most fats or carbohydrates, or greatly increasing protein intake, in the diet. However, nutritional research shows that these approaches are not only *not* optimal for disease prevention, but may actually be *harmful* to your health.

Let's now look at several of these popular diets and some of the misinformation and misconceptions commonly associated with them.

Low-Fat Diets

Different Apo E genotypes need varying amounts of fat, and *no one* should remove *all* the fat from their diet. There are good fats and bad fats. The good ones are unprocessed polyunsaturated and monounsaturated fats that have a positive reaction on the cell. They include nuts, seeds, olives, and avocados. Overexposure to the bad ones—trans fats, especially, and too many saturated fats—causes cellular inflammation, which in turn leads to disease.

If you remove the wrong amount and kind of fat from your diet, your long-term fuel supply becomes unbalanced. The recent epidemic of type 2 diabetes may have partly occurred because our country has been encouraged to eat a low-fat diet for many years. Based on the popularity of programs like *Dr. Dean Ornish's Program for Reversing Heart Disease,* some of our major health organizations encourage a low-fat diet for better health. However, now that we know more about the importance of fats, it is clear that not everyone can benefit from a low-fat diet. But changing widespread misconceptions is difficult. Fat has been given such a bad name that a study conducted by the American Dietetic Association discovered a major misunderstanding that people have about it. They found that many people thought they should delete *all* fat from their diet to have good health, believing that the more fat they remove, the better health they will have.[2] This is extremely dangerous.

If we don't eat healthy fats (particularly the essential fatty acids), we cannot survive because fat is part of every cell membrane in the body. Because the brain has a fat content of about 60 percent, the fat content of a healthy brain cell is important for your brain to work correctly.

---

2   *ADA's Nutrition and You: Trends 2002 Survey.* Survey results are based on telephone interviews with a nationally representative sample of 700 adults conducted in April 2002 by Wirthlin Worldwide. The survey has a confidence interval of plus or minus 5 percent in 95 out of 100 cases.

A Patient's Story: Scott

When Scott was first diagnosed with slightly elevated total cholesterol of 219 and an LDL cholesterol of 128, plus a slightly elevated blood-glucose level in the low 100s (which could mean the onset of diabetes), he preferred not to take any medications. Instead, he wanted to use diet and exercise to bring the numbers down and improve his health. His family doctor agreed, encouraging Scott to eat a low-fat diet and exercise.

Scott enthusiastically followed this advice. He joined a gym and worked out diligently. He changed his diet so that he ate very little fat. He was confident this strategy would do the trick—wasn't it the method all the experts recommended?

But within a short time, Scott started to feel worse and returned to his doctor. Tests revealed that his total cholesterol had jumped to 271 and his LDL to 189. His HDL was low at 43. His blood pressure was also elevated, at 138/80, and his blood glucose had also increased. Since Scott preferred not to take medications, his doctor recommended a switch to a high-protein diet, along with continued exercise. That didn't help, either: Scott's total cholesterol remained about the same, while his LDL increased to 197. His triglycerides had risen to an alarming 220 (triglycerides are blood fat and the optimal number is less than 150), and his small LDL cholesterol factor called LDL Pattern B was an unhealthy 44 percent. Even so, his doctor recommended that he continue the high-protein plan. After several months with no improvement in his cholesterol and a worsening of his blood glucose to 164, Scott agreed to try medications—eventually he was taking six different drugs, some twice a day. Not only did his cholesterol and blood sugar not improve, he also began having constant stomach and intestinal problems. His family doctor referred Scott to a gastrointestinal specialist, and he underwent tests to check for a stomach or colorectal problem, but nothing was discovered. His inflammatory diet and medication were most likely the problem.

Finally, after three years of misery with multiple medications and a continued low-fat, high-protein diet with daily exercise, Scott's total cholesterol dropped to 140 and his LDL to 80. However, his glucose level was 132 and another cholesterol factor called HA1c, a long-term look at blood glucose, was too high at 7.0. And he still didn't feel energetic or healthy. Tired of feeling so poorly and hoping to wean himself from at least some of his medications, Scott came to see me.

After a thorough physical and medical history, I recommended that Scott have more lab testing, including, an Apo E gene test, and he quickly agreed. He is an Apo E 3/3, the "normal" Apo E genotype that cannot tolerate either a low-fat or a high-protein, low-carb diet. We discussed his diet options for his genotype, and he agreed to eat a diet with moderate healthy-fat content, eager to be healthy and to feel good once again. He began making slow dietary changes so that his body could easily make the adjustment, eating anti-inflammatory fats rather than inflammatory ones, whole grains rather than highly refined carbohydrates, and plant and fish proteins. He continued to take his medications.

Scott started to feel better within a few weeks. A new cholesterol test revealed that his total cholesterol was 151, and his LDL was 83. Four months later, his total cholesterol was 135, his LDL was 69, and his HDL was 53—all excellent numbers. His triglycerides had improved and his Pattern B had dropped from 44 percent to 16 percent, becoming a healthy pattern A. Best of all, Scott was feeling healthy and vigorous again.

We reduced his cholesterol medication at first by half, and he was eventually able to quit taking it. Since his blood pressure was normalizing, continuing that medication was causing his blood pressure to drop too low and making him dizzy, so we slowly reduced that medication as well until he finally did not need it any longer. Scott is still slowly weaning himself from his diabetes drugs.

Scott's overall health has improved dramatically since he began following the correct Perfect Diet and exercise plan for his Apo E 3/3. All his numbers have improved: body fat 15 percent, total cholesterol 177, LDL 99, HDL 63, and blood sugar in the high 80s to low 90s. He has lots of energy and says his golf game has improved.

"It doesn't get better than this," he told me during one of our visits.

I had to agree with him.

However, it is extremely important to know what type of fat you are eating. Avoid inflammatory fats such as trans fats and excessive exposure to saturated fats, as well as highly processed polyunsaturated oils and omega-6 fats. This will be covered in more detail in later chapters. At the same time, you must also have the correct amount of inflammatory-reducing fats from a monounsaturated and polyunsaturated omega-3 source. The correct ratio of fats for all genotypes is very important, as we will see in the pages ahead.

Another critical misconception is not realizing that fat generally comes "packaged" with protein. For instance, beef protein comes with beef fat, and beef has the highest inflammatory fatty acid percentage of any of the animal-protein foods. You can't get one without the other, unless it's in an unhealthy, highly processed product.

You need also to be aware of the source of fats in your diet. Most fats don't just come as a simple fat source like cooking oils, so you need to know what types of fats come packaged with what proteins:

- Animal proteins (meat and dairy) come packaged with saturated and trans fat
- Plant proteins (nuts, seeds, beans, rice, and soy) come packaged with mono- and polyunsaturated fats

Most foods are usually a combination of fats, carbohydrates, and/or proteins, yet people generally see foods as belonging to just one of these main categories rather than being a combination. This means that if you succeed in removing all fats from your diet, you're also removing other important nutrients. You need protein, and it's very difficult to get good protein without getting fats. You need to eat good sources of fat with good protein, such as fish and soybeans, two excellent sources of protein with anti-inflammatory fats.

Not knowing these facts can, in time, cause health problems for anyone on a low-fat, high-protein, low-carbohydrate diet.

Low-Carbohydrate Diets
Another alarming fad is the low-carbohydrate diet. While certainly successful for weight loss, the problem is that most of the weight loss is water and lean mass. Carbohydrate is a short-term fuel. Since the brain, intestines, and other organs function only on glucose, which usually comes from carbohydrates, if you are not eating them at every meal, your liver takes on the extra job of making glucose—gluconeogenesis. While making the glucose that you didn't get from carbohydrates, your body is paying a high cost—stealing proteins from your tissues by breaking them down as a source of energy. This can put added stress

Popular Diet Review

Before we look more closely at a healthy diet, I want to share my view on a few popular diets that I encourage you to review carefully before deciding to follow.

Dr. Atkins Diet Revolution

Theory: Metabolic imbalance, not calories, causes people to be overweight. Carbohydrates are responsible for some of our most modern diseases. A high-protein, low-carbohydrate, low-calorie diet can cause rapid weight loss.

Truth: There is an initial rapid weight loss; however, it comes mainly from water loss. The diet is very dangerous to your health because it is very high in artery-clogging fats.

Dr. Dean Ornish's Program for Reversing Heart Disease

Theory: An extremely low-fat (fewer than 10 percent of total calories come from fat or long-term fuel) diet is said to reverse heart disease.

Truth: This diet is extremely difficult to stick to, specifically because it is very low in fat, which provides taste and helps you feel full and satisfied longer. I find that most people don't continue with this type of diet for very long.

South Beach Diet

Theory: Fewer carbohydrates, with good fat, not bad fat, are best for everyone.

Truth: This diet, like the Atkins Diet, showed the public a different side of the diet world. It is much better than most. However, it still focuses on the "one-size-fits-all" dietary approach.

The Zone

Theory: High-carbohydrate diets are largely responsible for the rise in obesity in Americans. This diet claims that 75 percent of Americans have a genetic defect that leads to high insulin levels when a high-carbohydrate diet is eaten. The "Zone" targets a ratio of 40 percent carbohydrates, 30 percent proteins, and 30 percent fats at every meal.

Truth: No studies or references exist, just testimonials from satisfied dieters.

Sugar Busters!

Theory: Sugar is toxic. While it is suggested that calories do not count, it offers 1,200-calorie plans and asks you to limit portions. It suggests three meals a day, minimal snacking, no eating after 8:00 P.M., and reasonable quantities that fit nicely on a plate. No seconds.

Truth: This is a low-calorie, low-fat, low-carbohydrate, high-protein plan that is high in cholesterol and low in calcium, iron, vitamin A, and folate, yet supplements are not recommended. Conclusions such as "sugar causes resistance to insulin and then obesity" are not supported by scientific evidence. Most researchers believe insulin resistance is a *result* of obesity, not the other way around. Other unsupported statements include "inactivity may not be significantly harmful" and "dietary sugar is recognized as an independent risk factor in heart disease."

on your kidneys and liver because the nitrogen from the amino acid by-products must be processed by the liver and excreted by the kidneys. The result is rapid weight loss, but in addition to burning fat, you also lose some of the body's engine (muscle mass). This means that your ability to burn fat in the future is reduced because your muscle mass, your body's fat burner, is also reduced. It's like killing the goose that laid the golden egg.

The Atkins Diet is the most popular low-carbohydrate diet. One of its primary shortcomings is a failure to distinguish between "good" fats (olive oil and other monounsaturates) and "bad" fats (corn, safflower, sesame, and other processed polyunsaturates and saturates). Another shortcoming is that since few fruits and vegetables are included, you get very little of the all-important fiber, vitamins, minerals, and health-protective phytochemicals these foods contain. And, even though a few carbohydrates are allowed, this diet makes no distinction between the healthy low-glycemic load carbs (Chapter 8, page 94) and the less healthy high-glycemic load carbohydrates.

While some studies have shown that short-term use of Atkins-type diets may be safe and effective for weight loss (but what is being lost?), many physicians are concerned about its long-term health risks. And I hope you will be, too! With any diet we need to consider results—are you losing fat, or losing weight in the form of fluids and muscle?

You only need to stand at the checkout line of any major grocery store and read the headlines of a tabloid to know that there are hundreds of diets out there all claiming to help you lose weight fast. While the proponents of these diets claim "one size fits all"—that their diet will work for anyone and everyone—recent research is beginning to put a damper on these claims. Keep in mind, research indicates that these "one-size-fits-all" diets may actually be harmful to your health.

The number one principle of any diet should be "do no harm" to the body. I never recommend short-term, quick-fix, weight-loss diets because of their costs to your health in the form of chronic disease. By eating the correct diet and engaging in the right levels of physical activity for your genotype, you can maintain a healthy body weight and reduce your risk of developing diet-related chronic illnesses, from heart disease to cancer.

Today we know that how our body processes fats, proteins, and carbohydrates is genetically guided. Given this knowledge, my book is about recommending and implementing a comprehensive plan based on the advances in the field of cholesterol science, metabolism, and your individual Apo E genotype. It is specifically tailored to work in harmony with your own body chemistry. This plan recognizes that while food is a critical element in your health, other environmental factors—such as exercise and relaxation practices—are also of real significance and must be tailored to suit your individual genotype.

While this program includes recommendations for optimizing the health of your entire environment—mind, body, emotions, and spirit—in this book I emphasize your food environment. This is the area that I have found to be the most confusing and complex for people to grasp, largely because there is so much misinformation and so many misconceptions surrounding what is a "good" food and what is a "bad" food.

Even for those not following a faddish, one-size-fits-all diet, danger lurks for the uneducated consumer in the thousands of processed foods that contain artificial fats and other substances that our bodies cannot easily assimilate. Everyone should avoid highly processed and preserved foods. The farther away from its source that a food has been processed, the more likely it is to be harmful to the body. Let's look at why.

Chapter Nine

GOOD FOOD, BAD FOOD

Eating the right diet for your Apo E genotype is one of the best health investments you can make; therefore, it is worth your serious attention.

We have all heard the saying "You are what you eat." Now more than ever, research shows how it could be closer to the truth than we ever thought. The food we eat today becomes the cellular makeup of our human tissue tomorrow—our food goes from our plates to our cells.

Consider this statement: "There are no naturally bad foods." I first heard this from a doctor during my integrative-medicine fellowship. My first reaction was one of denial—there *must* be bad foods! Our system is loaded with them! Walk into any supermarket and you are bedazzled with all types of substances we call food but that are so highly processed only a trace of any "whole" or "natural" food remains in them. Some people call this the SAD—Standard American Diet.

However, as I reflected on this and began to learn more, I decided that the doctor was right. There are no naturally bad foods. It's what's done to them that makes them bad. In addition to across-the-board bad—highly processed— foods, different Apo E genotypes require differing amounts of fat, carbohydrate, and protein. I believe our genes have been selected by the lifestyles and environments of our past, largely as a survival mechanism.

Highly processed foods are a relatively recent addition to the human diet. Prior to their introduction, we ate whole grains, nuts, and fruits; and we occasionally consumed meat from wild or free-roaming animal sources that fed on native vegetation and provided more omega-3 fats than the omega-6 fats in our foods today. The local environment delivered these foods according to the season, and we ate the fruits and vegetables that grew in our villages and the wild animals that were indigenous to the area.

In today's mega-technological and rearranged world, it is important to ask: Has the integrity of my food intake diminished from that of my ancestors? Is my daily food intake good or bad for me? Do I even know what's good or bad for me?

Mega-Fake Food World

Whole food is usually good food. Take wheat, for example. Whole-grain wheat is an exceptionally good food, containing bran and germ, which are the parts richest in nutrients, including B vitamins, folic acid, calcium, phosphorous, zinc, copper, and iron.

Wheat is one of the most common ingredients in bread—bread being one of the oldest forms of prepared food, dating back to prehistoric times—when Stonehenge was built. Now roll forward 9,500 years. Take that ancient recipe of whole-wheat, coarsely ground grain; add a little water and salt to it; then bake in a hot stone oven.

However, what happens to wheat if it is highly processed or genetically modified? After it has had the bran and germ removed, washed with unknown chemicals, steel milled (producing high heat), bleached, had synthetic fats and preservatives added, left to rise, and then baked, it ends up looking like fluffy white sponges. After all this processing, the fluffy white sponges are put in plastic bags with eye-catching colors and compelling, but misleading, marketing messages, and placed on a shelf in the supermarket. We call this *bread*. This is not a whole food by any definition.

What happened? How and why did we decide that these new recipes were better for the human body? Why did we get so bored with the original recipe? Why didn't we consider that this new way of creating bread by manipulating grain could harm the human body?

Have you ever wondered if there could be a possible connection between the present epidemic of food allergies and chronic illnesses, and the practice of converting whole food into processed food? We now *know* that processing food causes chronic illness, and we must stop pretending otherwise.

Bread manufacturing is only one example of intensive food processing. The food industry is out of control, wantonly adding more and more harmful additives to an ever-growing range of foods. Where did this processing mania originate? I think it is largely the profit motive of megabusiness and its ability to apply technology to our food without considering the ramifications to our health. And as long as we buy the foods, the corporations get the message that we want them, and continue to expand their repertoire of processed foods.

The U.S. food supply has largely been taken over by a few huge multi-national corporations, focused entirely on maximizing their profits. One of their means of maximizing profits is to "refine" natural foods by taking out their most nutritious components (because they spoil more quickly), adding back some of what was removed artificially, calling the product "enriched," and adding preservatives and other chemicals. The end result is good-looking, "tasty," but nutritionally deficient pseudo-food that will have a long shelf life and sell well.

Some of the common methods of food preservation—drying, pickling, and curing—are almost as old as humanity. Before the advent of commercial operations, canning and preserving foods was done at home in America and other parts of the world. As the commercial canning and preserving industry grew in the 1950s and processed foods got cheaper, a family tradition lost its appeal.

We began to make changes in how we stored our food years ago. With the advent of technology, we became much more efficient at preserving and processing through the use of various chemicals and radiation. Most recently on the scene is genetic manipulation via genetically modified organisms (GMO). This means that the genes of plants are being genetically engineered to delay ripening and make them last longer, among other things.

Even before GMO technology, plant breeders were creating hybrids that are resistant to the usual bruising of shipping and handling, such as the now-ubiquitous "taste-free" tomato that can be stacked 12 deep in a shipping crate without damaging the ones on the bottom. Consumers' willingness to buy into this lower-cost system has made it increasingly difficult to access natural, whole foods, because they are grown by relatively more expensive labor-intensive methods.

Our natural food sources have given way to a world of highly processed, adulterated foods with multiple human-made substances and chemicals added to them. We do not know the full impact of many of these materials on the human body, but what we do know is not good.

Toxins and Processed Foods

Besides the food itself being toxic and the huge number of chemicals being added to it as it is processed, most commercially grown foods come to us with residues of pesticides.

Consider the food chain where animals, including humans, are eating other animals. We are familiar with how mercury concentrates in fish as it moves from those lower on the food chain up to the fish we eat. The same is true with farmed animals, whose food source has been highly manipulated through changed farming practices at all levels. Whenever we consume conventional meats and fish, our bodies are being exposed to the toxic substances in that animal flesh. For many people, this may be as often as two or three times a day. The risk of chronic disease through the ingestion of toxic animal flesh can be greatly decreased both by switching from a diet high in animal protein to one of organic plant-based foods with some organically produced meats if desired.

Say No to These Substances!

Our planet's environment has been severely manipulated and is completely different from that of just two generations ago. Of course, the same is true of the food we eat. These altered foods have been implicated as causative factors to a host of illnesses, from the escalating rates of obesity to heart disease. Identifying toxic ingredients in our food is a big job and can be a very confusing process— even for medical professionals, scientists, and nutritionists. The first line of defense: Read the food label. If you don't know or recognize the ingredients, don't eat the food! Another helpful tip is to not purchase anything in a box or container that lists unpronounceable ingredients or has more than four chemical additives. A third consideration is to eat unprocessed foods as often as possible. Fourth, consider the source of *everything* you eat and drink, not only foods, but also your fluids, including water.

Our foods contain many harmful chemicals that can seriously damage our health if consumed frequently over long periods of time. The body can handle an occasional exposure, but with more than this it becomes very tired while trying to clear these chemicals. Some of us have the ability to clear these abnormal toxins more easily than others, but they still add up and take a toll.

There are many toxic chemical substances that should be avoided. The following partial list provides a good starting point:

- synthetic fats, especially hydrogenated vegetable oil
- any food containing heavy metals, such as fish with high mercury content
- agricultural pesticides
- hormones
- herbicides
- fungicides
- insecticides
- artificial foods
- artificial colorings (especially Blue #1 and 2, Green #3, Red #2, 3 and 40, Yellow #5 and 6)
- potassium bromate
- processed vegetable oil
- artificial flavorings
- MSG (monosodium glutamate)
- all artificial sweeteners, including aspartame, saccharin, sucralose (Splenda), and cyclamate
- hydrolysate invert sugar
- lactitol
- maltitol
- sorbitol
- brominated vegetable oil
- butylated hydroxyanisole (BHA)
- butylated hydroxytoluene (BHT)
- highly refined corn syrup and corn oil
- dextrose (corn sugar, glucose)
- high-fructose corn syrup
- hydrogenated starches
- mannitol polydextrose

So What Can We Do?

Now that we have created a huge range of health problems for ourselves by learning to process, preserve, and genetically alter food at high levels, how do we get back to finding and eating healthy, whole food?

Should we be processing what we eat as much as we do, even altering the genetic makeup of the food itself? While some of us are debating whether or not changing food at the genetic level is a good idea, most people are not even *aware* that they are buying and eating genetically altered food.

I encourage you to educate yourself, your friends, and your family with regards to processed and GMO products. Moving beyond the processing and preserving of food into changing the genetic makeup of the food itself is a big, scary step for humankind. I believe that invading the genes of plants to alter an entire food source is putting the health of the world at risk, since there is no definitive research on what these genetic modifications do to the person consuming them.

Alternatives to these chemicals are natural herbs and spices; and food colorings from plants, flowers, fruits, and vegetables. In addition, staying with organic, unprocessed whole foods can help eliminate the ingestion of the above harmful chemicals.

Whole food should stay whole, unrefined, unprocessed, and unaltered genetically until we are sure that it is not bad for us. The lack of evidence of harm does not equal evidence of no harm.

While it is true that whole food, in its raw state, can taste bland compared to highly seasoned and augmented processed food, this is because the bland has become familiar. Once your taste buds have become accustomed to processed food, you must adapt back to the taste of natural whole foods to maximize your health. This will take some time, on average three to four weeks, or maybe a few months— and then you will wonder how you ever ate all that highly processed stuff!

Here are some Websites where you can learn more about the impact of, and options in, food preserving and processing:

www.centerforfoodsafety.org

www.thecampaign.org

www.seedalliance.org

www.ecoliteracy.org

www.saynotogmos.org

www.thefutureoffood.com

www.cropchoice.com

www.ucsusa.org

www.organicconsumers.org

www.calgefree.org

Your health is everything! Although the intention behind modifying, processing, and preserving foods may initially have been a good one, the food industry has taken these practices to the extreme. Why? Because they can, and because they want the profits, which gives them more money to develop the technology and machines to take it to ever more extreme levels. As long as megabusiness knows we will buy their "foods," they will be produced and the standard American diet will persist. We each have a responsibility to vote "No!" to these foods with our every food purchase.

Always keep in mind that there are no naturally bad foods. It is what commercial entities are doing to natural foods, and how we expose those foods to our body, that makes them bad or good. Food processing and modifying may now be costing us more in disease treatment than the time and money it was supposed to save.

A "Normal" Day's Diet

At this point I want to highlight commonly eaten foods that we don't normally associate with disease. Let's assume for a moment that you are a typical person who eats breakfast, lunch, and dinner. Most of the foods you eat are from your local supermarket, and you buy the "regular" food, nothing fancy. Here, then, is a typical food and supplement log of one of my own patients:

Breakfast   cereal with banana and milk
                    toast and coffee
                    1 vitamin
                    one over-the-counter, slow-release niacin tablet

The cereal is likely to be low fiber and processed, containing some form of preservatives. The regular milk contains antibiotics and hormones, and its saturated fat content can often be higher than people realize—2% milk is not 2 percent fat, it is 38 percent fat by volume, and whole milk is much higher in fat (see page 120). The banana (unless it's organic) probably contains some form of chemical sprayed on it as a pesticide. The toast (usually highly processed white bread) contains preservatives, and the coffee (unless grown organically) could contain added harmful chemicals. The over-the-counter, slow-release niacin tablet, to help with high cholesterol, was found to contain trans fat to slow the absorption of the niacin. We'll talk more about trans fats, but for now, believe me, this trans fat causes far more harm than the niacin does good.

Decaffeinated Coffee May Increase Disease Risk

Drinking a few cups of decaffeinated coffee every day may increase the risk for metabolic syndrome, a group of several conditions that occur together and may increase risk of heart disease, stroke, and diabetes. Metabolic syndrome is the combination of increased blood pressure, elevated insulin levels, and excess body fat around the waist, all of which can lead to abnormally high cholesterol levels. Having just one of these conditions increases risk of heart disease, and having more than one makes that risk even greater.

A 2005 study funded by the National Institutes of Health and conducted by Robert Superko, M.D., showed that decaffeinated-coffee drinkers had higher levels of the laboratory marker for metabolic syndrome called Apo B and for nonesterified fatty acids (NEFA), which have been identified as playing a role in heart attacks.

The three-month "Coffee and Lipoprotein Metabolism Study" showed that only drinkers of decaffeinated coffee, and not those who abstained from coffee or those who drank only the caffeinated type, had an 8 percent increase in Apo B levels and an 18 percent increase in NEFA. In short, the cholesterol levels of the decaffeinated drinkers rose.

Superko said the difference could be related to the beans used for decaffeinated and regular coffee. Harsher beans are used for the former so that they can retain enough flavor in the process used to remove the caffeine. The harsher beans contain more of a substance called deptines, which may cause the rise in NEFA, which then results in more Apo B.

Snack   candy bar

soda

Candy bars typically contain large amounts of trans and saturated fats as well as sugar and high-fructose corn syrup, artificial food colorings, and preservatives. The soda contains artificial flavorings and coloring, plus either loads of sugar or artificial sweeteners; and the coffee contains caffeine and any chemicals used to process it, plus any sweeteners and fat from cream or creamer.

Lunch   chicken sandwich and chips

soda

The chicken was likely fed GMO food, and hormones to make it fatter. Other chemicals, drugs, and pesticides were likely added to its diet as well. Potato chips are processed potatoes fried in a wide variety of fats. Many of these go rancid quickly, making normally healthy fats toxic to the body. The chips are also typically loaded with salt and preservatives. Soda usually contains corn sweeteners or artificial sweeteners, artificial flavorings, and coloring.

Dinner   hamburger, fries, and a salad

soda

ice cream

Much of this meal's nutritional content depends on whether it was home cooked or from a fast-food outlet. The beef can contain saturated and trans fat, the fries are usually fried in trans fat, and the soda contains the same toxic brew mentioned above. While the salad can be healthy if organic vegetables and a healthy dressing are used, it's likely that this isn't the case, particularly if the salad comes from a fast-food restaurant. The ice cream usually contains saturated fat from full-fat cow's milk or cream, sugar, plus artificial flavorings and colors.

The above diet can be extremely toxic to the body, yet it's very common with many people. Just seeing the type and amount of fat alone in this one-day food log is cause for concern. It reveals a very high exposure to inflammatory fats, which cause inflammation in the body's cells.

As already noted, if you are an Apo E 4, clearing this type of toxic fat is very difficult. While it may take many years of chronic exposure to these toxins to develop disease, an individual who takes in a moderate to high level of these unnatural foods will likely develop disease much sooner than someone who doesn't. On the other hand, *with a diet of completely natural foods, the risk of disease is greatly reduced, or even eliminated.* Knowing this, we, as a society, must ask ourselves some crucial questions:

- What does defective food do to the minds, emotions, bodies, and spirits of our growing children?
- How do these toxins affect us, the adults?
- Are the long-term effects now showing up in the older members of the population?

While we don't have complete answers to these questions, we do know that the body can handle occasional exposure to these toxic chemistries. It is when we expose our bodies to them over and over again that we put ourselves in distress, which leads to disease. If the intake of toxic food continues for a long time, the body can accumulate so much damage that it may have a difficult time recovering.

The human body can be very forgiving and can also change from dis-ease to ease, if given the right fuel. Many patients recover from chronic illness by giving their bodies what they need (natural, whole food), and leaving the rest to their 100,000-year-old internal healing system.

Toxins, Genotype, and Toxin-Clearing Abilities

One man's meat is another man's poison. — Anonymous

First, let's define what I mean by a toxin. A toxin is a chemical or substance that brings imbalance to the body's cells, creating an adverse environment. Toxins are a poison, but not the same as arsenic or strychnine. Rather, they can be ordinary foods that act as poison to a particular genotype over a long period of time, simply because the foods are wrong for that type. There are many different kinds of food and food sources that can cause harm to the body, if your body is so predisposed.

The standard American diet delivers high amounts of inflammatory fat, usually more frequently than once in every 24- to 48-hour period. These fats, when eaten in excessive amounts, cause long-term inflammation that block the normal functioning of cells by limiting the delivery of nutrition into the cell membrane. The resulting cellular imbalances can bring about many major chronic illnesses.

Each Apo E genotype differs in its ability to clear toxic substances from the body. Educating ourselves to the capabilities of the different genotypes enables us to be more aware of our vulnerabilities to various food toxins. We can then use this information to better protect our bodies.

As we saw earlier, we each have one of the six possible combinations, or genotypes, of the Apo E genes we inherited from our parents. Our genotype determines our body's specific ability to handle toxins from our food: the Apo E 2 genotype provides the most ability to clear them; the Apo E 3 has a more limited ability; and Apo E 4 has a very limited to no ability at all, to clear toxic substances absorbed from our diet.

The Apo E 4 gene prevents the body's systems from processing certain fats in the diet in a regular and consistent manner. If there are two copies of the Apo E 4 gene present, then you should follow the rules for the 4/4 gene, which includes not exposing your body's cells to any inflammatory fat and proteins that cannot be cleared. As we have seen, bad fat, such as trans fat and saturated fat, causes an accelerated inflammatory response in the body, especially with an Apo E 4.

Many people with Apo E 4/4 have cholesterol levels in the high 300s to high 400s, with some reaching the 500s. Adhering to the correct diet, and allowing time for the body to recover between exposures, lowers those high cholesterol levels.

The Apo E 3/3 is considered the "normal" Apo E genotype, with an unhindered ability to clear and use most fats and proteins, but even the Apo E 3/3 has difficulty clearing excessive exposure to saturated and trans fats. Too much exposure to these fats in a 24-hour period may pose problems for the body. As we will see in Chapter 10, it definitely increases bad cholesterol (LDL) and lowers good cholesterol (HDL). However, by applying the correct diet for this genotype, and allowing ample time between meals containing inflammatory fats and proteins for them to be processed, a person's LDL and HDL will become normal.

It has been proven repeatedly that individuals with any of the Apo E 4 combinations will respond better to dietary changes than the other genotypes will. Also, people with the Apo E 2/2 or 2/3 combination are more likely to respond better to moderately higher fat diets, while Apo E 4/4 and 4/3 respond better to low-fat diets. The right balance needs to be provided for each genotype. Keep in mind that:

- The toxicity of our body can be influenced by the individual Apo E. This means bodies differ in their ability to clear toxic chemicals and substances.
- The Apo E 4/4 is limited to almost no ability to eliminate processed foods and toxic chemicals.

Enhancing the Body's Toxin-Clearing Abilities

The following list contains recommendations for behaviors that will enhance your body's ability to clear toxins:

- Avoid foods contaminated with chemicals.
- Avoid refined and processed vegetable oils.
- Avoid processed grains in snack foods.
- Avoid margarine, vegetable shortening, and products made with partially hydrogenated oils.
- Avoid any toxic chemicals and substances that can cause cell inflammation and increase toxic tissue levels.
- Avoid a contaminated water source (including chlorine, heavy metals, and pesticides).
- Identify your body's ability to clear toxic foods and chemicals by knowing your Apo E genotype.
- Help your body clear toxins by getting regular exercise and not consuming excessive calories.
- Always ask questions about the food that is going into your mouth—and body.
- Avoid excessively large portions.
- Choose organic foods and organic farming processes.
- Support the whole-foods industry.
- Support school-system education regarding healthy foods.
- Support accurate nutritional education for doctors, pharmacists, teachers, and the representatives of the food industry.
- Believe that whole, healthy food can be a way of life again—safe, delicious, convenient, and affordable—and a win-win for all.

Chapter Ten

FAT CITY

There are many types of fats in our food—ranging from the essential to the disease promoting. The fats we choose to consume are a primary factor in determining our state of health, and yet we are very confused about fats. So, here is a full chapter looking at this element of our diet. It also includes information on how bad fats cause inflammation and how to prevent it.

Sources of fats in our diet include:

- nuts and seeds
- fruits and vegetables
- fish
- dairy products
- animal proteins

As we just saw in The Big Three, fat is an excellent source of long-term fuel because of its biochemical complexity. Fat is involved in cell protection and communication and is also a major component of cell membranes, which serve as storage tanks for our fatty acids. These storage tanks are important in the production of our hormone messengers that direct the body's immune system responses. They may contain either inflammatory or anti-inflammatory fats, and if we do not eat healthy fats that can be stored, we may die of disease.

Essential fatty acids are vital to health. They cannot be made in the body, so they have to be eaten regularly. If you attempt to remove all fat from your diet, you will become very sick in a relatively short period of time. If you consume too much fat, your body is more than likely to become overfueled and overfed, and much of it will probably cause chronic low-grade inflammation.

When the body is fed a fat it doesn't recognize, or that it has to work very hard to break down—processed, saturated, and trans fats—it produces biochemical waste and inflammatory proteins. It must then deal with this waste because it is toxic to the cells. Forced into a state of toxic stress overload, the body is also deficient in the essential fatty acids it needs to operate properly—not a healthy situation.

The common types of fats found in our diet (grouped by inflammatory level with apologies to Clint Eastwood) are:

The Good

- monounsaturated fats
- polyunsaturated fats

The Bad

- excessive saturated fats
- excessive cholesterol

The Ugly

- trans fat

Fats, Inflammation, and the Immune System

For optimal cellular health and functioning of our immune system, we need to consume mainly fats that don't trigger an immune-system response of inflammation—what I call the anti-inflammatory fat sources, such as unprocessed monounsaturated and polyunsaturated. Consuming fats from a source the body can recognize and use promotes a proper immune response to:

- physical trauma
- viral, bacterial, and fungal infection
- allergies
- toxic chemical exposure

How well our immune system works depends partly on the type of long-term and short-term fuel sources it has presently, and what was stored in prior times. Inflammation is a natural part of the body's internal healing system, but when it becomes chronic, the body has a difficult time clearing the inflammatory substances and, as a result, produces a chronic reactive immune response such as:

- increased fever
- increased pain response
- increased tissue fluid retention
- narrowing of the blood vessels
- decreased circulation
- increased blood clot formation

A standard American diet of pro-inflammatory fats, carbohydrates, and proteins can easily be translated into coronary artery disease, vascular disease, psychological diseases such as mood disorders and depression, autoimmune disease, and even cancer. All Apo E genotypes are prone to disease states from pro-inflammatory fat, carbohydrate and protein intake, but Apo E 4s show a greater risk. On the other hand, a diet of anti-inflammatory nutrients, such as those of the individual Apo E diets, encourages normal cell function, normal immune system function, decreased inflammatory response, and total well-being.

With a better diet we see improved body functions such as breathing and lung function, relaxed blood vessel walls and better circulation, reduced clot formation, improved joint function, normal stomach and intestinal functions, and better muscular movement with reduced musculoskeletal pain.

APO E GENE AND DIET
Dietary Environment with Immune System Response

Human cells are made up of fat, and fat is essential for healthy cell function and life. Fat plays a role in cell protection, communication, nutrition intake, and waste removal. In addition, the brain is approximately 60 percent fat. Humans require fat from their diet.

The Apo E gene can provide either:

CELL "DIS-EASE": Gene-unsupportive environment (GUE—the common Standard American Diet—SAD)

Some saturated and all trans fats impair good health by providing cells with the wrong long-term fuel source. This creates a gene-unsupportive environment (GUE).

Immune System Environment Stimulus

Injury

Infection

Allergies

Chemical Exposure

CELL "EASE": Gene-supportive environment (GSE)

Omega 3 and monounsaturated fats support good health by providing cells with a source of long-term fuel they can recognize and use. This creates a gene-supportive environment (GSE).

When the immune system is activated by brief or chronic inflammation, allergic reaction, cellular injury, infection, or chemical exposure, fatty acids are released and changed into immune system messengers or cytokines called eicosanoids. If the correct fatty acids are not available or the body doesn't recognize the type of fat, the body produces inflammatory eicosanoids. When essential fatty acids are available, the body produces anti-inflammatory chemistry that helps optimal immune function.

Human Cell

Inflammatory fats

Anti-inflammatory fats

Human Cell

Lox Enzyme	Cox Enzyme	Cox Enzyme	Lox Enzyme	Cox Enzyme	Cox Enzyme
LTB-4	**TXA-2**	**PGE-2**	**LTB-5**	**PGE-3**	**PGE-1**
• Increases amount and length of inflammation, especially in the lungs and airways.	• Narrows blood vessels. • Decreases circulation. • Increases blood clot formation.	• Increases tissue fluid retention. • Increases pain response. • Narrows airways. • Decreases circulation. • Increases blood clot formation.	• Increases blood vessel functioning and improves circulation. • Increases airway relaxation.	• Increases blood vessel functioning and improves circulation. • Reduces pain response.	• Improves muscle function. • Reduces blood clot formation. • Improves gastrointestinal functioning.

PRODUCES INFLAMMATORY CELLULAR CHEMISTRY

PRODUCES ANTI-INFLAMMATORY CELLULAR CHEMISTRY

The Good: Fats That Decrease Inflammation in the Body

Certain fats, namely unprocessed monounsaturated and polyunsaturated fats, have been shown to decrease inflammation in the body. The body easily recognizes and uses these fats.

Monounsaturated Fats

Monounsaturated fats are the simplest of fats. They are anti-inflammatory if they have not been processed.

Sources of monounsaturated fats include:

- olives and olive oil
- avocados
- canola oil
- palm fruit
- peanut oil

Polyunsaturated Fats

Polyunsaturated fats are also anti-inflammatory, as long as they have not been processed. The essential polyunsaturated fat groups are primarily the omega-3s and 6s.

What Are Omega-3 Fatty Acids?

Omega-3 fatty acids are polyunsaturated fats the body cannot do without. They are a good source of long-term fuel and need to be included in the daily diet.

When you move from a diet of saturated and trans fat to a diet of unprocessed polyunsaturated and monounsaturated fats, the body becomes much more efficient at using fat and produces a lower cholesterol level.

When you change to a diet of unprocessed monounsaturated and polyunsaturated fats, you need to consider eating good fat at most meals. Why? Since your body is now able to recognize and use these essential fats, they get used more quickly, hence the need to eat the correct fat percentages for your Apo E genotype with most meals.

Omega-3 fats come mainly from fish and meats. Additional food sources include:

- canola
- walnuts
- soybeans

- flaxseed
- ocean-borne algae
- whole grains
- very dark green leafy vegetables

If you take it in supplement form—capsule or liquid—know the quality and source. Consider only a fish oil source from wild fish and avoid highly processed supplements. Always follow a medical provider's dosage recommendations for omega-3 fatty acid. I currently recommend omega-3 supplements in dosages ranging from 0.133 grams per day to just over 2 grams per day, but prefer that people get their omega-3s directly from fresh food. Further, I recommend a customized combination of EPA and DHA. Your customized dosing should be discussed with your medical provider.

What Are Omega-6 Fatty Acids?

Just like omega-3s, the omega-6 fatty acids are vital to health. They are usually found in our diet in large amounts and are really not difficult to obtain from common food sources.

Sources of omega-6 fatty acids include:

- nuts
- seeds
- corn
- soy
- safflower
- palm fruit
- canola
- cottonseed
- meats

What Are Omega-9 Fatty Acids?

Omega-9 (oleic acid) is another form of important fatty acids also vital to health. Omega-9 is a monounsaturated fat and can be found in safflower, pumpkin, flaxseeds, and black currants.

The optimal balance between omega-3 and omega-6 fatty acids appears to be a ratio of 1:1 to 1:3–4. Practically speaking, it can be difficult to translate those ratios into our daily food consumption. However, if you stay with non-processed foods, you'll get a more balanced ratio of omega-3 to 6s since higher amounts of omega-6s come from processed foods and cooking oils.

The Bad: Saturated Fats

Primarily found in animal proteins and some vegetable sources, saturated fats can be a powerfully damaging food, more so from some sources than others. However, given the fact that human breast milk contains saturated fat, I do not think that all saturated fat sources have negative effects on the body. Saturated fat is a very concentrated source of fuel, and different types of saturated fat, especially those from animal sources, have been linked definitively to very high levels of inflammation and disease, especially when our bodies are overexposed more than once in a 24-hour period.

High amounts of saturated fat can cause a rapid increase in the inflammatory process soon after the fat is eaten. Beginning in the mouth and moving all the way through the digestive tract, this inflammation can end up in the smallest systems of the human cell.

Sources of highly concentrated saturated fat include:

- cream and all milk except skimmed
- cheese
- lard
- butter, regular ice cream (made from cow milk fat)
- meats (beef, chicken, turkey, pork, lamb)
- processed meats
- coconut oil
- cottonseed oil
- palm seed oil (not the palm fruit)
- chicken fat
- ghee (used in Indian food)

Cholesterol

A related type of lipid, or fat, in our diet is cholesterol, which is found in many foods that also contain fats. We need cholesterol but should avoid excessive amounts of it. Cholesterol occurs naturally in the body and is also absorbed from food. An average body produces around 800–1,000 mg of cholesterol and takes in an additional 200–300 mg from food. We need this cholesterol to create and maintain cell membranes, break down fats, and absorb vitamins (especially vitamin D).

Cholesterol also plays a role in the production of bile and of hormones such as cortisol, aldosterone, progesterone, estrogen, and testosterone. In the brain, cholesterol assists in the maintenance of nerve synapses. Cholesterol also plays an important role in our immune system.

Sources of highly concentrated cholesterol include:

- eggs
- dairy products
- animal meats, both lean and fat
- organ meats
- lard

The Ugly: Trans Fats

The trans fats in the standard American diet are especially damaging. These mostly man-made fats actually begin as an unsaturated fat, usually a vegetable oil, which is mixed with hydrogen gas and platinum catalysts, then heated to temperatures in excess of 500°F to make it more solid and to give it a longer shelf life. This recipe results in changing the molecular makeup of healthy fatty acids into disfigured, twisted molecules—trans fats—often listed on food labels as hydrogenated fats or oils. Serve them hot or cold, and your body will deliver this toxic, inflammatory mixture to every cell in your body, including your brain cells. Chronic exposure to the man-made trans fats that are found in thousands of processed foods from salad dressings to snacks, and from margarines to cake mixes, can be very toxic to everyone, but extremely toxic to Apo E 4s. It is very difficult for the body to get rid of these types of molecules once they are incorporated into its cellular structure, and this can cause severe chronic disease states.

One of the reasons we have so much trans fat in our diet is due to a very powerful consumer interest group that campaigned to remove saturated fat and palm seed oil from our food. The drive in the early 1980s to remove saturated fats led to the food processors using something even worse—trans fat. In the early 1990s we began to realize the damage it causes. In January 2006, we saw even more subversive uses of trans fat via legislation with a labeling loophole allowing foods with less than 0.5 mg per serving of fat to be labeled *nonfat*. This means that you can still get a dose of trans fat in your "0" trans fat-labeled food. Best read the label and the ingredients!

While trans fat has been produced and used in food for more than 100 years, we still have much to learn about its effects on the development of cell membranes, brain cells, arterial inflammatory plaque development, and growing fetal brain tissue. We do know that our body manufactures cell membranes from the fats we eat, so if our diet is high in inflammatory fats, we are creating defective cell membranes, hormones, and brain cells.

Could this be why we have so much brain pathology, with severe neurological diseases such as Alzheimer's disease and Parkinson's disease? We do not yet have conclusive evidence, but logic tells us this could be a cause. Once again, we need to take precautions by removing these fats from our diet. Remember that no evidence of harm is not equal to evidence of no harm.

The food-processing industry is very powerful. As long as using trans fats saves money, increases food shelf life, and provides more flavor, they will continue to use the hydrogen process, unless forced to stop.

As a medical practitioner on the front lines, I say let logic prevail! We all need to learn more about food so we can make better food choices. Education is our best weapon. Toward the end of your life, it will be your long-term food choices that determine whether you will be playing with backpacks or bedpans. As a consumer, you can change the way the food industry produces the foods you purchase. The choice is simple—don't buy foods with inflammatory trans fats in them. As Marion Nestle, Ph.D., M.P.H., author of *Food Politics: How the Food Industry Influences Nutrition and Health* and *What to Eat,* says, "Vote with your fork." I agree with Marion, because behind your fork is green power—money!

Important sources of trans fat to avoid include:

- stick margarine
- deep-fried fast food
- commercial cookies
- crackers
- commercial dessert pastries such as pies and cakes
- sports drinks (a popular brand added a "Z factor," which turned out to be trans fat)

How to Avoid Trans Fat

Knowing that trans fat can be hidden, read the ingredient list, not just the percentage of fat on the front. Choose foods that do not contain "vegetable shortening" or "partially hydrogenated" or hydrogenated fats and oils. Avoid deep-fried foods from restaurants, fast-food chains, and school kitchens.

Students may want to do a small research project where they ask the cooks in their school cafeteria what kind of oil they use in the deep fryers and how often they change it. Is it healthy oil, like canola, or not, like shortening? Do the cooks change it once a day, once a week, once a month, or once a semester? Any cooking oil will oxidize and become rancid (toxic to the body) when exposed to light and heat, but the more unsaturated it is, the more quickly this happens. Therefore, while the cafeteria should be using healthy oils, these oils also need to be changed frequently. You may find that the oil your lunch is cooked in is being changed a lot less often than you think—possibly once a month or even once a semester. Shocking, isn't it! Request that the oil be changed daily.

Consciously purchase lower-fat baked chips and trans fat–free crackers, cookies, pastries, and other processed foods. Use olive or canola oil instead of butter, margarine, or shortening. Foods that are marketed as "cholesterol free," "low cholesterol," "low in saturated fat," or "made with vegetable oil" are not necessarily low in trans, hydrogenated, or partially hydrogenated fats. Once again, read the label and be informed.

In 2004, one of my patients showed me a very popular sports drink bottle and said, "Pam, does this drink have trans fat in it?" My response was, "No," but I had never read the label. The bottle he handed me, with "0" fat grams in the nutritional facts, listed partially hydrogenated vegetable oil plus many types of preservatives and artificial dyes. The brand is now being marketed under a new name with flavors such as lemon-lime and strawberry. Their market is our children, and the ads imply "drink enough of this drink and you will look like a professional sports player."

This patient, a world-class triathlete, had made a trip to my office to bring me this information and was understandably very upset. His concern was that this company, involved in every sport as a major drink supplier for better sports performance, is now using trans fat in its products and marketing it to athletes and parents, who give it to their children.

The moral of the story is: *read the label,* for both the nutritional facts and the ingredients. If you find inflammatory ingredients on the label, don't buy them!

Garbage In = Garbage Out (GIGO)

When any digested food enters the intestines, the body is smart enough to recognize the quality of the nutrients and decide if those nutrients should be used, stored, or excreted. A little-known fact about fats is what happens after they are stored and then later removed from the body's internal storage tanks to be metabolized as fuel.

Often a person will wise up to the bad fats they've been eating, clean up their diet, and begin to lose weight. What will happen, often unexpectedly, is that all the stored toxic fats with their inflammatory components are released into the body and metabolized, causing the same negative effects as when they first entered the body. It can take many months before all these stored inflammatory fats are removed, so be patient with any symptoms that persist after you have removed the bad fats from your diet. Remember, the garbage you ate and stored will still be garbage on its way out of your body. Keep in mind, though, that it is a finite amount and will be gone when you've emptied those storage tanks. The reverse is true if the stored fats are anti-inflammatory (mono- and polyunsaturated); they will be released and help reduce any inflammation present.

The American Heart Association (AHA) recommends that saturated and trans fat intake not exceed 10 percent of total calories each day for healthy people and 7 percent for those with cardiovascular disease, diabetes, or high cholesterol.

How Much Protein Do We Need?

We can thank Dr. Atkins for his contribution to nutritional medicine, but think twice about his popular diet, especially if you carry an Apo E 4 genotype. Even if you are an Apo E 3 or Apo E 2, I recommend avoiding a high-protein, low-carbohydrate diet because this diet is pro-inflammatory. Keep in mind that animal protein comes packaged with inflammatory fats. You can avoid producing inflammation in your body if you stay away from a diet that consists of excess inflammatory protein and the "bad" fats.

As an integrative health-care practitioner, I recommend that people who have liver or kidney disease consume a low-protein diet. In addition, the type of protein should come from milder vegetable sources (see below).

A normal person involved in a routine exercise program needs only 1.2–1.6 grams of protein per kilogram (2.2 pounds) of body weight. That translates into just 3–4 ounces of protein for a 160-pound person. Very few athletes need more. The reality of most protein sources is that they include fat—either inflammatory or anti-inflammatory, as follows:

- Beans have protein and mostly *anti*-inflammatory fat.
- Nuts and seeds have protein and mainly *anti*-inflammatory fat.
- Fish has protein and mainly *anti*-inflammatory fat.
- Meat has protein and mainly inflammatory fat.
- Dairy contains protein and inflammatory fat.

The first three are ideal proteins with good anti-inflammatory fat, which the body can use and eliminate easily.

The body does much better when its protein comes from vegetable sources that provide monounsaturated and polyunsaturated fat. Vegetable protein is better than animal sources because plant protein is a "weaker" form that the body can handle more easily. Does this mean you shouldn't ever eat protein with saturated fat? No, but you need to be very careful how much and how often you do consume these complex sources. Depending on what Apo E genotype you are, this general rule can be defined even more closely:

Apo E 4s will do much better with plant protein and monounsaturated fats than with animal protein and saturated and trans fats. This is doubly important because you need more time to clear (eliminate) fats, no matter what type of fat it is.

Even the most intense athletes require only a small amount of protein compared to what some fad diets recommend.

Milk Protein

What about milk? Milk is a food that contains protein, yet in its natural form, it's loaded with saturated fat, despite those low-sounding 1%, 2%, and 4% fat numbers. Let's look at the real fat content, while not forgetting that milk contains animal saturated fat that is difficult for the body to clear, and that this type of animal fat has been found to cause inflammation in the human body.

Nonfat milk is not without fat. The dairy industry has dubious standards for what can be called skim or nonfat milk. Many people think it has "no" fat. This is not true, as it is very difficult to remove all the fat from a product. Even skim milk is not totally devoid of fat, but because it is below the level requiring labeling (0.5 gram/serving), it is reported as fat free. This is terribly misleading!

Whole milk is advertised as 4 percent fat by volume, but since most of the volume is water, this means that with all the fluid removed, what remains is 48 percent animal fat! What is called "2% milk" is actually 37.5 percent animal fat.

Chapter Eleven

INDIVIDUAL MEDICAL AND NUTRITIONAL RECOMMENDATIONS BASED ON APO E GENOTYPE

Now, let's look at some specific information on the benefits of a diet related to your Apo E genotype. Not all foods are created equal. Certain foods create disease faster in some people than in others. Knowing how to feed your body based on your specific genotype is crucial to your good health. Remember, the Apo E gene directs your body's use of cholesterol and blood fat, so I strongly recommend you have your cholesterol and triglycerides evaluated at the same time that you are tested for your Apo E genotype. As we saw in Chapter 2, you should consider being tested for the seven subtypes of LDL (bad) cholesterol and the five subtypes of HDL (good) cholesterol. Then a complete advanced panel can be done to see the full picture of your blood chemistries, not just the tip of the iceberg that we commonly see in routine screening. Here we will look at recommendations for the six Apo E genotypes. Note that, along with differing nutritional needs, genotypes vary with respect to recommended exercise programs, outlined in the following guidelines:

Recommendations for the Apo E 2/2 Genotype

Fat 35%   Protein 15%   Carbohydrate 50%

With a poor nutritional intake and unhealthy environment, this genotype can develop very high levels of cholesterol, triglycerides, and very low-density lipoproteins (VLDL). A specific cholesterol condition called Type III high cholesterol is seen in this genotype. Typically, unless a person has a triglyceride level above 150 mg/dl, this genotype has no problems. A high triglyceride level is likely to develop with 1) abnormal eating behaviors such as meal skipping or 2) a high body-fat percentage from excessive calories and saturated/trans fat intake. In addition, overexposure to saturated fats and high exposure to polyunsaturated oils and margarines, coupled with excessive omega-6 sources, contribute to elevated triglyceride levels. When combined with excessive simple carbohydrate calorie intake along with little exercise, poor health will result. Alcohol is also a significant negative factor for this genotype. This genotype requires a very specific exercise program.

Use the following guidelines:

- Make dietary changes slowly.

- Work with your medical provider to check your basic and advanced blood cholesterol and triglyceride levels.

- Be aware that a gene-supportive environment can prevent many chronic diseases, especially neurological ones.[1]

- Have a body-composition test to evaluate your percentage body fat and lean mass (pages 246–251).

- See the exercise recommendations for this genotype in Chapter 12.

Recommendations for the Apo E 2/3 Genotype

Fat 30%   Protein 15%   Carbohydrate 55%

This genotype is considered a variant combination. We tend to see little dietary influence on bad cholesterol (LDL) levels unless the diet is high in calories from processed foods, inflammatory trans and saturated fats, and processed polyunsaturated fats. A highly inflammatory diet and lack of exercise increase the risk of heart disease. A significant negative risk factor for alcohol can also be seen with this genotype.

---

1   Keeping in mind that protein and fat usually come packaged together, pay close attention to the recommended serving sizes, and leave an adequate amount of fat clearance time (24–48 hours) in between eating fish or any animal protein with high saturated fat content.

Use the following guidelines:

- Make dietary changes slowly.

- Work with your medical provider to check your basic and advanced blood cholesterol and triglyceride levels.

- Be aware that a gene-supportive environment can prevent many chronic diseases, especially neurological ones.[2]

- Have a body-composition test to evaluate your percentage of body fat and lean mass (pages 246–251).

- See the exercise recommendations for this genotype in Chapter 12.

Recommendations for the Apo E 3/3 Genotype

Fat 25%   Protein 20%   Carbohydrate 55%

This genotype is considered the normal or neutral genotype and cannot tolerate either a low-fat or high-fat diet. Avoid excessive inflammatory fats. Wait 24 to 48 hours between meals of saturated fats to allow them to be cleared from your body. This genotype needs balance in both short-term (carbohydrate) and long-term (fat) fuels. Remember, all excess calories are stored as fat. Calories should match the body's ability to clear its fuel source. We tend to see metabolic disease when Apo E 3/3 patients fail to keep to a normally balanced diet and exercise.

Use the following guidelines:

- Work with your medical provider to check your basic and advanced blood cholesterol and triglyceride levels.

- See the exercise recommendations for this genotype in Chapter 12.

---

2   Keeping in mind that protein and fat usually come packaged together, pay close attention to the recommended serving sizes, and leave an adequate amount of fat clearance time (24–48 hours) in between eating fish or any animal protein with high saturated fat content.

Recommendations for the Apo E 4/2 Genotype

Fat 25%   Protein 20%   Carbohydrate 55%

For Apo E 4s it is critical to limit all inflammatory trans fats and overexposure to saturated fats, polyunsaturated oils and margarines, and excessive omega-6 sources, utilizing instead monounsaturated and omega-3 fats.

Due to the combination of the 2 and the 4 genes, this genotype must balance between the contrasting needs of the two. With the presence of the Apo E 2, carbohydrate intake must be strictly limited to complex carbohydrates with a low glycemic load. Fat and protein sources should be mainly monounsaturated and polyunsaturated fats. Plant protein should be considered over animal protein. It is extremely important for people with this genotype to use aerobic exercise to reduce stored body fat levels. These people should work closely with a medical practitioner who is trained in advanced lipid disorders as well as exercise science or sports medicine and be regularly evaluated for all types of cholesterol and triglyceride markers. See specific aerobic versus anaerobic exercise recommendations for this genotype.

Use the following guidelines:

- Make dietary changes slowly.

- Work with your medical provider to check your basic and advanced blood cholesterol and triglyceride levels.

- Be aware that a gene-supportive environment can prevent many chronic diseases, especially neurological ones.[3]

- Have a body-composition test to evaluate your percentage body fat and lean mass (pages 246–251).

- See the exercise recommendations for this genotype in Chapter 12.

---

3   Besides the risk of cardiovascular disease, research shows an increased risk of developing Alzheimer's disease with the presence of the Apo E 4 gene, but the gene alone should not be used to predict Alzheimer's disease risk. Research has not shown that Apo E definitely causes Alzheimer's disease. Many other factors are involved in the development of disease in this type, especially the nutritional environment. It appears to be not the gene that encourages a disease, but the environment. Creating a gene-supportive environment is key to lowering risk.

Recommendations for the Apo E 4/3 Genotype

Fat 20%   Protein 25%   Carbohydrate 55%

With a higher caloric level (greater than 2,800 kcal), the percentages change due to the body's inability to use more protein:

Fat 20%   Protein 20%   Carbohydrate 60%

Clearing fat and cholesterol from the body is hindered, so exposure to excess amounts of dietary fat and cholesterol causes stress that in turn pushes the body to produce too much LDL. Fat should come mainly from anti-inflammatory monounsaturated and polyunsaturated sources—those the body can recognize and use effectively.

It is extremely important for this genotype to use aerobic exercise to reduce stored fat levels. These people should work closely with a medical practitioner who has had additional training in advanced lipid disorders as well as exercise science and sports medicine. These people should be regularly evaluated for all types of cholesterol and triglyceride markers. See specific aerobic versus anaerobic exercise recommendations for this genotype.

Use the following guidelines:

• Make dietary changes slowly.

• Work with your medical provider to check your basic and advanced blood cholesterol and triglyceride levels.

• Be aware that a gene-supportive environment can prevent many chronic diseases, especially neurological ones.[4]

• Have a body-composition test to evaluate your percentage of body fat and lean mass (pages 246–251).

• See the exercise recommendations for this genotype in Chapter 12.

---

4   Pay close attention to the recommended serving sizes and leave adequate clearance time (24–48 hours) when a saturated fat has been consumed. This genotype combination contains an Apo E 4, so you need to be mindful when making fat and protein choices.

Recommendations for the Apo E 4/4 Genotype

This gene pattern of two 4s is a critical combination.

Fat 20%   Protein 25%   Carbohydrate 55%

As with the Apo E 4/3, with a higher caloric level (greater than 2,800 kcal), percentages change due to the body's inability to use more protein:

Fat 20%   Protein 20%   Carbohydrate 60%

This genotype contains two variant 4s. Clearing fat and cholesterol from the body is hindered in the extreme, so any exposure to dietary fat and cholesterol causes stress that pushes the body to produce too much LDL. Fat sources should be primarily monounsaturated and nonprocessed polyunsaturated.

It is extremely important for this genotype to use aerobic exercise to reduce stored fat levels. These people should work closely with a medical practitioner who has had additional training in advanced lipid disorders as well as exercise science and sports medicine. These people should be regularly evaluated for all types of cholesterol and triglyceride markers. See specific aerobic versus anaerobic exercise recommendations for this genotype.

Use the following guidelines:

- Make dietary changes slowly.

- Work with your medical provider to check your basic and advanced blood cholesterol and triglyceride levels.

- Be aware that a gene-supportive environment can prevent many chronic diseases, especially neurological ones.[5]

- Have a body composition test to evaluate your percentage body fat and lean mass (pages 246–251).

- See the exercise recommendations for this genotype in Chapter 12.

Up-to-date information and self-education, coupled with good common sense, are important when considering any nutritional recommendations. As our body of knowledge grows, it is likely that dietary recommendations will change. The best defense against those that would have us believe that we cannot take care of our own health is a good arsenal of facts. The one thing that will not change is the importance of common sense in any behavior change plan.

---

5   Pay close attention to the recommended serving sizes and leave adequate clearance time (24–48 hours) when a saturated fat has been consumed. This genotype combination contains an Apo E 4, so you need to be mindful when making fat and protein choices.

Diet, Hygiene, and Dental Health

The right diet based on your Apo E gene contributes to healthy teeth and gums.

Gingivitis and periodontitis are conditions of tissue inflammation affecting the gums that cause pain and bleeding. These are commonly found with advancing age, but we are beginning to see this in younger people. I believe this is due to the worsening of the standard American diet. The majority of dental disease, specifically gum disease, can actually be prevented by:

- practicing good daily oral hygiene
- obtaining regular professional dental care
- eating the right diet based on your Apo E genotype

Chapter Twelve

MOVEMENT AND EXERCISE

It's time to move our focus from the dining table to moving our bodies! In this chapter I will identify the common elements of a safe and healthy exercise program. As with dietary guidelines, there are general guidelines. However, one plan does not fit all. If you know your Apo E genotype, ask for a personalized exercise prescription for your profile. It is important, whenever possible, to have the correct exercise routine prescribed for you based on your Apo E genotype, taking into account your current fitness level.

Sometimes it seems that I can't open a magazine, watch a television program, or do a search on the Internet without hearing of new "guidelines" for exercise and movement. It can get confusing. But researchers do agree that you should exercise most days, if not every day. The latest recommendation by the American Heart Association is to exercise a minimum of 30 to 60 minutes, four to seven days a week.

When we look at the makeup of the physical body, we can see that it was built to move. Most of us move, in some way or other, every day. Not all of us move in the same way or at the same level. I will use the word "movement" here as an umbrella term to refer to activities of daily living or physically changing the position of the human body. I define "exercise" as a subset of movement, to mean the vigorous movement required of certain sports, the rare job requiring extensive physical effort, or a formal exercise routine.

We know that if the human body moves on a regular basis, it will be healthier. The health benefits don't just apply to the physical body but also to the emotions, mind, and spirit. I could easily include five full pages on the benefits of movement and exercise, but I think by mentioning just a few of these, you will agree that movement of the physical body is good for you.[1]

A Patient's Story: Lilian

Lilian was referred to me by her primary-care doctor. She was 5'4", weighed 103 pounds, and had high cholesterol and osteopenia (the precursor to osteoporosis). Several years earlier, she had received a diagnosis of fibromyalgia and depression, for which her doctor prescribed an antidepressant. However, Lilian did not like to take medication and so was not following her treatment plan.

After having many tests performed on recommendation of her primary-care doctor, Lilian decided she was done with tests. But then she heard about the Apo E gene test and decided she wanted to know her Apo E genotype.

When she came to my office, I did a complete medical history and a physical. I asked her to keep a diet log for a week, and it revealed only minimal food intake, mostly at dinner, with some coffee and water during the day. Lilian told me she didn't like to eat during the day because she felt uncomfortable eating before exercise, which she did from two to five hours a day.

I suggested that her first step should be to try a normal anti-inflammatory diet. But she was adamant—she would make no changes in her diet or her exercise patterns. She just wanted to know her Apo E genotype. I gently tried to educate her further about this test and how it relates to diet and exercise, but she insisted that she would not make any changes to accommodate the results of the test.

Lilian suffered from depression and anxiety, not to mention some deeply rooted, abnormal dietary patterns that were more than likely contributing to her illnesses. She was eating too little in any case,

---

1   An excellent resource for learning more about the benefits of physical activity is the American College of Sports Medicine: **www.acsm.org**.

which stressed her body, and then her over-exercising only made the situation worse. When the human body is pushed to these extremes, it's very common for extreme disease to develop.

I recommended some psychological counseling to help her discover the reasons for her extreme eating and exercise patterns, but Lilian was not interested. She continued to demand an Apo E test. In good conscience, I could not order it. What if she was an Apo E 4/4 and then was not willing to make any of the appropriate changes? I think such an outcome would have worsened her condition. With her mind-set regarding diet and exercise, she could have begun an even more extreme routine, which would have caused further harm.

Since I knew Lilian would not listen to me, I recommended she return to her primary-care doctor for further direction. She clearly needed help with a sensible alternative-eating pattern. I recommended to her doctor that she not be tested for her Apo E genotype but instead that she learn how to begin normal, healthy eating and exercise patterns through a consultation with an exercise physiologist and a registered dietitian with special training in alternative eating patterns. I also recommended that Lilian begin working with a psychological counselor and continue taking her antidepressant.

Perhaps Lilian would become a good candidate for Apo E testing later, but she clearly was not when I saw her.

Health Benefits of Exercise

Exercise keeps the body functioning at its best by increasing its muscle mass. Additionally, stored fat and carbohydrate consumption occurs at higher rates even after exercise ceases because they are used to create more protein in the muscle (so the body can perform more exercise next time), which increases metabolism. Movement helps the body function with ease. If we do not engage in enough movement, our body becomes susceptible to "dis-ease" and illnesses such as cardiovascular disease, dementia, Alzheimer's disease, hypertension, diabetes, obesity, and the high multi-level inflammation process of arthritis.

Exercise helps prevent the loss of cognitive abilities by increasing the body's internal brain chemicals, such as the morphine-like endorphins. The nervous system's performance is enhanced by the increase of blood and oxygen flow, and by increasing growth factors that assist in the generation of new nerve cells. Many common chronic illnesses can be helped with just a small amount of regular movement and exercise. It has been shown that as little as ten minutes of walking each day can help with the prevention of disease!

Regular exercise can help prevent:

- premature death
- heart disease and stroke
- high blood pressure
- high cholesterol
- cancers, such as colon and breast cancer
- diabetes
- non-insulin-dependent diabetes
- depression and anxiety
- sleep problems
- arthritis
- back pain, osteoporosis
- ADD/ADHD

Regular exercise can also:

- reduce or maintain body weight or percentage of body fat
- build and maintain healthy muscles, bones, and joints by decreasing inflammation
- improve psychological well-being
- enhance work, recreation, and sport performance

As you can see, the benefits of exercise extend far beyond the usual weight-loss goal. As a health-conscious nation, we need to understand and appreciate the many benefits of regular physical activity and know that the right movement and exercise program can help reduce our risk for chronic illness, which will in turn yield an overall improved quality of life.

Now that we've seen the benefits of exercise, I hope you're ready to get involved! Let's look at the elements of a safe and healthy exercise program.

Elements of a Safe and Healthy Exercise Program

A safe and healthy exercise program is multifaceted, sometimes requiring new clothing and shoes, learning new exercises, and establishing a new routine. This section describes the following 12 elements:

- Professional Evaluation and Guidance
- Physiologic Changes Associated with Exercise
- Exercise, Clothing, and Shoes
- How Often to Exercise
- Exercise Intensity
- Program and Progression Plan
- Warm-up and Cooldown
- Aerobic Exercise: A Walking Program
- Strength Training
- Flexibility and Stretching Exercises (Yoga or Pilates)
- Logging Behavior Changes
- Avoiding Exercise Program Dropout

Professional Evaluation and Guidance

I strongly recommend that when beginning an exercise program, you be evaluated and guided by a professional with knowledge of sports medicine. The providers most effective at exercise prescriptions are either licensed exercise physiologists, nurse-practitioners, sports-medicine physicians, or physical therapists who will probably work in collaboration with your primary-care provider. The goal is to make sure your cardiovascular and muscular skeletal systems can tolerate increased activity and still provide excellent health.

I recommend that you consult a licensed exercise-support person for a minimum of six months when beginning a new exercise program. They can be a vital component for exercise success and will:

- provide your exercise prescription
- guide your exercise progress
- deliver whatever exercise education is necessary to improve fitness
- encourage you in times when exercise motivation is low

Exercise Warning Signs

Before beginning an exercise program, learn some important warning signs. Stop exercise immediately and seek medical care if you experience any of these symptoms:

- palpitations (irregular or rapid heartbeat)
- sudden increases in your stress levels
- disorientation or vision disturbances
- nausea or vomiting
- sudden clamminess and perspiration
- chest pains, aches, or pressure
- shortness of breath
- dizziness
- upset stomach

To determine the optimal exercise program for you, consider getting an evaluation for any of the following areas that are relevant to you:

- complete health history
- evaluation of current lifestyle
- supplement use
- psychological questionnaire
- dietary evaluation
- exercise history
- physical exam—all systems
- weight
- blood pressure
- heart rate
- strength test
- flexibility test
- BMI (body mass index) (see Chapter 18)
- body-composition test (see Chapter 18)
- routine lab testing
- advanced genetic cholesterol tests (see Chapter 5)
- EKG

- VO2 max test
- cardiovascular test
- stress test

The above evaluations are highly recommended and may include some other screening tests as well.

Evaluating Your Overall Health

When you evaluate your overall health, you need to consider your current psychological health, sleeping patterns, stress level, eating patterns, cholesterol levels, body composition (percent body fat and lean mass), Apo E genotype, and inflammatory markers such as elevated C-reactive protein, fibrinogen, Lp-PLA2, glucose levels, and insulin levels. Medical screening is strongly advised, including an evaluation of family history, a full physical with special attention to the body's energy, metabolism, and musculoskeletal and cardiovascular system. Until you have been completely examined and clinically evaluated, you will not know your level of risk for any potential or existing disease process—low, medium, or high risk. When evaluating body composition, it is very important to consider the human body's blood chemistry at the same time because an abnormal body composition can produce abnormal blood chemistries.

Physiologic Changes Associated with Exercise

There are many different types of physical exercise, but they can be grouped into three general categories: aerobic (cardiovascular), anaerobic (strength training), and flexibility. Each yields different physiological changes in the human body. Performing any or all of these different types of exercises daily, as determined by your Apo E genotype, changes the body's chemistry and affects the human cell in a positive way, by building better human tissue and yielding improved cell health, tissue health, and organ health. This translates into improved health, not only of the physical body, but also the mind and the spirit.

Aerobic Exercise

Aerobic exercise increases a person's heart rate and sustains it for a specific amount of time. Cardiorespiratory endurance exercising is a specific type of aerobic exercise that has the capacity to carry out large-muscle, active, higher-intensity exercises for longer time periods. Cardiorespiratory exercise is directly dependant on the condition and functioning state of the respiratory, cardiovascular, and muscular skeletal system. Walking, bike riding, running, and swimming are examples of aerobic exercise.

Physiological changes that occur with aerobic exercise include:

- increased maximal cardiac output
- increased blood volume and ability to carry oxygen
- reduced workload on the heart for any given submaximal exercise intensity
- increased blood supply to muscles and ability to use oxygen
- lower heart rate and blood pressure at any level of submaximal exercise
- lower resting systolic and diastolic blood pressure in people with high blood pressure
- increased HDL cholesterol
- decreased blood triglycerides
- reduced body fat and improved weight control
- improved glucose tolerance and reduced insulin resistance

Anaerobic (muscular strengthening and endurance) Exercise

Anaerobic exercise increases and sustains a person's heart rate for short periods of time. Anaerobic exercise refers to the capacity of the muscular system's movement and performance ability. Muscle strength or weakness is directly related to the maximum power or force that can be created by a specific muscle or group of muscles. Muscle endurance is muscle contraction repeated multiple times to produce muscle stress or fatigue, thereby producing a state of maximum voluntary contraction for a tolerated period of time. Weight lifting repetitions and sprinting are examples of anaerobic exercise.

Physiological changes that occur with anaerobic exercise include:

- improved flexibility
- decreased risk of musculoskeletal injury
- increased musculoskeletal performance
- improved postural stability/decreased risk of falls
- decreased muscle soreness with activity
- decreased risk of lower back pain
- improved muscle coordination

Flexibility Training

Flexibility training gives the body a greater range of movement. This type of exercise refers to the body's ability to move a joint and all related tissue connected to a specific joint—tendons, ligaments, muscles, etc. Joint movement has a specific capacity of movement referred to as a range of motion (ROM). Human flexibility is dependent on multiple factors—hormone levels; bone structure; joint capsule distensibility; and size, length, and strength of ligaments and muscles. Age and gender are also important factors, especially in muscle strength and distensibility.

Physiological changes that occur with flexibility training include:

- improved flexibility
- decreased risk of musculoskeletal injury
- increased musculoskeletal performance
- improved postural stability/decreased risk of falls
- decreased muscle soreness with activity
- decreased risk of lower back pain
- improved muscle coordination

No matter where you are in your life—young or old—take time each day to move your body. If you devote as little as ten minutes to moving your body, it will respond in health and happiness. Note that the best type of movement and exercise program for you can only be determined when you know your Apo E genotype.

Exercise, Clothing, and Shoes

Clothing and footwear should be correctly sized and comfortable. Dress according to the weather and temperature. If you think the temperature could change during your exercise session, dress in layers. Personally, I like to dress as warm as possible in the beginning phases of my exercise session and shed clothing as I go.

With every type of activity, having the proper equipment is an important factor in reducing your chances of injury. Have your exercise specialist or a good podiatrist evaluate your natural foot position. This ensures that you get the correct type of shoes for your feet. Some shoe stores offer a foot evaluation, but I would go to a person who is well educated in exercise and exercise shoes.

How Often to Exercise

This needs to be determined by you, your Apo E genotype, and your exercise specialist. However, the new general recommendation is 30 to 60 minutes of moderate physical activity 4 to 7 days a week. Start with 5 to 10 minutes a day and slowly work up to the 30 to 60 minutes.

Guidelines for Beginning an Exercise Program

Start slowly: Consider very low-intensity exercises that you can gradually increase in intensity over time. Walking and swimming are among the best exercises to begin a program. Not everyone has access to a pool, but everyone has access to walking.

Schedule exercise time: Exercise needs to be part of your schedule. If you wait for free time to just show up, it is likely your exercise program will never happen. Why? Because we always have something else we can do. Ask any busy person. Exercise should be on the same priority level as taking a shower or eating a meal. You must make time for movement.

Stay focused on what you want: Time, family, weather, and work can all be barriers to a regular exercise routine. Recognize the problems that you know will get in the way of a routine exercise program and develop a plan to overcome them. Do not allow anything to come between you and what you want to accomplish.

Consider a support system: Having a support system in place to encourage you in your daily exercise is extremely helpful. It is part of the exercise prescription. Your support person can be a medical professional, spouse, family member, friend, or co-worker. Choose someone you feel comfortable with and whom you know will help you over the difficult times. Choose support people who already have good health-promoting habits in their lives—or who want to develop them with you!

Exercise Intensity

The exercise intensity of an activity or movement indicates how much power or force is used in performing that exercise. The intensity of an activity determines how much, and what type, of fuel is needed to provide the energy required for that exercise.

Fuel Needs

As we saw in Chapter 3, the body utilizes two types of fuel—short-term and long-term.

- Anaerobic exercise uses carbohydrate or fast, immediately available short-term fuel.

- Aerobic exercise requires a constant supply of oxygen and a combination of fuels—first carbohydrates, then fatty acids and glycerol (fat), which is a longer-term fuel. The amount of fuel used depends directly on the demands on the heart to pump and deliver oxygen and fuel. Aerobic exercise has a positive effect on the circulatory system. In fact, it has a beneficial systemic effect on the whole body if the body is properly fueled. Aerobic activities are best when practiced for extended periods of time—say 30 minutes or more—and use the large muscles in the lower part of the body (buttocks, thighs), which have an excellent whole body effect. As we age or as the body becomes more or less fit, the demands on the heart for oxygen and fuel change.

- Yoga or stretching at low intensities utilizes glucose for fuel, and some more high-intensity forms of yoga will start utilizing fat for fuel as long as a heart rate is maintained at an aerobic level.

These three types of exercise have different effects on the human body's chemical state and the way it uses fuel. The body adapts to both aerobic and anaerobic exercise by producing more or less of different enzymes inside the muscle, which utilize either blood glucose or fat for fuel. If you are an active aerobic exerciser and not a weight/strength exerciser, your body will produce aerobic enzymes in your muscles instead of the anaerobic enzymes, and vice versa. My goal is to provide an exercise guideline for your Apo E genotype. I will update this information as new research becomes available.

Calculating the Appropriate Heart Rate

Here is a general formula to help determine a general target heart rate. You can use this calculation if you cannot get the information with a VO2 max testing method (see below).

220 minus your age = your maximum heart rate.

For example:
220 - 40 years = 180 (a 40-year-old's approximate maximum heart rate).
or
220 - 60 years = 160 (a 60-year-old's approximate maximum heart rate).

Then, depending on fitness and current levels of exercise, multiply by 60 percent or 85 percent to get your estimated maximum heart rate. Use 60 percent if you are just beginning to exercise, and gradually increase to 85 percent as your stamina increases.

For example:

60% of maximum heart rate
220 - 40 years = 180 x 60% = 108
220 - 60 years = 160 x 60% = 96

85% of maximum heart rate
220 - 40 years = 180 x 85% = 153
220 - 60 years = 160 x 85% = 136

Calculating the Appropriate Heart Rate

Keep in mind that this "target heart rate" is a general guideline that focuses on the general population, rather than a specific individual's ability. Again, I recommend that you work with a medical professional trained in exercise physiology who can give you a personalized exercise prescription and program.

An exercise physiologist will probably use a testing method called "VO2 max." This test can give you a far more specific measurement of your body's ability to exercise by measuring how fast your body uses oxygen while exercising.

As you exercise in your currently tolerated Apo E zone for a given amount of time—days and weeks—your body will adapt, and its internal fuel-consuming enzymes will rise to a higher level, increasing your exercise tolerance level as long as the same amount of exercise is carried out every 48 hours.

The Apo E Exercise Zone Scale

Studies show that our own personal estimate of effort, or *our own view of how hard we are exercising,* is highly correlated with our actual heart rate and oxygen consumption during exercise. This means we should pay more attention to our inner warning mechanisms to guide our bodies during an exercise session. If a certain type of exercise feels too difficult, it probably is. If you have not exercised in a long time, you are not conditioned to have the muscle engine capacity to tolerate or perform the exercise type or pace of someone who exercises regularly for extended periods. The beginning exerciser may rate a given exercise as "very hard," but after you have been performing the same exercise for a longer period of time and have developed your muscles, you may find the same level of exercise fairly light. Your experience of the effort used in doing any particular exercise is directly related to your intramuscular exercise equipment.

The Apo E Exercise Zone Scale shown below can be adapted to every possible level and type of fitness. Following this scale will help you begin to trust your personal exertion abilities, instead of an impersonal generalized formula. Beginning exercisers are instructed to walk one mile at their own pace. After they have completed the exercise, they can look at the exercise zone scale and evaluate at what level they were exercising. Did they feel as if they were exercising at Zone 7 or was it at Zone 2? If they were at Zone 2, they need to pick up the pace a little until they feel they are operating in the moderate zone for them—not too easy and not too hard. In my experience, most people don't know what their correct zone is and tend to overdo it when they start out. Their rating for Day 1 is probably going to be a Zone 6 or even a Zone 7. Learning to pace themselves at about Zone 3 or 4 is an important first stage of an aerobic exercise program.

Exercise Zone Scale

Zone 1	Zone 2	Zone 3	Zone 4	Zone 5	Zone 6	Zone 7
Very, Very Easy	Very Easy	Fairly Light	Somewhat Hard	Hard	Very Hard	Very, Very Hard

Exercise Effort Level

When exercising, ask yourself, "How do I feel?"
Rate your current exercise level.
What exercise zone are you currently exercising in?

- Are you exercising too hard?
- Are you exercising too light?
- Are you exercising just right?

Exercise Effort Level

Use the Apo E Exercise Zone Scale, where appropriate, to answer the following questions:

- What is my current level on the exercise zone scale?
- Am I exercising within my current prescribed zone?
- When I exercise, am I asking myself, "How do I feel?"
- Does my exercise feel too hard?
- Does my exercise feel too easy?
- Am I making exercise progress?

Consider the following general guidelines:

- When exercising, you should be able to carry on a conversation.
- You should have easy, regular breathing, and not be gasping for air.
- You should not feel exhausted during or after exercising.

12.1 Percentage of Nutrients Used by Genotype for each Recommended Exercise Plan				
	Exercise intensity (% MHR)[a]	Heart rate range	% carbs[b] burned	% fat[c] burned
Apo E 4/4 75% aerobic, 25% anaerobic	60–65	120–125	35	65
	65–70	130–140	40	60
Apo E 4/3 75% aerobic, 25% anaerobic	60–65	120–125	35	65
	65–70	130–140	40	60
Apo E 4/2 50% aerobic, 50% anaerobic	70–75	140–150	50	50
	65–70	150–160	65	35
Apo E 3/3 50% aerobic, 50% anaerobic	70–75	140–150	50	50
	75–80	150–160	65	35
Apo E 2/3 55% aerobic, 45% anaerobic	70–75	140–150	50	50
	75–80	150–160	65	35
	80–85	160–170	80	20
Apo E 2/2 55% aerobic, 45% anaerobic	70–75	140–145	50	50
	75–80	150–160	65	35
	80–85	160–170	80	20

a. Exercise intensity as defined by a percentage of maximum heart rate (MHR).
b. The percentage of carbohydrates used during exercise.
c. The percentage of fat used during exercise.

Type of Muscle Fibers[2]

Muscle is the body's engine and makes up about half of all body mass. Muscle is composed of three main types of fiber.

Type I: Slow-contracting fibers use the body's aerobic metabolic pathways.

Fuel used: Glucose first and then free fatty acids

Type II: Faster-twitch fibers use anaerobic metabolic pathways.
Fuel used: Glucose

Type III: Intermediate-twitch fibers use both aerobic and anaerobic metabolic pathways.
Fuel used: Equal balance of glucose and free fatty acids

Different Apo E genotypes have different dominant types of muscle fibers that prefer different types of fuel:

Apo E 4 dominant in muscle Type I

Apo E 2 dominant in muscle Type II

Apo E 3 dominant in muscle Type III

Garbage In = Garbage Out—Again

This is so important that I'll remind you again of what happens when a person has eaten excessive inflammatory fats from saturated and trans fat sources that are now stored in the body's cells. When you begin an exercise program to reduce body fat, *you are now asking your body to mobilize and use these stored inflammatory fats as fuel.* This can elicit an inflammatory response and you may need medical support until the excessive stored trans and saturated fats have cleared from your body, which can take from 9 to 18 months.

Program and Progression Plan

An exercise program consists of three phases, each having different goals. Each phase builds on the previous one, with the end result being a healthy physical body:

---

2 Growing evidence suggests that human exercise performance phenotypes could be polygenic, e.g., Apo E, ACTN3, ACE. However, when considering an exercise prescription, a gene-supportive environment (GSE) related to the individual Apo E gene should remain a priority.

Initial Conditioning Phase
- Duration: 4–6 weeks
- Goal: increase frequency (sessions/week)

Improvement Conditioning Phase
- Duration: 7–11 weeks
- Goal: increase the duration (minutes/session)

Maintenance Conditioning Phase
- Occurs after 12–24 weeks of regular exercise
- Goal: maintain the exercise regimen (and your cardiorespiratory fitness)

Lifelong exercise behaviors usually can be maintained if initiated for more than 24 weeks.

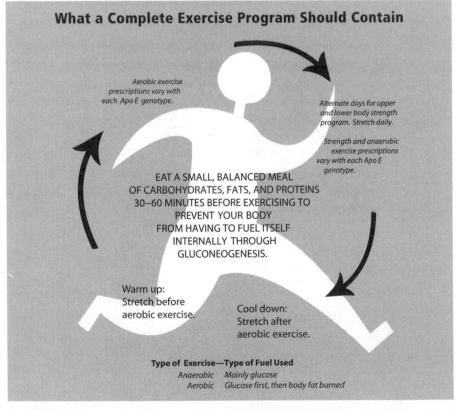

What a Complete Exercise Program Should Contain

Aerobic exercise prescriptions vary with each Apo E genotype.

Alternate days for upper and lower body strength program. Stretch daily.

Strength and anaerobic exercise prescriptions vary with each Apo E genotype.

EAT A SMALL, BALANCED MEAL OF CARBOHYDRATES, FATS, AND PROTEINS 30–60 MINUTES BEFORE EXERCISING TO PREVENT YOUR BODY FROM HAVING TO FUEL ITSELF INTERNALLY THROUGH GLUCONEOGENESIS.

Warm up: Stretch before aerobic exercise.

Cool down: Stretch after aerobic exercise.

Type of Exercise—Type of Fuel Used
Anaerobic   Mainly glucose
Aerobic   Glucose first, then body fat burned

I recommend that everyone consider a consultation with a licensed exercise specialist to create your individual exercise prescription plan.

Warm-up and Cooldown

Warm-up and stretching

Preparing for exercise is important at any age and fitness level. The key to preventing exercise injuries is to warm up beforehand. This helps increase blood flow to the muscles, including the heart; ligaments and tendons are less likely to tear or be strained if they're warmed up first. A warm-up includes a slow increase of activity to help increase blood circulation. Some of my very sick patients with chronic arthritis actually go into a hot tub or spa to warm up and stretch, and I have noticed that Apo E 4s like to warm up the same way.

Flexibility is a must when performing any exercise. Flexibility training teaches your ligaments and tendons to stretch and retract appropriately, which helps prevent injury to the muscles and fractures to the bones. After your warm-up, stretch slowly, without forced bouncing movements, and hold each stretch for 20 to 45 seconds. Never stretch to the point of pain.

The stretching exercises can be either static or dynamic. Static stretching involves slowly stretching a muscle to the point of mild discomfort and then holding that position for an extended period of time. Dynamic stretching involves the active stretching of the muscles by slow, controlled movements through the full range of motion.

You can stretch as part of your warm-up and cooldown routines, and even between resistance training sets or exercises.

Cooldown

The cooldown period provides a gradual recovery from the aerobic (endurance) phase and includes exercises of diminishing intensity. Static stretches are more appropriate to the cooldown since they help muscles to relax and increase their range of motion. Cooldown should consist of the following:

- 5 to 10 minutes of low-intensity, aerobic-type activity (to decrease body temperature and remove waste products from the working muscles)

- 5 to 10 minutes of static stretching exercises (to increase range of motion)

Flexibility Training Prescription

Stretching exercises should include three or four exercises for the major muscle groups of the upper and lower body. Start slowly. If you are only able to do these exercises once, then do them only once. Don't overdo any exercise because overexercising leads to injury. Increase the amount of exercise as you can tolerate it.

Stretching Exercises[3]

Improving Your Flexibility
Stretching exercises give the human body freedom of movement to do the things you need to do in your daily life.

Hamstring Stretch
For back of thigh muscles

- Sit sideways on a flat, hard surface.
- Keep one leg stretched out on surface, toes pointing up.
- Keep other foot on floor.
- Straighten back.
- Hold stretch 10 to 30 seconds.
- To feel a greater stretch, lean forward from hips.
- Repeat up to 5 times on each side.

Calf Stretch
For lower leg muscles

- Stand with hands supported on a table, arms outstretched and elbows straight.
- Keeping knee of one leg slightly bent, with toes of other foot slightly turned inward, move it back 12–24 inches and place flat on floor. Stretch is felt in calf muscle.
- Hold stretch for 30 seconds.
- Repeat with each leg, up to 5 times.

Ankle Stretch
For front ankle muscles

- Sit toward front edge of a chair and lean back, using a cushion to support back.
- Stretch legs out in front of you.
- With heels on floor, bend ankles to point toes toward you, then away from you.
- Hold position for 2 seconds.
- Repeat up to 5 times.

---

3   Adapted from The National Institute on Aging, U.S. Department of Health and Human Services (HHS). www.nia.nih.gov/HealthInformation/Publications/ExerciseGuide/chapter04c.htm

Triceps Stretch

For back of upper arm muscles

- Hold one end of a cloth in one hand.
- Raise and bend that arm to drop towel behind head.
- Reach behind you with other hand and grasp bottom of towel.
- Move hand higher up towel, which also pulls other arm down. Continue until hands come close together or touch.
- Repeat on each side up to 5 times.

Wrist Stretch

For wrist and hand muscles

- Place hands together.
- Slowly lower hands as far as you can, keeping flat against each other.
- Hold stretch for 30 seconds.
- Repeat up to 5 times.

Quadriceps Stretch

For front of thigh muscles and knees

- Lie on side on floor, hips aligned one directly above the other.
- Place head on hand.
- Bend knee that is on top.
- Reach back and grasp leg or heel (use belt loop if necessary).
- Slowly pull leg until you feel a stretch in front of thigh.
- Hold stretch for 30 seconds.
- Repeat up to 5 times with each leg.

Double Hip Rotation

For hip and thigh muscles

- Lie on back, knees bent, feet flat.
- Keep shoulders flat on floor at all times.
- Keeping knees bent and together, slowly lower legs to one side as far as comfortable.
- Hold stretch up to 30 seconds.
- Return legs to upright position.
- Repeat on each side up to 5 times.

Single Hip Rotation

For pelvic and inner thigh muscles

- Lie on back, knees bent and feet flat.
- Keep shoulders flat on floor at all times.
- Lower one leg slowly to side, keeping other leg and pelvis in place.
- Hold stretch for up to 30 seconds.
- Repeat for each leg up to 5 times.

Shoulder Rotation

For shoulder muscles

- Lie on back, stretch arms out to each side. Shoulders and upper arms remain flat on floor throughout exercise.
- Bend elbows so hands point toward ceiling.
- Let arms rotate backward/upward so hands point above head.
- Hold stretch up to 30 seconds.
- Slowly lift arms back up again to point toward ceiling.
- Let arms roll downward, pointing toward hips.
- Hold stretch for up to 30 seconds.
- Rotate arms back up toward ceiling.
- Repeat up to 5 times.

Neck Rotation
For neck muscles

This exercise can be done standing or on the floor.
- Rotate head slowly from side to side (you may need to place a thick phonebook under head if on floor).
- Hold stretch for up to 30 seconds on each side. Don't tuck in chin or angle head upward while rotating head. If lying down, keep knees bent.
- Repeat up to 5 times.

Strength Exercises[4]

Exercise either upper or lower body—not both—every day.

Arm Lift
Strengthens shoulder muscles

This exercise can be performed sitting or standing.
- If sitting, sit on an armless chair with back well supported by chair—feet remain on floor.
- Hold hand weights straight down by sides, with palms facing inward.
- Slowly raise both arms to side, as high as you can toward shoulder height.
- Hold for 1–2 seconds.
- Slowly lower arms back to resting position. Relax.
- Repeat as tolerated, up to 15 times. After a rest, repeat up to an additional 15 times.

Floor Lift
Strengthens abdominal and thigh muscles

- Slowly lift upper body as shown.
- Repeat up to 15 times. Rest in between repetitions.

4   Adapted from The National Institute on Aging, U.S. Department of Health and Human Services (HHS). www.nia.nih.gov/HealthInformation/Publications/ExerciseGuide/chapter04a.htm

Biceps Curl
Strengthens upper-arm muscles

This exercise can be performed either standing or sitting.
- Keep feet flat on floor, shoulders even.
- Hold hand weight down at sides, with palm facing inward.
- Slowly bend elbow, lifting weight toward chest. (Rotate palm toward shoulder while lifting.)
- Hold for 1–2 seconds, then slowly lower arm to resting position.
- Repeat with each arm, up to 15 times. After a rest, repeat up to an additional 15 times.

Plantar Flexion
Strengthens ankle and calf muscles

- Stand straight, feet flat on floor, holding on to a support.
- Slowly raise heels off floor onto tiptoes, as high as you can go. Hold for 1–2 seconds.
- Then lower heels back to floor.
- Repeat up to 15 times. After a rest, repeat up to an additional 15 times.

Triceps Extension
Strengthens muscles in back of upper arm

Support arm with your other hand throughout the exercise.
- Sit with back supported.
- Keep feet flat on floor, even with shoulders.
- While holding a weight in one hand, raise that arm toward ceiling, palm facing in.
- Support this active arm, below elbow, with other hand.
- Slowly bend raised arm at elbow, bringing hand weight down toward same shoulder.
- Slowly straighten arm back up toward ceiling.
- Hold for 1–2 seconds.
- Repeat up to 15 times with each arm. After a rest, repeat up to an additional 15 times.

Knee Flexion
Strengthens back of thigh muscles

- Stand straight, feet flat on floor, holding on to a support.
- Gently bend back knee, lifting foot off floor as far as possible. Hold for 1–2 seconds.
- Slowly lower leg down and pause.
- Repeat with other leg.
- Alternate legs up to 15 times. After a rest, repeat up to an additional 15 times.

Hip Flexion
Strengthens thigh and hip muscles

- Stand straight, feet flat on floor, holding on to a support.
- Slowly lift one knee toward chest, without bending waist or hips. Hold for 1–2 seconds.
- Slowly lower leg down and pause.
- Repeat with other leg.
- Alternate legs for each leg up to 15 times. After a rest, repeat up to an additional 15 times.

Shoulder Flexion
Strengthens shoulder muscles

- Sit in an armless chair with back supported by back of chair.
- Keep feet flat on floor, even with shoulders.
- Hold hand weights straight down at sides, with palms facing inward.
- Raise both arms in front of you (straight elbows, palms upward) to shoulder height. Hold position for 1 second.
- Slowly lower arms to sides and pause.
- Repeat up to 15 times. After a rest, repeat up to an additional 15 times.

Knee Extension

Strengthens front of thigh and shin muscles

- Sit in chair with only balls of feet and toes resting on floor. Place a rolled towel under knees, to lift feet, if desired. Place hands on thighs or on sides of chair.
- Extend one leg in front of you as straight as possible.
- Flex foot to point toes toward ceiling. Hold for 1–2 seconds.
- Slowly lower leg and pause.
- Repeat with each leg up to 15 times. After a rest, repeat up to an additional 15 times.

Side Leg Raise

Strengthens hip and thigh side muscles

Use weights if ready.

- Stand behind a chair for support, feet slightly apart.
- Slowly lift one leg 12 inches out to side. Keep back and both legs straight with toes pointing forward. Hold for 1–2 seconds.
- Slowly lower leg and pause.
- Repeat with other leg.
- Repeat with each leg up to 15 times. After a rest, repeat up to an additional 15 times.

Aerobic Exercise: A Walking Program

Walking is an excellent form of aerobic exercise. I chose walking because it is a very flexible activity. Regardless of fitness level, walking is something nearly everyone can do.

Aerobic exercise is a continuous movement at a moderate intensity level so that your lungs and heart can provide enough oxygen to prevent lactic acid from building up and creating anaerobic conditions (no oxygen) in your cells. Each of us has our own unique aerobic level depending on how fit we are. If you are out of shape, you do not have much aerobic capacity in your muscles that pull in the fuel used by aerobic exercise—oxygen and free fatty acids. This type of exercise uses glucose first, then switches over to fat—the long-term fuel—for sustained periods, which makes aerobic exercise the fat-burning exercise for the body.

When preparing for aerobic exercise, it is extremely important to warm up slowly and stretch the muscles, ligaments, and tendons that will be used during the session. This prevents injury and ensures a productive exercise program. A walking program has many benefits, such as:

- It's free.
- It's available to nearly everyone.
- No equipment is needed.
- It's convenient.
- No training needed, unless you are 9 months to 1 year old.
- You can change the pace whenever needed.
- It's flexible; walking can be increased to a jog or run or decreased to a slow, gentle pace.

Use the Progressive Exercise Schedule on the next page to help you plan and follow a regular exercise program. As you get to week 6, you might want to refer back to pages 145–146 and review the information about each of the conditioning phases.

Progressive Exercise Schedule

Week 1

EXERCISE ACTIVITY	Stretch	Warm-Up Walk	Aerobic Walk	Cooldown & Stretch	Strength Exercise	Total Time
DAY 1	5 min	5 min	5 min	5 min		20 min
DAY 2	10 min					10 min
DAY 3	5 min	5 min	5 min	5 min		20 min
DAY 4	10 min					10 min
DAY 5						0
DAY 6	10 min					10 min
DAY 7						0

Week 2

EXERCISE ACTIVITY	Stretch	Warm-Up Walk	Aerobic Walk	Cooldown & Stretch	Strength Exercise	Total Time
DAY 1	5 min	5 min	5 min	5 min		20 min
DAY 2	10 min					10 min
DAY 3	5 min	5 min	5 min	5 min		20 min
DAY 4	10 min					10 min
DAY 5	5 min	5 min	5 min	5 min		20 min
DAY 6						0
DAY 7						0

Week 3

EXERCISE ACTIVITY	Stretch	Warm-Up Walk	Aerobic Walk	Cooldown & Stretch	Strength Exercise	Total Time
DAY 1	5 min	5 min	5 min	5 min		20 min
DAY 2	10 min					10 min
DAY 3	5 min	5 min	5 min	5 min		20 min
DAY 4	10 min					10 min
DAY 5	5 min	5 min	5 min	5 min		20 min
DAY 6						0
DAY 7	10 min					10 min

Progressive Exercise Schedule

Week 4 (initial conditioning phase)

EXERCISE ACTIVITY	Stretch	Warm-Up Walk	Aerobic Walk	Cooldown & Stretch	Strength Exercise	Total Time
DAY 1	5 min	5 min	5 min	5 min		20 min
DAY 2	10 min				10 min	20 min
DAY 3	5 min	5 min	5 min	5 min		20 min
DAY 4	10 min				10 min	20 min
DAY 5	5 min	5 min	5 min	5 min		20 min
DAY 6	10 min					10 min
DAY 7	5 min	5 min	5 min	5 min		20 min

Week 5 (initial conditioning phase)

EXERCISE ACTIVITY	Stretch	Warm-Up Walk	Aerobic Walk	Cooldown & Stretch	Strength Exercise	Total Time
DAY 1	5 min	5 min	5 min	5 min		20 min
DAY 2	10 min				10 min	20 min
DAY 3	5 min	5 min	5 min	5 min		20 min
DAY 4	10 min				10 min	20 min
DAY 5	5 min	5 min	5 min	5 min		20 min
DAY 6	10 min				10 min	20 min
DAY 7	5 min	5 min	5 min	5 min		20 min

Week 6 (initial conditioning phase)

EXERCISE ACTIVITY	Stretch	Warm-Up Walk	Aerobic Walk	Cooldown & Stretch	Strength Exercise	Total Time
DAY 1	5 min	5 min	15 min	5 min		30 min
DAY 2	10 min				10 min	20 min
DAY 3	5 min	5 min	15 min	5 min		30 min
DAY 4	10 min				10 min	20 min
DAY 5	5 min	5 min	15 min	5 min		30 min
DAY 6	10 min				10 min	20 min
DAY 7	5 min	5 min	15 min	5 min		30 min

Progressive Exercise Schedule

Week 7 (improvement conditioning phase)

EXERCISE ACTIVITY	Stretch	Warm-Up Walk	Aerobic Walk	Cooldown & Stretch	Strength Exercise	Total Time
DAY 1	5 min	5 min	20 min	5 min		35 min
DAY 2	10 min				10 min	20 min
DAY 3	5 min	5 min	20 min	5 min		35 min
DAY 4	10 min				10 min	20 min
DAY 5	5 min	5 min	20 min	5 min		35 min
DAY 6	10 min				10 min	20 min
DAY 7	5 min	5 min	20 min	5 min		35 min

Week 8 (improvement conditioning phase)

EXERCISE ACTIVITY	Stretch	Warm-Up Walk	Aerobic Walk	Cooldown & Stretch	Strength Exercise	Total Time
DAY 1	5 min	5 min	20 min	5 min		35 min
DAY 2	10 min				10 min	20 min
DAY 3	5 min	5 min	20 min	5 min		35 min
DAY 4	10 min				10 min	20 min
DAY 5	5 min	5 min	20 min	5 min		35 min
DAY 6	10 min				10 min	20 min
DAY 7	5 min	5 min	20 min	5 min		35 min

Week 9 (improvement conditioning phase)

EXERCISE ACTIVITY	Stretch	Warm-Up Walk	Aerobic Walk	Cooldown & Stretch	Strength Exercise	Total Time
DAY 1	5 min	5 min	25 min	5 min		40 min
DAY 2	10 min				10 min	20 min
DAY 3	5 min	5 min	25 min	5 min		40 min
DAY 4	10 min				10 min	20 min
DAY 5	5 min	5 min	25 min	5 min		40 min
DAY 6	10 min				10 min	20 min
DAY 7	5 min	5 min	25 min	5 min		40 min

Progressive Exercise Schedule

Week 10 (improvement conditioning phase)

EXERCISE ACTIVITY	Stretch	Warm-Up Walk	Aerobic Walk	Cooldown & Stretch	Strength Exercise	Total Time
DAY 1	5 min	5 min	25 min	5 min		40 min
DAY 2	10 min				15 min	25 min
DAY 3	5 min	5 min	25 min	5 min		40 min
DAY 4	10 min				15 min	25 min
DAY 5	5 min	5 min	25 min	5 min		40 min
DAY 6	10 min				15 min	25 min
DAY 7	5 min	5 min	25 min	5 min		40 min

Week 11 (improvement conditioning phase)

EXERCISE ACTIVITY	Stretch	Warm-Up Walk	Aerobic Walk	Cooldown & Stretch	Strength Exercise	Total Time
DAY 1	5 min	5 min	30 min	5 min		45 min
DAY 2	10 min				15 min	25 min
DAY 3	5 min	5 min	30 min	5 min		45 min
DAY 4	10 min				15 min	25 min
DAY 5	5 min	5 min	30 min	5 min		45 min
DAY 6	10 min				15 min	25 min
DAY 7	5 min	5 min	30 min	5 min		45 min

Week 12 (maintenance conditioning phase)

EXERCISE ACTIVITY	Stretch	Warm-Up Walk	Aerobic Walk	Cooldown & Stretch	Strength Exercise	Total Time
DAY 1	5 min	5 min	35 min	5 min		50 min
DAY 2	10 min				20 min	30 min
DAY 3	5 min	5 min	35 min	5 min		50 min
DAY 4	10 min				20 min	30 min
DAY 5	5 min	5 min	35 min	5 min		50 min
DAY 6	10 min				20 min	30 min
DAY 7	5 min	5 min	35 min	5 min		50 min

Progressive Exercise Schedule

Maintenance Weeks _____

EXERCISE ACTIVITY	Stretch	Warm-Up Walk	Aerobic Walk	Cooldown & Stretch	Strength Exercise	Total Time
DAY 1						
DAY 2						
DAY 3						
DAY 4						
DAY 5						
DAY 6						
DAY 7						

Strength Training

Strength training causes the muscles to adjust to the stress or resistance placed upon them. If you stress a muscle with anaerobic exercise, the body will accommodate with additional strength in that muscle. Strength training increases a person's consumption of short-term fuel because it creates an increase in the enzymes that use glucose. More muscle equals more muscle enzymes, which in turn equals a higher metabolism, glucose need, and fuel use.

There are two types of strength exercises:

- weight resistance (such as sit-ups, push-ups)
- machines or free weights

If you are new to strength exercise, consider first using only your body weight as a resistance to accomplish the specific movement. This helps you prevent injury as you increase your fitness level. After you become stronger, you can incorporate free weights and then move to a weight machine.

Important: For each strength training session, begin with a warm-up and stretching session as described above. At the end, cool down slowly to allow the body to gradually come back to a normal movement level. The heart rate should be allowed to gradually decrease to help balance blood delivery and prevent blood pooling or possible fainting.

A Patient's Story: James

James, 38, was a determined exerciser: 40 to 50 minutes of hard bike riding every morning, an hour of aerobics plus strength training at lunch, and more riding in the evening. But until he had chest pains and shortness of breath one day during a bike ride, he had never suspected he had coronary artery disease.

After a screening stress test with his primary-care doctor produced more chest pain during the test, James was referred to a cardiologist, who immediately placed a stent in his coronary artery to open up his artery and help clear the blockage. Shortly afterward, James returned to his usual exercise routine and continued his strict low-fat diet, following the typical advice for such patients. He was also referred to me for additional care, but did not appear for his appointment.

Within five weeks of the first stent being placed, James again experienced chest pains and shortness of breath. His cardiologist discovered that coronary plaque had already overgrown the stent, once again blocking the coronary artery and causing chest pain. So James had a second type of stent inserted.

Frightened about the poor condition of his health at such a young age, he kept his next appointment with me. He clearly wanted to know why he had such aggressive heart disease and what he could do to stop or reverse it. He had never had any significant health problems before the chest pains began, but his medical history revealed a strong family trend of heart disease at early ages, which had been the motivation behind his extreme exercise routines. His daily caloric intake was on the low side, and it was split between only breakfast and dinner; he rarely ate anything in between, which left his body with insufficient fuel for a good part of the day. His main source of protein was meat, and he ate little in the way of good fats. With his intense exercise routine, he had only 7 percent body fat. With a happy marriage and an enjoyable job, his only real source of stress was his heart condition.

A complete cholesterol test showed his total cholesterol, LDL, HDL, and triglycerides well within normal numbers, thanks at least in part to the statin medication he had begun taking after the chest pains began. But after I evaluated all 13 different types of cholesterol, we discovered he also had an abnormally high amount of what are called small dense LDL particles. These very tiny particles of bad cholesterol slip through artery linings twice as fast as the larger LDL particles and encourage artery inflammation—this was most likely the reason for his artery disease as well as the rapid re-blockage around the first stent. He also had a trait called LDL pattern B, which also encouraged his artery disease. Finally, James's gene test revealed him to be Apo E 2/3. This is a gene type that does not seem to do well with a very low-fat diet. Taken together, all these traits combined to produce a rapid growth in his heart disease.

We looked at James's risk factors and his behaviors, including diet, exercise, and work, as well as his personal mission and life's journey, including what he could learn from this experience. Then we created a plan to address his entire being—body, mind, and spirit, plus his physical environment. He had begun exercising so often and so hard and drastically reducing his fat intake because he feared dying at a young age from heart disease, as many of his relatives had done. He believed this to be a logical path to follow, based on his doctor's recommendations and the generalized advice in the media. Unfortunately, it was the wrong path for him.

James was very anxious and nervous about having two occasions of chest pain and having two stents inserted in such a short time period, and wanted to prevent another episode. So in addition to the proper diet and exercise for his genotype, along with necessary medication, we focused on the ultimate outcome for his total health, defining that as a healthy physical, psychological, and spiritual body with no diseases whatsoever. We also explored the positive factors of his experience and what he might learn from it all. I explained some effective tools for relieving his stress and anxiety, including meditation, prayer, yoga, and a relaxation breathing technique he could do anywhere, anytime.

Finally, we reviewed James's plan of care, and he said he had already begun to feel better, knowing he could improve his health. He was ready to begin his new lifestyle, in partnership with three main support people: his primary-care doctor, his cardiologist, and me, his integrative-medicine provider. He would be the judge of all our advice. Feeling as if he had some control over his life once again, James now felt hopeful and determined to follow his clear plan of action. Within a very short time, he felt much better and more energetic. Lab tests showed that all his cholesterol numbers improved.[5]

Flexibility and Stretching Exercises (Yoga or Pilates)

You may be reluctant to start exercising regularly because it involves pain, strain, special equipment, other people to work out with, or travel. If this is true for you, then a gentle form of exercise called yoga may be just the approach you need to get started on the road to overall fitness. Yoga not only focuses on the alignment of your outer body but also encourages awareness of your inner self. It can be very restful to the mind as well as something to stretch and strengthen the body.

The word "yoga" means "union." It is a discipline that seeks to unite the body, mind, heart, and spirit. It consists of a series of physical postures along with breathing exercises that are easily learned. Regular practice increases flexibility; strength; balance; grace; breath control; endurance; and overall health and integration of mind, emotions, and body. The exercises also provide special stimulation of the endocrine glands and thus promote a rebalancing of your energy. Many people experience a greater serenity about life in general, as well as improved circulation; a firmer, trimmer body; and less illness.

You are advised to move slowly and with concentrated awareness to avoid strain or pain, and to coordinate your breath with your movements. Yoga exercises can be done almost anywhere. It helps to wear loose clothing to make stretching easier, and to have a mat or cloth under you, something that marks this spot as your yoga practice space. You can teach it to yourself simply by following a book or set of instructions, although a trained teacher is highly recommended, especially as you advance into more difficult postures.

Here is a simple yoga posture called the Lion: Inhale deeply, then forcefully exhale through your mouth. While exhaling with mouth wide open and eyes

---

5   *ADA's Nutrition and You: Trends 2002 Survey.* Survey results are based on telephone interviews with a nationally representative sample of 700 adults conducted in April 2002 by Wirthlin Worldwide. The survey has a confidence interval of plus or minus 5 percent in 95 out of 100 cases.

wide and staring, thrust out your tongue and stretch arms down with fingers stiff and spread tautly apart. Hold the breath for a few seconds. Then close your mouth and inhale deeply through the nostrils, expanding the abdomen. Exhale again slowly through your nostrils and relax. Repeat three times.

Yoga classes are widely available, as is a popular Westernized variant, called Pilates (puh-LOT-eez). If a book or DVD is not enough for you, check your local community bulletin board. Be aware that yoga comes in many flavors, some much more strenuous than others, so sample as many as you can and pick your favorite.

Logging Behavior Changes

What Is a Health Log?

A health log is a tool designed to help you establish and follow a new behavior. The behaviors most frequently observed with these kinds of logs are exercise and eating patterns, fluid intake, and sleeping patterns, though they may also support new behaviors ranging from personal hygiene to a spiritual practice. Logging your daily thoughts about whether you are embracing or struggling with the new behaviors can help you sustain your new behaviors.

Research has shown that keeping a health log is an extremely important part of a person's success with developing a new behavior or changing an established behavior. Some of the best Olympic athletes, triathletes, cyclists, swimmers, and runners keep detailed records of their daily performance that includes not only their physical performance but also a psychological component—their thoughts and feelings.

Getting a Logbook

Logbooks are available in most bookstores or on the Internet. I have always enjoyed going to my local bookstore to find a new logbook. For me, the cover can be important. If I like it, I'm more apt to use my logbook. And because my logbook helps me record all my thoughts and behavior changes in one place, I am able to refer to my positive changes when I need encouragement.

General Exercise Log

You can create a general log to document the type of exercise you are doing. You will log the amount of time you spent exercising, your beginning heart rate and your mid-exercise target heart rate, and how you felt before and after the exercise (rating 1–10).

Now let's look at two examples of logging—one for a walking exercise and one for a nutritional change.

Pedometer Program Log

The Pedometer Program Log on the next page is for those who would like to keep track of their progress with a walking program, by counting the number of steps taken during an exercise session. If such a program is of interest, you will need to use a walking pedometer to be able to keep track of your steps.

A pedometer is a little machine about the size of a cell phone. It is usually worn on a waistband or belt and counts the number of steps a person takes by measuring body movement. Some pedometers are simple tools that just measure steps. Some are a little more complex and can track steps, calories, and distance walked. I am not sure how accurate the calorie count and distance tracking are, but they sure are fun to use. A pedometer can be worn during a given exercise session or worn all day.

A goal is to walk as many steps as you can in the beginning. For example: 400 steps. Then slowly increase your steps on a daily basis to 410, 425, and so on. Once you have finished your exercise session, log your steps on an exercise log sheet or in your exercise journal.

My patients have a lot of fun with the Individual Pedometer Program. School children especially love pedometers; they become very excited about getting in their quota of steps during the day.

Pedometers are available for purchase in many stores. However, they vary in quality, so invest in one that will last. In addition, consider buying a pedometer with a safety strap; pedometers are famous for ending up in the toilet. You can go to our Website **www.ThePerfectGeneDiet.com** for some information about our online pedometer program.

Daily Food Log

Use the Daily Food Log on page 167 to log your food and fluid intake for seven days using a new sheet for each day. Write in the type, amount, and time you ate the food. This will help you see whether you are missing meals or successfully supporting good eating habits.

Pedometer Program Log

NAME: MONTH:

MON	Steps:	Steps:	Steps:	Steps:	Steps:	Notes:
	Goal:	Goal:	Goal:	Goal:	Goal:	
TUE	Steps:	Steps:	Steps:	Steps:	Steps:	
	Goal:	Goal:	Goal:	Goal:	Goal:	
WED	Steps:	Steps:	Steps:	Steps:	Steps:	
	Goal:	Goal:	Goal:	Goal:	Goal:	
THU	Steps:	Steps:	Steps:	Steps:	Steps:	
	Goal:	Goal:	Goal:	Goal:	Goal:	
FRI	Steps:	Steps:	Steps:	Steps:	Steps:	
	Goal:	Goal:	Goal:	Goal:	Goal:	
SAT	Steps:	Steps:	Steps:	Steps:	Steps:	
	Goal:	Goal:	Goal:	Goal:	Goal:	
SUN	Steps:	Steps:	Steps:	Steps:	Steps:	
	Goal:	Goal:	Goal:	Goal:	Goal:	

Daily Food Log

	Breakfast		Morning Snack		Lunch		Afternoon Snack		Dinner		Evening Snack	
	Food	Amount	Food	Amount	Food	Amount	Food	Amount	Food	Amount	Food	Amount
MON												
TUE												
WED												
THU												
FRI												
SAT												
SUN												

Avoiding Exercise Program Dropout

Many people who begin an exercise program drop out within the first few days, weeks, or months. Even regular exercisers, on occasion, have to triumph over obstacles that can prevent them from staying with a regular exercise program. Stopping or taking a break from exercise is normal—this is the body's natural break time. Fortunately, an exercise support system can keep these breaks from becoming permanent.

People who *do not* get advice from a licensed exercise physiologist or certified sports-medicine professional may set unrealistic goals for themselves. They may try to do too much too quickly and often become frustrated or injured, at which point they give up. In fact, the major causes of people giving up their exercise program are frustration, being overwhelmed, and not having first been through a pre-planning exercise process.

Exercise and movement are basic to life. The human body needs to move, and move often. This is simply a part of our genetic and physical makeup. Just because our lifestyles have become more sedentary in recent years doesn't mean our bodies no longer require lots of movement to be healthy. We didn't always have the supermarket where we could buy our food. Once, we had to work really hard to grow and produce our own food, or at least walk to buy it. Moving our bodies every day to just eat and survive was much more common even 50 years ago than it is today. Unless you are extremely active in your work or leisure (with an activity, such as extreme sports), consider doing your body a favor by exercising regularly.

Chapter Thirteen

HEALTHY FOODS AND OTHER NUTRIENTS

It's common to think that our bodies grow until a certain age, then stop. But in reality, the human body is in a constant state of growth and repair. To best handle these tasks, the body should receive an optimal diet from optimal food sources. This means that our food choices in both the major categories of carbohydrates, proteins, and fats and the quality of them (purity and supply of vitamins and minerals) should not only follow a general guideline, but should also be tailored for our Apo E genotype. For example, we should receive a certain percentage of fat, carbohydrates, and protein, based on our particular Apo E genotype. However, it appears that some foods are beneficial for everyone. Here are some of the foods that I suggest you consider when adding new ones to your diet. Enjoy!

Water

About 70 percent of the human body is made up of water. Most of this is found in the body's muscles, bones, blood, and lymph. Water is an essential body component, involved in every function, including regulating body temperature, assisting in respiration, transporting nutrients, circulating body fluids, absorbing nutrients, and removing waste from cells. A good daily intake of water is essential if your body is to function optimally, and it needs to be spread over the course of the day, since it is being continually lost through many bodily functions. It is difficult to give an exact recommendation of how much water you require each day, since individual needs differ and the external environment also plays a big role in the body's fluid requirements. A general guideline is six to eight glasses each day, although there seems to be no research to support these figures (and the custom of people carrying bottled water everywhere was perhaps was just good marketing from the bottlers).

Even more important than quantity is quality. The water you drink needs to be as pure as possible. If you drink water from a source that contains cell-damaging chemicals, the result will be high cell stress and this, in turn, can give rise to cell and tissue damage and disease. This is particularly important for the Apo E 4s, as this genotype has very low tolerance for toxic chemicals.

Tap water run through a good filter is often of better quality than water obtained in bottles, is one-tenth the cost, and is far less costly to the planet than the huge costs of manufacturing the plastic bottles (made from dwindling petroleum supplies), transporting them (more petroleum), and finally hauling them to landfills when they are not recycled (and many are not). In addition, the plasticizers in plastic bottles can leach into the water inside, with unknown future health effects, so carry your water in glass bottles whenever possible. Daily doses of leached plastic are not good for anyone and especially not good for the Apo E 4s.

Water quality can vary greatly, and when you find what you think is a pure source, have it tested by an independent lab. If your water does not get an A+ result, consider installing a water filter. Remember, toxic substances chronically interfere with the normal processes of the body and can cause disease. The body can tolerate an occasional imbalance or interference, but when it becomes chronic, the body becomes overwhelmed and then sick.

Chlorine and lead are the two most common toxic contaminants in water. While chlorine kills bacteria and viruses in water, it is not healthy for human cells. It may increase the risk of heart disease and has been linked to some kinds of cancer and birth defects. Lead is particularly damaging for fetuses, infants, and children—and probably for everyone else, since it can result in organ damage and stunt nervous system growth. Water with more than ten parts per billion of lead is a health risk.

Mercury is also toxic to the developing brain and nervous system of an unborn fetus, but currently research is very limited on mercury's chronic effects on adults, especially on effects resulting from the levels now found in most seafood.

Other toxic contaminants in drinking water may include, but are not limited to, microorganisms (viruses, bacteria), disinfectants, heavy metals, fertilizers, pesticides, herbicides, a host of other inorganic and organic chemicals, and radionuclides (low levels of naturally occurring radioactive contaminants). Some experts also view fluoride as a toxic chemical, but consensus is lacking, so I suggest you educate yourself about fluoride, especially if you are an Apo E 4.

Dr. Andrew Weil suggests that if you use tap water for drinking or cooking, let your kitchen faucet run for three to five minutes every morning to flush out the lead that can concentrate there. In short, your drinking water should be pure, with no toxic additives.

Apo E Gene Top 15 Healthy Foods

Below are the healthiest 15 foods and drinks according to many nutrition experts. I also recommend them for many reasons, including heart protection, phytochemical content (which may help reduce cancer risk), high fiber, low glycemic load (which helps to regulate blood sugar levels), cancer protection, nutrient density, great taste, versatility of food type in cooking, and good fat content, to name only a few benefits. This section will tell you more about some of them, but know that they are all healthy, delicious, and good for you.

- avocado
- broccoli
- extra virgin olive oil
- green tea
- red grapes
- whole soy
- garlic
- wild fish (Alaskan sockeye salmon, for example)
- berries
- dark chocolate
- flaxseed
- whole grains
- tomatoes
- fresh water (100% pure)
- nuts (walnuts, almonds, for example)

Garlic: Our Aromatic Friend

Garlic is a very interesting plant. A cousin of the lily, it contains a substance called allicin that is the active ingredient in garlic's distinctive flavor and smell. The aroma is released only when the garlic clove skin is broken, allowing an enzyme called alliinase to react with the odorless compound alliin, which creates the familiar allicin.

The use of garlic has been traced back to ancient times, as long ago as 4,000 years, when it was used not only for cooking, but also for a multitude of health benefits by the ancient Egyptians, Greeks, French, and Romans. Today, most cultures use garlic in cooking. People either love it or dislike it—or it dislikes them.

Garlic is the subject of considerable, ongoing research to evaluate its potential health benefits, particularly relating to cancer, cardiovascular disease, and viral infections. Although garlic's ability to improve health by reducing cholesterol has not been substantiated, early studies have shown some anti-platelet and circulation-improving qualities.

I recommend that you eat garlic in your food, or take a small serving of fresh garlic, each day. By keeping the amount small, you can reap the benefits while avoiding the distinctive (some might say overpowering) smell. If you are taking any anticlotting or blood-thinning medicines such as Coumadin, check with your medical provider before increasing your garlic consumption significantly.

Including garlic in your daily intake can be easy and delicious. Here are a few of my favorite dishes to which garlic can easily be added:

- soups
- roasted potatoes with olive oil
- roasted chicken and turkey with herbs and citrus juices
- tomato-based soups and pasta dishes
- salad
- roasted vegetables
- stir-fry fish and vegetables dishes
- omelets, scrambled egg whites or egg substitutes, and egg dishes
- roasted red pepper salsa

These are just a few. Be creative and add garlic to your favorite recipe. Who knows, you may end up liking garlic ice cream.

The Mysterious Mushroom

Most everybody knows what a mushroom is. Some of the oldest varieties can be found growing in circular patterns called fairy rings, which even today can be found right next to Stonehenge, in southern England. When I was a child living in Cornwall in the south of England, the common button mushroom grew wild in the fields behind our home. These little fungi held a mysterious, almost magical presence for me. I would go out with my family to pick mushrooms, and we would clear the field of these little white buttons one day, only to find just a short time later that they had grown back. As a child, this fascinated me. Later on, it was especially interesting to learn there is an entire world of mysterious mushrooms that hold immense health benefits just now being discovered by the Western medical community, even though the Eastern world has known about them for centuries.

Simply described, the mushroom is a fast-growing, spore-producing fungus that gains its food from anything that is decaying. There are many types of mushrooms—ranging from the delicious and nutritious to the exotic and deadly varieties. Leaving the toxic ones behind, mushrooms can benefit our health in very powerful ways by:

- stimulating the immune system
- helping fight and resist viral diseases
- helping treat certain cancers
- lowering cholesterol levels

Mushrooms provide the following nutrition:

- fiber
- protein
- vitamins (niacin, B12, vitamin C, thiamin, biotin)
- minerals (phosphorus, selenium, potassium, iron)

I see an exceptionally exciting use of mushrooms in the medicinal arena, as well as in the culinary arts. My advice is to keep your mind and palate open to new and interesting ideas for fungi and mushrooms. The mushroom is proving to be very versatile and can be easily grown by anyone, practically anywhere: outdoors or indoors in natural or controlled climate environments. They just might improve your health while at the same time adding a delicious complement to your next omelet or pasta dish.

Consider eating all mushrooms cooked. The following varieties hold positive health benefit.

- shiitake (lentinus edodes)
- oyster mushrooms (pleurotus ostreatus)
- nameko mushroom (pholiota nameko)
- lion's mane mushroom (hericium erinaceus)
- enokitake mushrooms (flammulina velutipes)

An excellent resource for mushrooms is **www.fungi.com**.

Tea Therapy

Tea is a popular beverage in many countries, ranging from England, Scotland, and Australia to China, Japan, and India. Although not yet as popular of a beverage here in the United States, a growing number of tea drinkers are taking advantage of recent research regarding tea's potential health benefits. In ways similar to red wine and chocolate, entire food industries are built around tea. The formal Japanese tea ceremony dates back to the early 1600s. Having grown up in Scotland and England, I have been a tea drinker for most of my life, so I was very excited when I learned that this familiar beverage might also provide a positive effect on good health.

Tea's health benefits are due to:

- an antioxidant effect that helps decrease general body inflammation
- a reduction in blood clotting in the arteries and improvement in artery-lining health
- a decreased heart attack risk, with as few as three 8 oz. cups of tea per day

These positive effects come from catechins—extremely powerful antioxidants, specifically polyphenols and bioflavonoids—that seem to be very beneficial to the human body and may help counter the effects of aging and chronic disease.

The most popular teas today come from a plant called the *Camellia sinensis.* Originating in ancient China, this tea became popular in England in the late 1700s, and teahouses there became social gathering places. *Camellia sinensis* produces most varieties of tea, ranging from the common black and oolong teas and the lesser-known white teas, to the now popular, highly beneficial green teas. The difference in color comes from how the leaves are processed; dried leaves become black tea, lightly steamed leaves produce green tea, and leaves picked very early and left unprocessed become white tea. If you are looking for a tea packed with an exceptional punch of antioxidants, you may want to try a green tea or one of the new varieties of white tea. Decaffeinated tea has also been shown to yield health benefits. A word of caution for those taking "blood thinners": green teas contain large amounts of vitamin K, which can counteract the decreased clotting effect desired.

One other benefit of tea drinking is the relaxation that comes from taking a break to sip this warm, delicious beverage. Tea drinking definitely produces relaxation in both the mind and the body. Does this come from the tea itself or the relaxing behavior related to drinking it? I believe it's a combination of both.

Take a Tea Break

Compare drinking your tea from a plastic or paper cup to sipping hot tea from an English bone china cup or iced tea from a Scottish or Irish cut-crystal glass—it's an experience well worth having. You may not have time to sit down with friends for an hour every afternoon, as we did in the "old days" for an English high tea with a sultana scone, fresh fruit, jam, and Cornish clotted cream (unfortunately, we didn't know clotted cream wasn't good for our health!), but you could take a 10- or 15-minute tea break (remember the fine china!) and have a small snack. (In fact, I encourage morning and afternoon snack breaks.) Take this personal reward of quiet time to reflect on your life or to chat with a friend. Bring some flowers into your day to add some beauty to your surroundings. It doesn't take much effort to bring the elegant quality of the past to the busy world of today. Happy tea sipping! I will think of you and send you positive energy for making a positive cultural change as I sip my tea from my English teacup each morning and afternoon. Remember: focus on what you want!

If you would like to search for your own special china teacup, here are some famous English china and crystal companies for you to explore.

Spode	www.spode.co.uk
Wedgwood	www.wedgwood.com
Royal Doulton	www.royaldoulton.com
Waterford	www.waterford.com
Edinburgh Crystal	www.edinburgh-crystal.co.uk

A few years ago I had the pleasure of participating in an old, very spiritual Japanese tea ceremony with a type of tea called matcha, which I had never had before. Matcha has a very organic taste, which many of us in the West are not used to. A Japanese colleague of mine, Yoshihiro Hotta, M.D., performed the tea ceremony and then shared his experiences of other tea ceremonies. This beautiful cultural experience can bring a renewed spirit and quality to a common beverage that many of us indulge in every day. The next time you get ready to drink your hot green or black tea, think about the centuries of culture behind just this one plant and feel some peace of mind as you sip it, knowing that your steaming drink will have positive effects on your health.

Ginger

The Latin name for ginger is *Zingiber officinale*. Its main beneficial ingredient is gingerol. Ginger provides many health benefits, the main one being its exceptional anti-inflammatory properties.

I've always liked ginger. As a child I enjoyed ginger pieces and also ginger cake and biscuits, and homemade non-alcoholic ginger beer. I can still remember seeing the homemade ginger brew in thick, old-fashioned bottles sitting in the parlor of our old country home, lined up against the cold, damp, cob walls for what seemed like forever. Once it was ready to drink, the ginger flavor was unforgettable.

I have been recommending ginger to my patients for many years. It is a very effective supplement for its anti-inflammatory properties and excellent flavor. I suggest adding ginger to Asian food such as stir-fry and wok dishes, as well as to fresh fish, sauces, salads and cold foods, fresh fruit, and cooked vegetables. Consider adding ginger to hot tea and iced drinks, and if you are adventurous, consider making some homemade ginger beer. Explore the use of ginger in your daily cooking and see if the delicious flavor of ginger could bring a touch of pizzazz back to your food or your (non-alcoholic) beer drinking!

Ginger Beer Recipe

Ingredients

2 oz. ginger root
1¼ oz. cream of tartar
1 packet yeast

8 pints water
10 oz. brown sugar
Juice of up to 2 whole lemons
     can be added

Directions

In a large pot, bring 8 pints of water to a boil. Add all ingredients, and mix well. Let sit for 24 hours. Bottle and allow to sit in a cool room for a few weeks to brew.

Dark Chocolate

Oh, for the love of chocolate! Did you ever dream a medical practitioner would encourage you to eat chocolate? Well, it's true, I do recommend it, since chocolate is proving to have some excellent health benefits.

Made from the seeds found in the pods of the *Theobroma cacao* plant, chocolate can be fun to give and fun to receive. For a long time, we have connected chocolate to happy occasions such as Valentine's Day, anniversaries, birthdays, Halloween, and other fun events. Dark chocolate seems just right for a romantic gift (and the addition of a dozen long-stemmed red roses can't hurt!). Yet sometimes eating chocolate leaves us feeling guilty because we know we're not supposed to eat candy.

Today, unfortunately, chocolate is often highly processed and mixed with many unhealthy products. But the more natural form of chocolate—cocoa, or cacao—has many beneficial qualities for protecting health. Certain forms of pure, dark chocolate with more than 70 percent cacao and less sugar provide benefits from flavonoids, just as tea does, including antioxidant effects and improving vascular and artery quality and blood platelet or cell stickiness (the latter is a quality chocolate shares with red wine). Milk chocolate or white chocolate (which is not chocolate at all) do not provide these benefits.

For me, the balance of sipping hot tea while nibbling a piece of pure, dark chocolate has magical properties—which could be why there is so much research being done to find out more about it. It shows such promise for promoting health that The National Center for Complementary and Alternative Medicine at the National Institute of Health is conducting studies regarding chocolate and how it can improve blood pressure and insulin resistance. So far, the research is telling us to include a wide variety of flavonoid-rich foods in our diet every day—including some high-quality dark chocolate.

Soy—An Excellent Food, with Cautions

Soy is a legume that contains a high-quality protein as well as isoflavones, which may protect against breast cancer, prostate cancer, menopausal symptoms, heart disease, and osteoporosis. Soy also contains a fat, but a type that does *not* seem to cause inflammation in the body unless processed. Therefore, I recommend eating only soy *protein* from its whole food sources—soybeans (edamame), tofu, tempeh, and soymilk—while avoiding any and all processed soy foods.

Processed soy food can come in many forms, including flour, oil, protein powders, soy concentrates, and the soy isolates added to many processed foods. The soy-processing industry has become a multibillion-dollar business, but since we do not yet know the effects of eating excessive amounts of soy protein, there appears to be cause for concern. Meanwhile, with recommendations about how much soy to eat ranging from a lot to a little, I think it's reasonable to eat only moderate amounts of soy and only from the natural, whole-food form.

Soy also contains a natural substance called phytoestrogen, which is shown to both reduce your risk of cancer and also increase it! For this reason, soy remains a controversial source of protein. While I think soy protein has great health benefits, it may take a while to learn to like it and adapt to the taste. I recommend first adding a small amount of a soy into a recipe, then trying a soy dish as your main protein source.

A note about soymilk: It often includes a thickening agent called carrageenan, which is derived from red seaweed. Carrageenan is in all sorts of foods, especially dairy products and toothpaste. It has been connected to gastrointestinal ulcerations and cancer, so my recommendation is to consider avoiding soymilk made with it. Brands of soymilk that *do not* contain carrageenan include homemade soymilk, Trader Joe's Organic Unsweetened, Westsoy, and Organic Vitasoy. Not all Vitasoy flavors are carrageenan free—check the label. One additional consideration with soymilk is to choose to buy organic, as some use chemicals such as aluminum in their processing. If you don't like taste of soymilk, try almond milk.

A Patient's Story: Jeff

In early 2004, Jeff, 54, went to his primary-care physician about an elbow problem. During the visit, he mentioned he hadn't had a cholesterol test in two years. His doctor sent him to me for those tests, and he had blood drawn for the standard cholesterol panel— total cholesterol, HDL, LDL, triglycerides—as well as for testing the subclasses crucial to understanding someone's entire cholesterol story. Jeff had known about this additional testing, but his doctor had never recommended it.

Jeff's results were substantially the same as they were two years earlier. While he said he was pleased, I was concerned: Even though his total cholesterol, HDL, and LDL were in line, his triglycerides and many of the cholesterol subclasses were outside the healthy range. Along with these warning signs, he was 45 pounds overweight, had been controlling his high blood pressure with medication for 15 years, and was also taking three drugs to lower his cholesterol. His diet consisted of lots of red meat and fast foods, with very few fruits and vegetables. He said he worked out "once or twice a week" and used wine to relax in the evening, usually three or four glasses, but sometimes more.

I knew from Jeff's medical history that his father had died of a heart attack at age 59. He said his father had been overweight all his life, smoked cigars, loved to eat steaks, never exercised, and was always stressed from running his business. Furthermore, his father's mother had died at a young age as well. Given all these indicators of poor health, I asked Jeff if he thought he could make some changes to improve his health.

"Sure, but why?" he asked.

I showed him some information about heart attacks and explained how they happen, explaining in detail the subclasses of cholesterol and how important they are to health. As his interest grew, I suggested a total program that included healthy changes to his diet, a better exercise program, readjusting his cholesterol medications, and the addition of several vitamins and minerals. Perhaps with fears of an early death in mind, Jeff agreed to this program, and in order to help him make the correct changes, he accepted an appointment with a dietitian and a physical therapist. I also gave him some books to educate him about this entire process: *Before the Heart Attacks* by Robert Superko, M.D., *8 Weeks to Optimal Health* and *Healthy Aging* by Andrew Weil, M.D., and *The Power of Intention* by Wayne Dyer, Ph.D.

Most important, though, Jeff also had a genetic test to determine his Apo E genotype. This would be the guide to his new nutrition and exercise program, which he understood was not a temporary "diet" but a new way of living that he could follow for the rest of his life.

Jeff eagerly embraced his new program, accepting my recommendations of sample meals and new foods, many of which he had never tried or heard of, and some of which he said "sounded downright weird," like soymilk. Accepting his program as a challenge, he plunged in and found that soymilk, especially the vanilla flavor, was "quite good." And when his extreme enthusiasm led to his being called the "food police," he discovered that "harmony requires flexibility."

"I've learned to like tofu and soymilk," he said, "but it's not something I brag about to my golfing buddies."

Jeff lost more than 45 pounds in 18 months, despite a few ups and downs. Since he takes a body-composition test (determining lean mass vs. body fat) every six weeks, he knows what he has to do to build muscle and keep the fat off. His exercise program was designed by a physical therapist and is modified frequently as he progresses. He works with a personal trainer since that keeps him motivated; otherwise, he admits that he tends to do the exercises he likes and drop the ones he's not so fond of. Now in a stable workout routine, Jeff gets his cardio exercise on an elliptical machine for 40 minutes and also weight trains an additional 30 to 45 minutes, each five days a week. As a former couch potato, he now looks forward to his workouts. "If I miss a session, I just don't feel the same that day," he said.

When his weight first began to go down as he increased his exercise, Jeff's blood pressure dropped, and dropped low enough so that he felt dizzy and had less energy. His cardiologist recommended cutting the dosage of his blood pressure medicine in half, but the problems continued even after a month of less medication. Then Jeff's primary physician told him to stop the medication completely, which Jeff did. When his cardiologist learned about this six months later, he wasn't comfortable with Jeff's decision, so Jeff agreed to have his blood pressure checked in another six months, at which time the cardiologist would make a decision about the medication. Jeff passed the test and has been off the medication ever since while maintaining normal blood pressure. He still takes niacin and a cholesterol medication because of a gene trait not connected to his diet or Apo E genotype.

In Jeff's own words:

"I am struck by the changes I have made and the results I have achieved. It's only now that I have made these changes that I can appreciate what they have done for me. They are based on integrated medicine, taking care of the whole person. The blood tests were the beginning, and certainly they pointed us in the right direction as far as medication was concerned, but without the lifestyle changes and the professional help that I received to make those changes, I do not believe I would have achieved the results that I have achieved so far. I am still making progress, still learning, still succeeding, and still failing, but it's been a great journey and one which I hope to continue with for the rest of my life."

Smart Foods

Smart foods, sometimes called functional foods, are a subclass of nutrients called phytonutrients. Phytonutrients provide not only nutrition but also biologically active compounds with significant protective and health-enhancing qualities.

Research on these phytonutrients is ongoing, and focuses on determining the true function of these beneficial nutrients. Do they support the immune system? Do they reduce inflammation? Do they protect human cells against immune system triggers such as allergens or viral and bacterial infections? Does their function extend beyond the immediate cell response to protect against long-term processes such as inflammation in the cardiovascular system and the precursors of cancer? We don't know for sure yet, but I believe we will find that these phytonutrients play a much bigger role in supporting the immune system than we have given them credit for in the past.

13.1 Key Types of Phytochemicals and Phytonutrients

Phytochemical	Food Sources
Alpha-linolenic acid	whole soy, flaxseed, and walnuts
Carotenoids	tomatoes and tomato sauce
Flavonoids	most berries, pears, apricots, tomatoes, onions, red cabbage, and pinto and black beans
Curcumin	Indian curry powder, mixed spice, turmeric, and cumin
Capsaicinoids	peppers (hot chili peppers), capsaicin is the active ingredient
Isothiocyanates	spinach, kale, broccoli, cauliflower, and cabbage
Indoles	brussels sprouts, turnip, and horseradish
Isoflavones	soy, flaxseed, grains, beans, and peas
Lignans	seeds and grains
Phenols	spinach, kale, broccoli, cauliflower, cabbage, brussels sprouts, peppers, tomatoes, celery, parsley, soy, oranges, limes, lemons, whole flaxseed, grains, and most berries
Terpenes	herbs, citrus, and red cherries

Alcohol—Good or Bad?

Is alcohol harmful or protective? Alcohol consumption is a controversial subject in medicine today because it has shown both positive and negative properties. Medical research on red wine has shown *some* positive cardio-protective effects, mainly an increase in HDL, the good cholesterol. However, this has led some medical providers to make blanket assumptions and statements about alcohol that patients can translate as, "Drink alcohol—it's good for your heart, so drink it and drink it often."

But let's stop and think about this for a minute. First of all, if there is a "good" amount for daily alcohol intake, it is a moderate amount—not all you can drink. The American Heart Association's definition of moderate alcohol consumption is no more than one drink per day for women and no more than two drinks per day for men, where one drink equals 12 oz. beer, 5 oz. wine, or 1.5 oz. distilled spirits. In addition, what about a person who has glucose intolerance, insulin resistance, or diabetes; and is on multiple medications or has very high triglyceride levels? A person with any one of these should stay away from alcohol, yet I have known practitioners to tell these patients to drink it because it's good for them. When I look at these patients' medication lists, I see statin therapy (LDL cholesterol–lowering medication), Niaspan (a slow release form of niacin), vitamin B3 (*reduces* LDL cholesterol and *raises* HDL cholesterol), diabetic medicines, and sleeping pills, all of which can make alcohol consumption dangerous. The benefits in these cases do not outweigh the risk. People taking cholesterol medications especially need to avoid alcohol because combining these medications with alcohol can cause serious harm to the stomach lining, liver, and kidneys. Even so, I've seen many patients who take high doses of cholesterol medication and also drink alcohol, with their doctor's permission—a dangerous mistake in my view.

So once again we see that a blanket health recommendation can't possibly apply to every individual. Alcohol has been shown to raise LDL cholesterol in all Apo E genotypes, and I see LDL increase even more in the Apo E 4s. Alcohol raises *all* cholesterol levels, as well as triglyceride levels, which have been shown to raise the most dangerous types of cholesterol (LDL). The only Apo E genotype that shows a promising effect from alcohol is the Apo E 2/3, but this genotype has a sensitivity to triglycerides with simple carbohydrates, and alcohol can elevate triglyceride levels.

I recommend that a patient with any active disease *not* drink alcohol. However, if you are in very good health and drink alcohol in a moderate fashion, here is a list of some positive effects of consuming small to moderate quantities:

- relaxation and stress reduction
- pleasurable taste
- romantic associations
- increase in HDL good cholesterol
- tannins, flavonoids, and antioxidants in wine
- possible increase in nitrous oxide production, potentially widening and improving flow in arteries

- potential improvement of antioxidant defense system
- reduction of platelet stickiness

Could the negative effects of alcohol outweigh the positive effects? Its negative effects include:

- immediate absorption into the circulatory system, causing rapid rises in triglycerides, blood sugar, and insulin, and reduction in reaction times (dangerous if driving)
- increased blood sugar levels even more quickly in diabetic and insulin-resistant people
- worsened diabetes
- increased "bad" LDL cholesterol in certain Apo E genotypes by as much as 300 percent
- hindered calcium metabolism and bone growth

With wine, is it the ethyl alcohol component that gives the benefit, or is it something in the grape juice? Grape juice alone has been shown to lower the risk of developing blood clots that may lead to heart problems. In addition, research has identified the antioxidant catechin as a major antioxidant in grapes, and catechin from grapes remains in a person's bloodstream more than four hours after consumption—longer than the alcoholic variety.

While there are lots of good qualities to alcohol when used wisely, it pays to think carefully when it comes to alcohol consumption.

Sodium in the Diet

Sodium—salt—is a must-have chemical element essential for good health. In the body, it is mainly found in the fluids around the cells—the blood and lymph. Sodium is very important for regulating fluid balance, and without it nerves and muscles do not function. With too little sodium, the body loses its ability to incorporate other major nutrients and cannot hold an adequate water-to-mineral balance. But when sodium intake exceeds what the body can handle, the kidneys have to work harder to remove it. A sustained buildup may cause the body to hold extra fluids in the blood and around the cells, which can contribute to a higher blood pressure from excess water retention.

Sodium is found naturally in many foods, and most of us, especially those with high blood pressure, should not consume more than 2,400 mg a day. However, the average American now consumes between 4,000 and 10,000 mg of sodium daily! Most of this excess sodium generally comes from eating too much processed food, which now makes up a large part of the average diet in the Western world. These foods nearly always have high levels of salt, partially because salt is a good, cheap preservative. In addition, the salt used in these foods replaces some of the tasty, valuable nutrients that were removed from them.

Consider a natural sea salt when ever possible—without any flavor enhancers and other additives. Read labels carefully when it comes to salt. An excellent benefit of a diet based on your Apo E gene is that the natural, whole, unprocessed foods it recommends are naturally low in sodium. A daily intake of unprocessed foods like fruits, vegetables, and plant proteins or fats contains far less than the recommended maximum of 2,400 mg sodium.

How well can you adjust to a low-sodium, whole-food diet after eating highly refined foods for a long time? Quite well, if you shift your diet gradually; your taste buds may go into shock if you attempt a rapid change. If 6,000 mg per day has been your average intake, you can gradually lower it to 5,000 mg per day by the end of the first week, continuing down to 4,000 mg the following week, then to 3,000 mg, reaching a goal of 2,000 mg per day by the end of the first month. The goal is to slowly make changes you can live with, while enjoying this new nutritional recommendation for the rest of your life.

A good place to start reducing sodium levels is by reading the labels for the sodium content in the foods you eat. Choose products labeled "sodium free," "low sodium," or "unsalted." In addition, the following general guidelines will help you make the transition from high sodium foods to natural whole foods:

- Buy fresh vegetables, poultry, fish, and lean meat.
- Use herbs, spices, and salt-free seasoning blends in cooking and at the table.
- Cook rice, pasta, and hot cereals without salt or preservatives.
- Remove all instant or flavored rice, pasta, and cereal mixes with added salt.
- If buying frozen or canned foods, choose those with labels that say "no salt added."
- Avoid all foods with preservatives.

In addition, cut back on frozen dinners, mixed dishes like pizza, packaged mixes, canned soups or broths, and salad dressings. Instead, choose low-sodium versions of:

- canned organic soups
- dried soup mixes
- organic bouillon
- canned vegetables and organic vegetable juices
- condiments like catsup and soy sauce
- crackers and baked goods
- snack foods like chips, pretzels, and unsalted nuts

Note: Rinse canned foods, such as water-packed tuna or vegetables, to remove some of the salt.

Micronutrients

As indicated by their name, micronutrients are necessary only in very small amounts to help the body run its normal functions. Mainly vitamins and trace minerals (micronutrients) help maintain the structure of the body, as well as regulate many internal processes. They can be obtained from a balanced and varied diet of whole foods, which, in today's world, can be difficult to obtain. When an optimal diet is not available, I recommend a high-quality daily multivitamin.

An important factor in aging is deterioration at a cellular level. As we age, the efficiency of our cells decreases, with the effect that our body operates at one-half to one-fourth of the energy it had in its younger days. Fortunately, a regular intake of micronutrients from whole food can help prevent this inner-cell deterioration.

The brain is the most important organ affected by aging, since it consumes more energy than any other organ of the body. An energy deficit in the brain and central nervous system affects the activities of all the organs throughout the body, as well as mental acuity and mood. This could be a key factor for diseases such as Alzheimer's disease. A regular, balanced supply of micronutrients from fresh fruits and vegetables, whole foods, and daily supplemental vitamins and minerals can be a huge benefit.

Choosing Dietary Supplements or Vitamins

How do you choose multivitamins and minerals? How do you know which are the best ones for you? The supplement industry is a fast-moving, multibillion-dollar operation not regulated by any government agency. While some products are very high quality and provide honest supplementation for a fair price, others are supercharged by gimmicky marketing schemes that play on the promise of extreme health claims.

Reputable supplements can be a very good insurance policy when you're not eating an optimal diet, but you need to understand the risks and benefits of any supplement. This is not easy. Supplements are not regulated, most medical providers are inadequately trained in their use, and the research is limited. So if you are going to purchase a vitamin, you may want to do a little research yourself. The best policy is education.

Talk to an integrative medical provider trained in the field of dietary supplementation. Ask questions of anyone recommending a particular supplement. Ask what type of training they have had, and their qualifications for recommending a certain vitamin or botanical supplement. These products are not harmless. The incorrect dosage of supplements can cause problems. Choose a formulation designed, selected, and approved by a team of trained experts (not just one person), and manufactured under strict quality control.

Check whether the ingredients are tested both prior to and after manufacturing to ensure the content and doses are correct. All should be free of any preservatives, artificial colors or flavorings, and nonessential additives. Avoid products connected to pyramid schemes.

The American Medical Association has a very strict policy regarding products that practitioners sell for profit in their examination rooms, so be wary of providers who do so. Also be aware of medical practitioners endorsing a product for profit.

Chapter Fourteen

SHOPPING AND DINING TIPS FOR HEALTH

I grew up in the small town of St. Austell in the south of England. Most of the local merchants had their shops and markets on the town's main streets, but they were nothing like the shopping areas we have today. The closest shop resembling a supermarket was the local market house, with small stalls where local tradesmen sold their goods. Every type of food was represented, and I can still remember many of them: butchers with different types of meat, a baker, Cornish pasty shop, dairy, fish, green grocer, hardware, wood and coal shop, and flower shop. My favorite was The Sweet Shop, which had the best sweets you could have imagined—licorice, fruit gum, and dolly mixture (a kind of soft fruity candy). My grandmother seemed to know everyone, and I usually didn't mind going shopping with her since I was allowed to buy sweets and sit on the steps of the market house watching the people come in and out.

Those days, and those kinds of shops, are long gone. In the "old days," people knew where their food came from and what it contained. This began to change in the early 1900s in the United States with the appearance of the large self-service stores called supermarkets, which now have become massive food suppliers. Often, they do not hold the intention of providing the best, most nutritious, high-quality whole food of the past. Luckily, specialty food markets have begun to reappear, and many supermarket chains are adding organic products and other healthy foods to their shelves in response to consumer demand.

Due to all the changes in food growing and manufacturing practices, we must now pay attention to how our food was grown—for example, with or without pesticides? Is it a "genetically modified organism" (GMO) or not? We must also pay attention to how it was processed and prepared. This section shows you how to choose your food wisely no matter where you shop or dine out. Not everyone will have the wide variety of choices that comes with living in California, but you can learn how to choose a supermarket or a restaurant wisely.

Common sense tells us that we need good, clean, appropriate food in order to provide our bodies with the building blocks of good health. We cannot possibly expect to remain healthy if we are not providing all the proper nutrients our bodies need. Remember that grocery store managers want to stock the products you will buy, so ask them to carry healthy products you don't already see on their shelves. Chances are, many other people who are also becoming more health-conscious want the same products. If you want to buy organic foods, then ask for them and tell your friends to ask as well. If you want to avoid genetically modified food, ask your grocer if a particular food has been modified in that way (although it may not be possible to tell, since there is currently no government regulation that requires the labeling of GMO foods). If you want meat and chicken grown without hormones or antibiotics, or fruits and vegetables grown without pesticides, ask for them. Don't buy foods with preservatives and additives. Finally, if you don't know what's in a food product, don't buy it. Grocery stores will stop carrying products that no one buys.

In the end, it is up to each one of us to make healthy and intelligent choices about the foods we buy and eat. You might consider buying locally grown food in season. Buying from local organic farmers usually means purchasing products from people who put a great deal of effort into supplying their customers with high-quality herbs, spices, fruit, vegetables, eggs, poultry, and meats.

It is up to each of us to make healthy and intelligent choices regarding to the food we purchase and consume.

Restaurants

Eating out is very commonplace in today's world. There are many reasons for this, but the most common is probably convenience. Anyone who has cooked a meal from scratch knows how long it takes to prepare and cook even a basic home-cooked meal, beginning with deciding what to eat, shopping for the food, cooking it, eating the meal, and then cleaning up afterward. Many families in America today just do not seem to have the time to do all this, and consequently, they eat in restaurants more often.

In addition, restaurant food tastes good. The average person is not a chef, and it's difficult to compete with great-tasting food prepared by a talented chef. Keep in mind, however, that the intention of most chefs is not generally focused on maximizing the customer's health but rather on presenting good-tasting food so that customers will return. More and more chefs are becoming health-conscious, but even they may still wish to slip a little something into the food that tastes great, but is not especially good for the customer.

Here's an example of that. I once attended a presentation in Arizona with Dr. Andrew Weil and Rosie Daley, Oprah Winfrey's chef. Both of them were in very funny form. As Daley was demonstrating how to prepare a heart-healthy dish, Dr. Weil sat in the audience, making an occasional comment. Every so often, Daley would share the contents of a recipe and then add, "If you want this dish to taste really good, add some real butter." She would look at Dr. Weil, who would reply, "Or not. It's delicious enough without the butter. Don't listen to Rosie." The audience loved these friendly disagreements, but keep in mind that even the best chefs who work closely with the best practitioners of integrative medicine are still focused on making food taste good, and are therefore tempted to use not so-healthy ingredients.

On the Menu: Nutritional Confusion

As a practitioner of integrative medicine, I have seen that one of the most powerful tools for reducing and alleviating disease is the diet. People are often reluctant to try this nutritional medicine because they've been utterly confused about diets and nutrition, thanks to what they see in the media. They ask, "What is the most popular diet of the day? Is it low fat, high fat? Low carb, high carb, high calorie, low calorie?" In addition, many people are satisfied with their diets and see no need to change, regardless of their current health status. And many people who eat frequently in restaurants and enjoy it, do not realize that they have lost control over what goes into the food they're eating.

This confusion is not surprising. The so-called experts can't seem to agree on the best diet for good health, so how can the average person have a hope of understanding? People tend to give up on a healthy diet after convincing themselves they have no time to understand the nutritional value of what they are eating. Nevertheless, a good start is to think positively and then, if you eat out a lot, acknowledge that restaurant meals do count. Start with a little education from a reliable source. The most unreliable nutritional information is usually the most accessible, particularly from ads (beware of infomercials touting health or diet foods!), but also from articles in popular magazines and newspapers, the Internet, and TV. On the other hand, researching reliable sources requires time and commitment. First, educate yourself. Seek out trusted, evidence-based information from a reliable source, such as a trained integrative-medicine provider who has been well trained in all fields of medicine, including M.D.'s, doctors of osteopathy, nurse-practitioners, or physicians' assistants. Then, focus on a commitment to visiting health-conscious restaurants and ordering healthful meals.

Another factor in healthy eating is to become a food detective, both when you're grocery shopping for yourself and when eating out. You may find it easier to eat out if you screen the restaurant's menu beforehand to determine if you can stick to your recommended diet. Locating healthy food choices for your Apo E genotype may not be easy at first, but learning about macronutrients and how they affect you can be good for your health. Remember that what is on your plate and goes into your body *becomes* your body.

Limit or even avoid certain foods, except perhaps on your birthday, which, you should note, happens only once a year. You can splurge occasionally, but like many of my patients, you might find that changing to a healthy diet means your stomach may no longer appreciate a splurge, thanks to all the positive changes the body makes when fed the right diet.

Foods to avoid in a restaurant (and elsewhere):

• rich sauces, including butter, cream, hollandaise, and béarnaise

• fried foods—pan-fried or deep-fried

• braised cheese, au gratin, or scalloped dishes

• hashes

• pot pies

One way to begin establishing your new nutritional habits when eating out is to get comfortable asking questions about the menu and how the food is prepared, and then making special requests that fit your diet. Most restaurants understand that many of their patrons have become more health aware, so the chef and staff are making more efforts to accommodate their requests. You can request that the server ask the chef how foods are prepared (the server probably will not know without asking), and you can also ask that your selection be prepared the way you want it done.

When I order in a restaurant, I want to have a meal both healthy and delicious, so I often do both of those things—which is when my family wishes they could crawl under the table and disappear. But since I'm paying for the meal and understand that the restaurant staff most likely doesn't care about my health, I simply ask for what I want to eat. In most restaurants, you can put together a healthy meal by doing the following:

- Order steamed, broiled, roasted, poached, or dry-broiled preparations.
- Choose red and stock-based sauces.
- Ask for salad dressing "on the side" and use sparingly.
- Try lemon juice, vinegar, olive oil, or buttermilk dressing as a low-fat alternative.
- Trim all visible fat from meat and the skin from chicken before eating.
- Hold off on the butter and margarine; use avocado instead.
- Practice portion control (many restaurants now serve one person with enough food for four people).
- Stay away from foods described as large, jumbo, supreme, king-sized, double, or triple.
- Order one 5-lb. lobster (hold the butter, bring the lemons) with lots of salad and veggies for the entire table.
- Search out smaller descriptions: petite, regular, small, single, appetizer, children's portion.
- Don't be tempted by offers of more food for less money.
- Share menu items with your dining partner.

Most important, if you are not served what you ordered or it was not prepared to your specifications, send it back to the kitchen. As a patron paying for the food you want, you have the right to send back food not prepared according to your request. The kitchen of a busy restaurant is fast paced, and a special meal request can get lost very quickly, so if your entrée comes to the table smothered in sauce that you requested on the side, it may simply have been an oversight. You can usually remedy this situation by politely asking your server to take it back and replace it with the correct item.

Also, be aware that many food portions in restaurants are getting larger and larger these days—much larger than healthy portion sizes. For instance, the recommended portion of steak is 3 to 5 oz., but the average petite filet in a steak restaurant today can be anywhere from 10 oz. to 18 or even 20 oz. Wow! Unless you're a lumberjack working in the frozen country up north and burning 12,000 calories a day, that's too much food to stuff into your body. What are you going to do with all that meat? Grow another arm?

I had to chuckle recently when I was ordering in a restaurant. I asked the server about the size of the lobster tail, and he replied, "They range from 2 lbs. to 5 lbs." Who on earth could eat 2 lbs., not to mention 5 lbs., of lobster at one meal? Needless to say, I did not order the lobster or the butter sauce. Remember: in order to eat less, you must order less.

Mindful Dining: Setting a Table Fit for a King and Queen

In these hectic times, eating nothing or grabbing something on the go are the two choices often facing us. Not eating when you need to is not healthy, but there is also a difference between consuming food and dining. Eating, ingesting, food intake, consumption, dining, snacking, eating on the run, fast food, convenience foods, and food "to go" are just some of the many descriptions for the modern culinary experience. As you can see, most of the latter descriptions are about saving time. For many of us, gone are the days of eating at home, or packing a small parcel of food prepared at home to take with us on a journey. In the not-so-distant past, there were few restaurants and no fast-food outlets, and the home-prepared meal was about all that was available. Home cooking was an art and displayed daily. Many times the meal served was a cherished event, especially the evening dinner, because it was a family's main social activity centered on a pleasurable dining experience.

Learning from Our Past

For many centuries, food preparation has been a primary activity at the center of daily life. Sometimes, it was also a major form of entertainment. It may have begun with the hunt of the day, which many times supplied the main dish.

Collecting flowers and vegetables from the garden or hothouse; and afternoon walks down to the local farmhouse or shops to get milk, meat, cheese, or eggs were all part of the meal preparation experiences of the past.

The English trend of entertaining with afternoon tea at 3:00 started in the late 1700s, when dinner typically was served from 7:00 to 8:30. Because people grew hungry during the long stint between lunch and dinner, it became common to serve a light afternoon snack with tea. Anna Marie Stanhope, Queen Victoria's lady-in-waiting, later began the practice of inviting friends for tea and is often credited with turning this practice into a social event for many middle- and upper-class households.

As the popularity of afternoon tea grew, the English china pottery industry began with the discovery of English china clay. This led to the growth of the china pottery industry by William Adams & Sons, Spode, Wedgwood, Denby, followed by such artistic delights as Edinburgh and Waterford crystal glasses and England's famous Sheffield sterling silver cutlery.

Formal gatherings that revolved around this afternoon tea, as well as the evening meal, became an established pattern, and the tea and dinner table were transformed into an art form. Eventually this major form of entertaining evolved into more of a family tradition. My family followed this tradition as I grew up in Cornwall, where afternoon tea had taken on cultural as well as economical importance. Besides being the home of the copper- and tin-mining industries and a strong and vibrant fishing industry, Cornwall is the major source of English china clay and is home of the high-class Cornish Cream Tea, "The Best Cream Tea Event in all of England."

The fashionable cultural event of the daily "high tea at three" included displaying your beautiful English bone china tea service with aromatic English teas in warmed china teapots. Exhibit plates were used to display and present dainty cucumber and watercress sandwiches and an array of Cornish pilchards or herrings on toast. There were Cornish buns and sultana scones, topped with wholesome local fruit jam and, of course, a mountain of unwholesome—but we didn't know that back then—Cornish clotted cream. This culinary experience was laid out on a white linen tablecloth, with fresh linen napkins and silver spoons, knives, and forks. In the center of the table was usually a small bouquet of delicate wild flowers. I can still remember fresh strawberries and cream, hot cross buns and jam—all culinary delights of Cornwall.

This formal, festive feasting, a great part of the English culture, spread around the world. It influenced some of the early Americans' traditions, encouraging, for example, an iced version of tea. Sadly, today's fast-paced lifestyle has diminished the once-daily ritual of high tea gatherings to something done only on a special occasion.

Today, most people are so busy they rarely find the time to experience some of these wonderful aspects of dining together that I knew so well as a child. There is no time to stop, reflect, and enjoy our family and friends, even our possessions. The attractions of the past's romantic dining experiences included the time spent with friends and family, savoring the food, not to mention the ritual of preparing the food and setting the table, and collecting roses from the garden or wildflowers from the meadow. Compare the elaborate dining experiences of the past to the dining experiences of today's fast-paced world. Today, there aren't many times that we bring out the good china, the special silverware, and the extra-nice crystal for a meal—maybe Thanksgiving, Christmas, and a birthday or two. It is no longer a daily ritual.

Many people still enjoy preparing a fine meal for a gathering of friends and families, complete with the excitement of a beautiful table laden with delicate china, sparkling crystal, shiny silver, and fresh white linens, but it is difficult for most of us to find the time to do this. In many households, daily meals have changed from home cooked to fast food, complete with plastic containers, forks, knives, spoons, and paper or plastic cups with straws. Even *I* resort to fast-food choices once in a great while. However, I know that the common dining experience can change, and with a little effort, a rich cultural tradition can return to our lives.

Here are some suggestions to enhance your dining experience:

- Light a candle on the table while eating breakfast in the morning.
- Put a flower in a vase to lift your spirits while drinking that cup of coffee or tea.
- Bring a flower home or to work for your table or desk.
- Choose a china cup instead of a paper version.
- Choose a crystal glass bowl instead of a plastic container.
- Take a minute before eating to give thanks with a song, grace, or even ten seconds of silence.
- Most of all, remind yourself that you and your family are worth the effort.

Families are connected through tradition and stories, which can help build trust and communication between their members. If you usually eat out, consider skipping the restaurant tonight. Cook dinner at home together. If you already cook dinner for your family, consider making this time together even more special. Leave the paper napkins in the drawer tonight and use cloth, or surprise the children by asking them to put flowers on the table. Light a candle, or use the china a little more often. And please, turn off the television. For those moms and dads who have little children, invite them to join you in setting the dinner table as if you were kings, queens, princes, and princesses. Imagine and talk about what it was like back in the "olden days" when family and friends entertained each other. The children will probably love it. They seem to always want to know the stories of the world, and the best people to tell them these stories are their moms and dads.

My husband and I often serve a mysterious dinner on the floor in our home for our children, under a rainbow of multicolored toile that serve as a magical Eastern desert tent. At a dinner such as this, your family can discuss past traditions, dining, and culture. You can also explore how to bring a little tradition into your family life today. If there are small children present, conversation may center on fairies, pirates, kings and queens—Robin Hood, King Arthur and his knights, or even Cinderella. You might want to use a little book I wrote for a school children's program called the *Cornish Fairy-Pixie Conference*. It is set in medieval Cornwall and contains artwork to guide children in a fun walking exercise and a diet program using a pedometer for each child and posters that can be put on the wall.[1] And consider some simple whole-food meals you can make at home. You can find lots of great books in your library or bookstore, even for "quick and easy" whole-food preparation. Begin with planning even one meal at home each week. If you can engage a friend in becoming a food detective, you can share the great recipes you each discover, or even get together to prepare a healthy meal each week. A little planning like this can help immensely with the long-term goal of better nutritional intake and enhanced health.

---

1   For a copy of this book, write to: The Harvest of Hearts Program
    4165 Blackhawk Plaza Circle, Suite 125
    Danville, CA 94506

    All proceeds go to "The Harvest of Hearts Program," which educates children and their parents about the benefits of healthy nutrition and exercise.

Chapter Fifteen

THE HARMONY OF MIND, EMOTIONS, BODY, AND SPIRIT

"I think, therefore I am."
— René Descartes

Does the way we think affect our physical body? Are our mind, emotions, and body connected, or are they completely separate entities?

The 17th-century French philosopher and mathematician René Descartes contemplated the philosophical question of how the world seemed to him, versus what the world actually was. He asked questions such as:

• Who am I?

• Where do I come from?

• What do I really know?

• What can I be certain of?

Descartes concluded, "I think, therefore I am," meaning, I am thinking, so my mind is real. We have physical bodies, we can touch the physical body and the world; therefore, our bodies are also real.

Reductionism emerged from this philosophical thinking process. It was based on the cognition that because we can actually see and measure the physical body, it is truly real. Medicine was on its way to full-fledged separation of mind, emotions, and body, as it focused on the physical realities of "If I can see it or touch it, I know it is real." Since the mental, emotional, or spiritual aspects of the physical body could not be touched, felt, or understood, they did not exist, at least according to the world of medicine. Hence, medicine took the responsibility for the care of the physical body alone; and the mind and emotions, as well as the spirit and soul, were left to the church for safekeeping.

This separation was not necessarily a bad thing, because it enabled medicine to focus on the physical realities of the body, which it could witness, dissect, measure, and weigh. As a result, medical scientists made amazing discoveries in the physical world of physiology, anatomy, microbiology, molecular biology, genetics, biochemistry, and pharmacology. Medicine thought it had arrived—until quantum physics entered the picture in the early part of the 20th century. The discoveries of quantum physics threw many previously held "facts" about the physical universe out the window. It showed that there was much more to understanding and treating the body than had been thought. Quantum physics defies description, even among the quantum physicists themselves, but an idea can be gotten from the popular movie *What the Bleep Do We Know!?*

Additionally, the work of Hans Selye, M.D., who uncovered the mechanisms of stress in the human body in the 1940s, laid the groundwork for what we now recognize as the intricate connection between the mind and the physical body. Medicine can no longer view mind, emotions, and body as three separate entities.

The power and potential of understanding the connections between the mind and body are quite incredible—*whole-body health involves caring for the mind, emotions, and spirit as well as the body.* With that in mind, I want to present a new perspective on how to both view and approach your health—and your life.

The bottom line is that the human body doesn't function on the physical level alone. It also functions on psychological, emotional, environmental, energetic, and spiritual levels. The way you think and feel, the state of your environment, and your relationship to spirit *all* impact—influence and shape—your physical body, all the way through to your cells and genes. Quantum science has proven this, and clinical medicine is now using this knowledge with patients, recognizing there is more to treatment than handing out pills and performing surgeries.

Have you ever asked yourself:

- How does my mind influence my physical body?
- How do my emotions influence my physical body?
- Does my environment influence my mind?

- Does my environment influence my emotions?
- Are my mind, emotions, and body connected, or are they three separate entities?

While a single theory rarely provides the whole answer, advances in science and technology have enabled us to understand more than ever before. Some of the answers to our questions regarding the power and potential of the mind-emotion-body connection can be found in the fields of psychoneuroimmunology and neuroendocrinology. From these disciplines, we know that certain thought patterns produce beneficial or harmful body responses, and that these in turn can produce corresponding positive or negative physical outcomes or states of health. This is real clinical science that we can apply to our lives, to bring us better health, joy, and happiness.

Perhaps one day we will be able to answer the question, "What is a thought made of?" Once we have a complete understanding of our physical selves, perhaps we can apply what we've learned to a deeper understanding of how thoughts affect the physical body. Possibly, one day, we can join the three arenas of mind, emotions, and physical body, and view them working interdependently as a whole, instead of as separate entities. This will enhance our efforts to be of service to humankind through science and medicine.

Evidence of the Mind-Emotion-Body Connection

Let's look at some common human experiences that typically produce negative or positive thinking states, and what research tells us about the chemicals the body produces in response to them. Here are some "negative" human experiences:

- loss of a loved one through death
- divorce or separation
- depression
- loneliness
- chronic stress
- chronic illness

The negative-thinking states typically associated with these experiences have been shown to reduce the immune system's ability to fight disease. If we perceive the world as stressful, we will continue to produce stress hormones generated by negative feelings. Here are some "positive" human experiences:

- fulfilling personal relationships and social support structures
- fulfilling your life's work
- humor and laughter
- guided imagery
- hypnosis
- relaxation techniques
- meditation
- aerobic activity and exercise

The positive states often associated with these experiences increase your number of white blood cells and other immune factors such as your T-cell count, elevate endorphin levels, and promote healing, and a feeling of well-being.

If we evaluate patients who report being happy and content in their lives and contrast their immune functions with those of patients who are chronically stressed, unhappy, or depressed, we find that the latter group are less well. So we can use the mind-emotion-body connection to improve our health and prevent disease.

It is useful to classify the different states of awareness available to us to see how each influences—even governs—our brain and central nervous system.

Levels of Awareness

The following model was adapted from many sources (it also correlates to the seven chakras; see page 223). It identifies seven levels of awareness that we, as humans, may operate on. As you read through these, consider which is the level or levels you operate on most of the time. An awareness of each level can be of use in helping you define who you are and what you want.

First Awareness Level: Fight-Flight-or-Freeze Response

The fight-flight-or-freeze response is an acute survival reflex mechanism that was programmed into our brains for millions of years. The oldest part of our brain on an evolutionary scale is called the "reptilian brain." This response is a necessary component for the survival of all animals with a central nervous system. Life-threatening events produce a specific type of acute stress response or chemical chain reaction in the body. These adrenal stress hormones are responsible for shutting off all non-necessary body systems and focusing on the systems essential to our survival, such as the brain, heart, and lungs.

We do not have to think about anything to generate this response. It just happens. Thanks to this, people have found themselves able to perform amazing things they ordinarily could never have accomplished, such as lifting a car to save another person or running faster than they had ever imagined possible.

While primitive humans often had to fight for food or survival and to flee from danger, humans in the Western world at least, rarely encounter actual life-threatening events. This doesn't stop activation of this inner-body protective warning system, however, and our brains are often imagining situations from the past or future that seem like they are life threatening but aren't.

The freeze component of this response has been largely suppressed by our "civilization." When other animals have survived a life threatening experience and are emerging from the freeze state, they literally shake it off. We humans tend to not do this, and that suppression of the unshaken-off fear remains in our bodies. It is now implicated in many post-traumatic stress conditions (PTSD), when stress is stored in parts of the brain and body.

Second Awareness Level: Spontaneous Action Response
The second level of awareness is the reaction response—an adaptation of fight-flight-or-freeze that evolved because the human mind, by using intellectual processing, concluded that we do not always need to fight or flee a situation of potential negativity or danger. If a situation is not really life threatening, we could theoretically avoid the intensity of the fight-flight-or-freeze response by using a different response: a controlled reaction response. This response, depending on our personality, may be expressed with a kind, mean, or indifferent demeanor.

The fight-flight-or-freeze reaction is still with us. We know that responses to stress come in many forms—as severe as a full-fledged panic attack, as gentle as what we call butterflies fluttering in the tummy, or even a hot flash. It can be as silent as an elevated blood-pressure reading. All are expressions of the fight-flight-or-freeze survival mechanism.

Today we know a great deal more about the environment produced by chronic stress within the body on a daily basis. Chronically stressed bodies produce a chain-reaction response, with stress hormones, glucose, and fat being dumped into our bloodstreams. Today we know that these reactions are generated by the negative-thinking states engendered by certain experiences.

Should you, could you, be using your mind in a more positive way? Should you be modifying how you view and react to the world? If your answer is yes, be aware that some of your reactions to life are difficult to change because they are learned behaviors, usually ingrained into your cellular chemistry at an early age. Receptor sites in the body feed off the chemistry generated by this stress response. Interestingly, if we do not feed those receptor sites, we can actually experience a withdrawal from not having them filled—the same as a drug addict on cocaine or heroin would experience, but not as strongly. This can make personal change more difficult than we might hope it would be.

Third Awareness Level: Calming Awareness Response

This tranquil response coincides with not having to work hard to survive, hunt, fight, or sleep all of the time. It arises when human beings have time to rest and think about and reflect upon life's ever-changing challenges. When humans have time to do this, they evolve into higher-functioning beings.

Some people might choose to classify this state as meditation, prayer, analytical thinking, or contemplative problem solving. How does this level relate to us in today's highly technological environment? In a chronically stressful life, few of us have the time or space to engage in reflection and questioning—we revert to the unconscious older patterns. And yet, it's more important than ever to reclaim this state if we are to develop and sustain a healthy, balanced life.

The bottom line is, don't be a caveman. Strive to step out of that primitive, reptilian-brain, spontaneous reaction and gain some tranquil time for yourself where you can explore questions such as, "What do I want out of my life?" "How are my relationships going?" or "Am I engaged in my life's work?" Shift yourself from the caveman mentality and focus on you and what you want.

Although it sounds simple, it's not always easy. Women, for example, tend to get lost in their husband's and children's lives, but some women are not cut out for a life of laundry, children, dishes, and household chores. On the other hand, men tend to focus on bringing in the income and providing for the family's physical needs. To both, I recommend taking a day off—or as much time as possible—to reevaluate your work and duties to focus on your desires. You might be amazed by what you find when you make the time to search deeply within yourself for what you really need and want. The next time you are performing your regular tasks, whether around the house or where you work outside the home, slip into your intuition within a restful state and ask, "Do I like my life the way it is? Is this what I imagined doing with my life?"

Fourth Awareness Level: Instinctive Response

Instinct, intuition, sixth sense, and one's source of spiritual intelligence can create higher thoughts than the rational mind is capable of generating. Instinctive intuition is not the same as rational thought. It is more of a knowing without knowing how you know it: you simply somehow feel it, sense it.

To answer the question, "Do we know we have a physical body?" we must do as René Descartes suggested and move into that spiritual, nonphysical essence of our being that we may sense but cannot see. Here we can connect with an experience of higher knowing—an experience of knowing that something is so, even though we may not know how or why we know. This state is not a feeling of gaining or losing; it is simply "what is"—the instinctive, intuitive knowing that something is right or wrong.

Perhaps some people can get to this level of knowing, but can you? The answer is an unequivocal yes. The fact is, you already have it inside of you, and you do not need to find what you already have. You just need to set the intention to access it. To do so, I suggest you do a breathing exercise or enter a silent state within yourself and ask your instinctive intuition to be activated and heightened. Then, ask a question. You will get an intuitive reaction, no matter what question you ask. To experience this is a powerful feeling, and the attempt has never failed me.

Fifth Awareness Level: Imaginary Response

This is the imaginative or visionary state. This is where you actually begin to know what is needed to generate what it is you want to manifest. This state evolves naturally when you are in sync with the purpose and mission of your life journey. I know this because I have been doing this visualizing my entire life, though I may not have always been totally aware of it.

My experience has shown me that once I become aware of what I want to manifest, the universe seems to show up with exactly what I need. You too will have an intuitive feeling that this—whatever it is you are drawn to manifest—is right for you. Sometimes others' intentions try to push you off your original mission, but it is up to you to stay true to your mission. If you are focused and keep tapping into what you truly desire in your life—what feels good and right for you—you will manifest whatever it is you choose.

Sixth Awareness Level: Innovative Response

At this level, you can gain an understanding that you can create something not currently present in your reality. I have had this experience in my life and have created many things I have never seen before. To understand that you can create something by recognizing the components that must go into it, and then create that something out of your own intention, is the creation response level in action. It doesn't have to be anything fancy at first, but just knowing that this creative process and response is possible is very important.

With every creative process, spirit is needed. You and your creative spirit need to be engaged if you are to create whatever it is you want. Spirit brings together the pieces.

Let's say you want to build or create something—a song, a book, a cake, a dress, or even a company. What do you need? Break the end product down to find what the whole is comprised of—many parts, many ingredients. But even having these, it takes the will and the intention to put those parts together to be able to make the dress, cake, song, or book. Once you actually take your desire and put something together, it is unique, it is your creation. You can say, "Well, lots of people make cakes or books or dresses, even companies," but it may never have been done in your way with your particular viewpoint. Focus on your mission, your awareness, your life, your creation. You are important, and your desire to build something is also important. Function at your own level of creativity. Believe that you count as a creator in this world—because you are one.

Seventh Awareness Level: Spiritual Response

The spiritual response is being aware of a higher source of spiritual "something." No matter how we paint this higher "something," if we reach this spiritual-response level, we ask some foundational questions of the universe. Most of us who experience this level at some point in our lives come to realize that we have a higher spirit level or higher divine source. We don't experience it as we do other, more physical levels; it's a completely unique experience and goes back to the foundation of creation where "the making" of something comes from spirit. This process goes all the way back to those fundamental questions that our French philosopher René Descartes asked: "Who am I? Where do I come from?"

We can ask the same of everything around us. Where do all the different varieties of cakes, songs, and businesses come from? Where do all the butterflies, birds, and flowers come from? Fundamentally, from the same place all other creations come from, but when you break down those creations into parts and follow them back to their source, you still come up with the same question and the same sort of an answer. You can't have the physical development of a pie, cake, or business without a spiritual wanting or desire to create.

So ultimately I do not think we know the answer to Descarte's questions because the source of formation is beyond our own understanding. We clearly do not have enough information to gain a cognitive understanding to answer these questions that were asked hundreds and even thousands of years ago, and are still being asked today. Some would define the starting place of physical formation as "God." Depending on where you live and what culture you live in, or at what stage of your life you are in, your definition of the ultimate being or creator will vary. I don't think it really matters, as long as you realize that you do have access to a higher spirit or higher divine source. That belief needs to have importance and belong to you, and only you.

Where Are *You* in This Model?

What does all this mean? Review these levels of awareness and try to understand where you operate: Are you operating in the first level of awareness from a fight-flight freeze response where you are constantly in the protective mode? This is a very stressful response to be living in. If you expend most of your energy trying to survive, not a lot is left for anything creative. If you are able to live beyond the first few levels of awareness, it is a lot easier on your body; and life is more productive, joyful, and creative. Be aware that moving up to higher levels is more difficult for some Apo E genotypes. While no one stays out of the fight-flight-freeze response all the time, the Apo E 2s and 4s seem to have a harder time getting to the higher levels if they are not in balance with their environment.

How Does This All Fit into a Diet Based on the Apo E Gene?

Our body needs the right nutritional ingredients for our genetic makeup in order to maintain cell balance and ease. Yet, as we've seen, our bodies do not get nutrition from food alone. The way we think, how we feel about our life, and the state of our environment, as well as how we deal with our environment, all affect this balance.

Depending on the level of awareness from which we're operating at any given time, we may produce the endorphins of love if operating on Level 5–7, or the chemicals of fear if operating in the fight-flight-or-freeze mode of Level 1. Operating at Level 1 requires a large and constant flow of blood sugar, so if you are in chronic state of fear and you are an Apo E 4, your body is constantly producing the stress hormone adrenaline. This in turn requires more fast-acting glucose fuel, which adds an additional demand for fuel—the body now has to work extra hard and is less able to attend to the growing and healing that occurs when it is supposedly at rest.

Not eating the correct food and otherwise creating a gene-supportive environment doesn't mean your body stops needing the right fuel. The brain will ask the liver to make some fuel (glucose) to feed it, and the body adapts to produce it, feeding itself from itself—becoming its own internal fuel source. That internal fuel production process is hard on the body, and can unbalance your body's cells and tissues. This process happens with the all Apo E genotypes, but not to the same degree as for the Apo E 4s.

Are you in a state of chronic stress? A typical answer is: "Sure! It's the nature of my work, and I can't change it." Focus on what you *can* do, not on what you *cannot*. If you cannot change your work, can you change how you react to it?

When operating on Levels 5–7, you are focusing on what you love and making changes to give yourself more of that, and you find the world supporting you. The more you practice being on the higher levels of awareness, the more you create a better life for yourself.

So it is important to focus on what you actually want *for you*. Stay focused and directed on your desire and needs. Identify what level of awareness you are operating at most of the time. If you are not happy with this, know that you can change levels. Make it a priority to take some quiet time each day to make change.

Knowing the levels of awareness you are on plus your Apo E genotype, you can begin to understand if you need to make changes or if you are all right staying at the levels of awareness that are familiar to you.

Of course, this is dependent on your knowing who you are and what you want. Consider your current level of awareness. Are you going about your life in a state of observation, living in someone else's intention—operating at a Level 1 or 2 of awareness? Or are you living in your own intention—a state of creation at an awareness Level of 6 or 7? You are the best judge of this.

We began this process in Chapter 2, but now we will look at this a little more deeply. I believe that who you are now, and how you perceive your state of health and happiness, will be different than when you first began reading this material. Let's see.

Learning Who You Are and What You Want

Most of us would like to have what we want and get rid of what we don't want. Yet sometimes we seem to argue for our own limitations, coming up with a host of reasons why we can't have what we want. The fact is, you can have exactly what you want and get rid of what you don't! You can create your perfect life— just the way you want it. Here's how:

First, you need to decide exactly what you want and do not want in your life. If you have never given this any thought, you may have to think about it for some time. When I ask my patients this very question, at least 80 percent have never taken the time to think about what it is they truly would like to have in their life. You may have been living in other people's worlds and doing what they wanted you to do for so many years that you have never taken the time to seriously think about what it is you actually like, need, or want. I did this for many years, until one day I got smart and said, "No, I don't want that. I want something else in my life."

While it is easy to say this, actually taking the steps to accomplish the change you want is another matter altogether. Let's look at how you can make it happen.

Map out very clearly, on paper, exactly what you would like to experience in your life. Then, work out just how you will accomplish each goal. You can review your work with a spouse or partner later, but initially you must do this by yourself. This exercise requires imagination (daydreaming, some might call it), and may involve meditation or prayer. We will look at these more closely in the next chapter. For now, you can get started with the checklist below.

Your map does not have to be perfect the first time around. Initially, you may want to work on naming only a few of the things you want, or changes you want to make. Starting small is best; do not try to make too many changes all at once. Your goals can be simple or complex, but putting your plan on paper is very important. Once your plan is completed, you can modify and refine any aspect of it that you care to.

Now, let's begin. *If you had all the time in the world and no restrictions on what you did with it, how would you spend your time? If you had endless monetary resources, what would your life be like?*

Ah, wait. I heard you say, "I don't have all the time in the world, or all the monetary resources." Don't focus on the information of the past. *Focus on the future of what will be.* The task involves mapping your life as *if* you have already accomplished your goals. For now, set your goals based on what you would like it to be—not on what it is not.

Now, I'm asking you to set aside some time to look over specific areas of your daily life to consider what is and what may be, and to write down what would be *ideal for you.* If you don't know what you want, you're unlikely to get it!

When I am creating in this way—I always like to place only the positive on my paper—I like to add: "All my life lessons will be learned through joy and happiness."

In Your Ideal World

Remembering that what goes into your body *becomes* your body, complete the following questions. If you need more room than the lines provided below, use a separate piece of paper to write down your responses to each of the following:

Breakfast and Morning Snack

In your ideal world, with a focus on your health:

- Who prepares your food? You or someone else? _____
- If others prepare your food, are they educated about the foods your specific Apo E type needs to eat daily to maintain good health? _____

What is your preferred type of (be as specific as you can):

- Carbohydrate:

    fruit _____

    vegetable_____

    grain/starch_____

- Fat _____
- Protein (plant or animal) _____

Exercise

In your ideal world, with a focus on your health:

- What are your preferred types of exercises?

    ☐ stretching

    ☐ aerobic—cardiovascular

    ☐ anaerobic—strength

    ☐ other _____

- When do you most like to exercise?

    ☐ morning

    ☐ noon

    ☐ afternoon

    ☐ evening

Work

In your ideal world:

- Do you work? (If not, skip to next section)_____
- What kind of work are you doing? _____
- Who do you work with, or do you work alone? _____
- What does your ideal workplace environment look like?_____

    _____

- How many days a week do you work?_____
- What time does your workday begin and end (choose from the following possibilities or write in your own at the end)?

All day—an 8-hour day:
7 A.M.–4 P.M.
8 A.M.–5 P.M.
9 A.M.–6 P.M.
10 A.M.–7 P.M.

Or: *Morning only*
6 A.M.–Noon
7 A.M.–1 P.M.
8 A.M.–Noon

Or: *Afternoon only*
Noon–4 P.M.
Noon–5 P.M.
Noon–6 P.M.

Or: *Afternoon and evening*
Noon–8 P.M.
Noon–9 P.M.
Noon–10 P.M.

Or: *Evening only*
6 P.M.–10 P.M.
6 P.M.–11 P.M.
6 P.M.–Midnight

Or write in your perfect work hours _____

Consider:
- Are you currently doing your life's work? _____
- How do you rate your work—"1" being you dislike your work, and "10" being the perfect work for you:

Dislike   Like
   1   2   3   4   5   6   7   8   9   10

- Are you comfortable with the noise level? _____
- Does the space support you in doing your best work?_____

- What can you do to make it better, now? This may be as simple as placing a photograph of a loved person (or place) on your desk or as complex as rearranging the furnishings. _____

_____

Lunch and Afternoon Snack
In your ideal world, with a focus on your health:
- Where do you eat—at home, in a park, or at a restaurant? _____

_____

- With others or alone? _____
- What is your preferred type of (be as specific as you can):
  » Carbohydrate:
    - fruit _____
    - vegetable_____
    - grain/starch_____
  » Fat _____
  » Protein (plant or animal)_____

Home Environment
In your ideal world:
- What would your home space look like? Consider the size, the furnishings, the colors, and whether the space is cluttered or uncluttered. Who do you share the space with? What are the smells—fresh or stale? What are the sounds? Do you have a personal, dedicated space just for you? What does the surrounding environment of your ideal home look like? _____
- What makes your home space very special for you? _____

_____

Consider:
- Do you care what your home space looks like? _____
- What is just one thing (or two, or three) you could decide to do now that would make your existing home space better for you?

_____

Hobbies and Interests
In your ideal world:
- What are your favorite hobbies and interests—sports, art, creative development, writing, reading, other?_____
- How much time do you spend on these? _____
- When do you like to do these? _____
- With other people or alone? _____

Family
In your ideal family experience:
- How do you and your family spend time together?_____

  _____

Consider:
- Do you spend more or less time than you presently do with a spouse or partner, children, pets, extended family? _____

Dinner and Evening Snack
In your ideal world, with a focus on your health:
- Who prepares it? _____
- Where do you eat it—at home, a restaurant, or some other special place?

  _____

- Alone or with others? _____
- What is your preferred type of (be as specific as you can):
  Carbohydrates:
  - fruit _____
  - vegetable_____
  - grain/starch_____
  » Fat _____
  » Protein (plant or animal)_____

Evening Activities
In your ideal world:
- How do you spend your evenings? _____

  _____

- Are you alone or with family, friends, or in group activities? _____

  _____

- Is every evening similar, or do you set aside some evenings for family, some for friends or personal-growth activities, and some alone or with someone special? _____

Sleep Pattern
In your ideal world:

- What time do you go to bed? _____
- What time do you rise in the morning? _____
- What are the optimal number of hours of sleep for you? _____
- What does your sleep environment—bed and bedding, furnishings, lighting, colors, temperature, sounds, scents—look and feel like?

  _____

- What does your sleeping pattern look and feel like? (e.g., "Early to bed and early to rise," or vice versa?)_____

  _____

Consider:

- When does your body want to go to bed? _____
- If you have difficulty sleeping, do you use any medications or natural alternatives? _____
- Does your existing sleeping environment nurture you? _____

Happiness
Circle your level of happiness on the following scale, with "1" being very unhappy and "10" completely happy.

Unhappy   Happy
1   2   3   4   5   6   7   8   9   10

Consider:

- If you are not happy, why? _____
- Can you identify some of the reasons you are not happy? _____

  _____

- Do you know what changes will make you healthier and happier, and bring you more peace and joy? _____
- How could you create your day, your way, remembering that your happiness is your responsibility and no one else's. What is even one small change you could make, today, to be happier? _____

  _____

If you think you cannot accomplish this alone, consider finding someone to support you. Enlist the help of a friend, family member, doctor, or counselor/ therapist. You can create your life and day the way you want it to be. Focus on what you want! Not on something you don't want.

Now let's look at some practical tools that can support you in manifesting your ideal life.

Chapter Sixteen

TOOLS FOR CHANGE

Now that you know what you want, let's look at some tools that can help you make your dreams come true.

Expressive Arts Therapy

Expressive arts therapy can support you in making the changes—psychological, physical, or spiritual—that you want to make in your life. While psychologists are not totally sure how this process actually manifests the desired changes, it does! Most of my patients really enjoy this expressive arts exercise.

With this exercise, you create a picture or "dream board" illustration of your ideal life. This process assists you in focusing on your innermost needs, desires, hopes, and dreams. It puts you a step beyond just feeling or thinking what your life is going to be like when you have it just as you want it, since it helps you actually see some physical picture or form of what your new life is going to look like. You can create this picture by cutting out words and pictures from magazines; as well as drawing, painting, and writing on it yourself. Make it your very own masterpiece. Are you ready? All you need to do is dream, and focus on what you want. See yourself as already having this new object or behavior in your life. Then be thankful for your new life, as if you are already living it: your newfound health, your new exercise program, your healthier eating habits, or your healthier relationships.

The goal is to include a drawing or picture of each aspect of your life you want to change. *Example 1:* if you are currently living in a certain town or home, yet you want to live in another, place a picture of the town or home you want to live in on your picture. *Example 2:* if you want to start eating healthier foods instead of fast food or poor-quality, unhealthy foods, add pictures of healthy foods. *Example 3:* if you want to become more active in your life, place a picture of the activity or exercise you see yourself doing every day. *Example 4:* if you are unhappy in your job, place a picture of the job you want.

Whatever it is—remember to dream from your heart. My patients have used any and all of the tools below to create their personal collage:

- a large piece of cardboard or paper to serve as your blank canvas
- crayons, markers, paints, or pencils
- magazines (with pictures you like)
- scissors to cut out magazine pictures
- sticky tape or glue
- photographs of anything you want to add to your life

Once you have all your tools, have fun and create your new life vision board. Then look at your collage every day and see yourself as already living this new healthier dream life of yours.

Mindful Breathing

Mindful breathing involves using the breath to release stress, calm your nervous system, and focus on what you want. Such a shift enhances your health on many levels, and it is a tremendous step toward realizing your dreams.

Most of us are so busy that we rarely find the time to sit calmly and just breathe. Busy lifestyles create an overactive nervous system, so such breathing is essential for relaxation, contemplation, and focus. It is important to take even a few minutes here and there throughout the day to simply breathe, with the intention of returning to a place of calm and focus within yourself—regardless of what is happening around you. Try it. You may be astounded at the gains you will reap.

Here is a simple anti-stress breathing technique you can try right now. If possible, remove yourself from physically being in contact with the stressor.

1. Sit quietly in a comfortable position, and close your eyes.

2. Take one or two deep cleansing breaths, breathing in through your nose and out through your mouth at a slow, regular rate.

3. Blow out all the air in your lungs through your mouth.

4. Take a deep breath in through your nose, hold it for a second or two, and then slowly exhale all your air through your mouth. Repeat three more times.

After you have completed the fourth deep breath, sit quietly for a few minutes and see how you feel. Do you feel less stressed and more peaceful? You can do this exercise again if you would like to feel even calmer, and do it anytime you feel stressed or anxious.

Remind yourself to do a stress-reduction breathing exercise a few times a day. When you practice this type of breathing, you are guiding and teaching your nervous system to become familiar with how it feels to be in a relaxed state. After practicing for only a few weeks, you can just think about relaxing, and your nervous system will follow in kind. The relaxing biochemistry will follow, and then your body will usually relax immediately if it has become familiar with the practice. Historically, it has taken my patients two or three weeks of doing this exercise just a couple of times a day to gain an automatic response so that when they begin to think about relaxing, their body follows.

Meditation

I used to have a problem with the concept of meditation. Having tried it many times over the years with no formal direction or even a belief in the technique, it seemed to be a waste of time, and I saw my efforts as a failure. But one day I was given some basic practical instruction that focused and shifted my mind and energy in a different way, giving me my first positive meditation experience. Having been instructed to meditate on a specific intention rather than on a general concept, I suddenly was able to connect with a higher feeling and get some clear direction and insight. Wow, what a difference!

Being the practical person that I am, I now see a real purpose for meditation and do it regularly. I no longer have a vision of a yogi sitting on a carpet for hours, seemingly wasting time. What is the purpose of my version of meditation? While I don't meditate in the same way or for the same reasons that yogis do, my purpose is to get valuable information and insights that help me excel in this journey called life. You can do the same.

I decided to put the "art of meditation" to the test. I chose to write this book as a way of documenting what I was learning on my life journey, but I needed all the help I could get. Meditation gave it to me. Suddenly, out of thin air came the information and direction I needed—more than I could have imagined. I got answers to questions and solutions to difficulties I would never have thought possible. I met people who provided me with content I could add to my own ideas for my book. The help I got was so great, it was as if I had tapped into my own personal computer database—a database with some, if not all, of the answers I needed.

I now have a whole new appreciation for meditation. If I can learn to meditate, you can at least try it. Keep it simple and short to begin with. You don't need any fancy stuff. There's nothing you need to buy—no special mats or clothes to wear. All it takes is you and the universe, relaxed and comfortable.

Practical Meditation with a Purpose

Find a place and time when you can have uninterrupted quiet. You *can't* meditate well in a busy room with people watching TV or any other electronic disturbances (radios, CDs, or telephones). Turn off your cell phone. You need peace and quiet so you can become still and centered.

Sit in a comfortable position. Sitting cross-legged in the middle of a room is not comfortable for me, so I choose to put my body in a comfortable, supported position. I most often lie on the ground with a couple of my favorite pillows. When I travel and stay in a hotel, I pull all of those lovely white fluffy pillows off the bed and get all the extra pillows out of the closet. Then, I lie on a sea of soft fluffy pillows and get quiet. You might try relaxing in your favorite chair in a comfortable position. Be sure that your legs and arms are not crossed.

Being comfortable is the key. Make sure you do not have to go to the bathroom. Invariably, once your body begins to relax, the body begins to function more effectively, and without fail you end up wanting to go to the bathroom after only a few minutes into your meditation time.

Once you are comfortable, look at your life and focus your thinking on something you would like to change or gain more information about. Here are some examples.

- How can I find an exercise partner to help me be successful in my fitness program?

- I would like some help and guidance with my finances. (Be specific about what you want: I need help paying a bill. I need help accomplishing a little saving each month. I need help to stay within my budget.)
- I would like some direction and help with a relationship.
- I would like to focus on being able to incorporate the right diet into my life.

Keep it simple and be specific, and then see what comes up for you. Remember, this takes practice, so don't expect to become an expert overnight. Use the breathing exercise above to turn off your fast-paced nervous system, which may have been racing all day. When your breathing is smooth and rhythmic, let all negative thoughts that flow into your mind flow right out again. Know that you can't turn off your thoughts, so just let them go once you notice that you're dwelling on something negative. Be prepared for information to flow to you. You might want to have a pen and paper ready so that after your meditation, you can write down the information that comes to you.

The Use of Sound in Meditation

"Om" and "Ah" are two ancient sounds used for meditation. These sounds are from a sacred syllable chanted in Hindu and Buddhist prayers and mantras, and are said to date back as far as 624 BCE. They are connected with creation and joy and are known to encourage information to surface in your conscious mind.

Using sound for meditation is a personal choice. Some people say sound helps; some say it doesn't. I use both the "Om" and "Ah" sounds. I don't decide to use a sound or not—if I start, that's fine, if not, I meditate quietly. Whatever happens at each meditation session is right for you. I have found that using one of these sounds encourages me to focus on creating my own sound and vibration, which brings an experience of clarity and creation.

Meditation and Visualization with the Chakras

The ancient Ayurvedic Hindu tradition, which has successfully taught the art of healing and prolonging life, tells us about chakras (see chakra chart, page 223). The chakras are the seven energy centers, running from the base of the spine to the top of our head, each connected to a major organ.

For your creative meditation exercise, you can begin with an energy-cleansing process to remove negativity and to provide a clear channel for energizing thoughts to enter your consciousness. Visualize energy flowing from the base of your spine and all the way up to the top of your head, then flowing out through the top of your head into the universe. The energy is drawn up from the earth through your first—or root—chakra (at the base of your spine), up along your spine, and out of your head through the seventh—or crown—chakra.

Does this information all sound a little "out there" to you? It sure did to me—for the longest time. Please consider trying it anyway. At worst you might get really relaxed and go to sleep. At best you could get clear direction and answers to the questions you have. At least try meditation once or twice before dismissing this practice.

Meditation/Visualization Chakra Chart

	Crown	Connected with the pineal gland in the brain
	Third Eye	Connected with the pituitary gland in the brain
	Throat	Connected with the thyroid gland in the neck
	Heart	Connected with the thymus gland and heart in the chest
	Solar Plexus	Connected with the liver and adrenal glands in the abdomen
	Sacral	Connected with the testes and ovaries in the pelvic area. This is the area of the body where procreation occurs
	Root	Connected with the uterus and prostate gland

Guided Imagery

As part of your meditation, you can also try a technique called *guided imagery*. It can be especially helpful if you find yourself in a situation for which you can find no cause, such as:

- an inability to experience good health
- chronic illness
- recurring depression
- chronic anxiety
- an inability to heal

I have found guided imagery to be immensely valuable. For example, for many years I had questions about my spiritual health and how it affected my work and my life, and it wasn't until I practiced guided imagery that I finally found answers to many of these questions.

Guided imagery is a form of focused relaxation combined with guided inner exploration. It has been documented to improve a person's physical and emotional well-being, and is used to facilitate healing of many illnesses. A very strong body of research is showing us that a high percentage of common medical conditions or problems respond positively to this gentle therapy.

I believe that everyone can benefit from guided imagery whether or not a health problem exists. The intent of guided imagery is to make connections between the body, emotions, and mind by using your thoughts and any associated images that encourage relaxation and desired changes in attitude. This usually produces beneficial changes in behavior.

My first experience of guided imagery was facilitated by a psychologist who is experienced in the technique. While I was aware that research showed that this mode of healing was generating good results, I knew little about the actual practice of it. So, at that time, I did not recommend it to my patients; our appointments were usually so short that I was not able to ask all the questions necessary to understand the state of their psychological and spiritual health. However, after studying guided imagery in my integrative-medicine fellowship, and experiencing sessions myself, I now have a full appreciation of what it is and the profound role it can play in the healing process. I now highly recommend guided imagery to my patients who would benefit from it.

Guided imagery supports whole health and healing. It accesses our subconscious, those inner realms where we hold memories of the past in the form of feelings and mental images, which, if negative or blocked, can cause thinking patterns that can obstruct our health. Guided imagery can access much of this stored material and guide the mind to understand the details of an event or occurrence in a way that releases or transmutes any negative associations and replaces these with positive, healing ones.

Guided imagery can be performed with a trained therapist or practitioner. You may also have success using a guided imagery audio CD or DVD. While there are many of these on the market today, I highly recommend you choose one that has been developed by a trained guided-imagery practitioner. These providers are qualified to guide you in the best possible way. Here are some recommendations that my patients and I have reviewed that have had excellent results:

- Emmett Miller, M.D., **www.drmiller.com**
- Health Journeys, Belleruth Naparstek, LISW, **www.healthjourneys.com**
- Andrew Weil, M.D., and Martin Rossman, M.D., CD: *Self-Healing with Guided Imagery,* available from **www.amazon.com**
- Andrew Weil, M.D., and Jon Kabat-Zinn, Ph.D., CD: *Meditation for Optimum Health,* available from **www.amazon.com**

Gratitude

An important element in any change process is *gratitude*. Thank your past life and now state that you deserve to move on to a healthier new life. Become grateful for all you have and all that you are going to have. For example, people with chronic illness can see themselves making healthier changes and being grateful for internal natural healing. I recommend that you find an object precious to you, something you can keep with you at all times, into which you can symbolically direct your gratitude. My favorite items for this are a stone I received during the opening ceremony of my integrative-medicine program; and a deep blue, glasslike stone resembling a sapphire given to me by a patient. Both have a very special attraction for me. Find an object that attracts you and which holds some special significance. You can then direct the strength of your intention and the gratitude you feel for your new life into this object. When you touch it, the feel of the object will be a reminder of the gratitude you feel for your new behaviors and life you are already living. As you grow with this object, it will become even more valuable as time passes.

A Day with God (Whoever/Whatever "God" Is to You)

Not everyone believes in the same god or even recognizes that God exists. Some people have no concept of what God is, yet they still have a concept of some higher power. I think it really doesn't matter if you believe in God or not; this exercise can still be valuable to you. If the term "God" interferes with your reading, please substitute any other term you would like.

Here, my entire focus is on positive thoughts. God and the concept of God reside in Love and Light, both positive concepts. I believe we are all here in service to some larger picture, and as part of that, we have an inherent need to create in our areas of interest. Coming to restful awareness and gaining inner direction from this source can be of exceptional value. Yet, if we don't give ourselves time to stop for one minute and listen to this inner voice or direction from our higher source, we can wander off the path we were born to walk. This method of connecting with a higher spirit of good or God is a form of meditation we can use to listen for that voice.

A Connecting Day with God

Welcome to your day with God. Some of us have never realized our gift or purpose in life. Very few of us take the time to ask for God's help or to listen to the guidance being given us. If you're a person who does not live your life to the fullest, and are not loving what you do and doing what you love, it may be especially important that you consider having "A Connecting Day with God."

Think of it as a day of connecting to an endless river of love and gentle guidance.

So who can benefit from a day with God or a higher spirit? The simple answer to this question is that every one of us needs time to connect in this way. Connecting on a regular basis offers us clear direction for identifying or developing our gifts of creativity and intentionality. Taking a focused day to be with God or your higher spirit so as to gain vision and direction for your life is one of the best things you can do for yourself and the people who share your life. It can be a magical day. The experience you can gain from this time is beyond words. It changes you and brings Love. You will get answers if you ask your questions. We all have equal access to the same Love. This is not going to be difficult at all. In fact, this will be a very exciting day for you.

Caution: Your experience may vary each time you take the time to connect with God. Have no expectations of what will happen. Enter the experience with an open mind and an open heart. See this time as if you are drifting on a calm, open sea, where God is guiding you. It may not turn out to be what you expected, but seek

out the underlying gift of the experience, even if you feel disappointed or didn't "get"
what you wanted. Some times will be more precious than others, but they are all
valuable. The important thing is to make it a practice to set aside time for connecting
with God and your higher spirit.

Preparing for Your Day with God:
Make a commitment to yourself and to your higher spirit, or God, to spend a
day together. Set the date for your day with God. Consider this your special day,
but keep it to yourself (for now). Mark it on your calendar and plan for that
date. Plan your day with God at least two weeks ahead of time.

Choose the place where you will spend your day with God, somewhere
comfortable and where you feel safe. Some examples of places to spend the day are:

- a beach or somewhere near water
- a secluded area in a park
- a scenic area where you have a beautiful view
- a scenic, secluded area where you can park your car for the day
- at home, if no one else will be around for the whole day
- a home rented or borrowed or where you can house-sit for the day
- a hotel room, with a beautiful view (hang the "Do not Disturb"
  sign outside)
- a quiet church

Your busy life has many technological ties that should be avoided during your
day with God. Do your best to disconnect yourself, it's just you and God, so:

- Turn off your cell phone and/or pager.
- Turn off the ringer on landline phones.
- Turn off the volume on your answering machine.
- Take no watches or clocks.
- Turn off the radio or television.
- Turn off the computer or e-mail.
- Make sure no one else is present.

Choose a specific amount of time to spend with God. See if you can
designate a large chunk of time. If you can, plan to spend an entire day. To be
safe, overestimate the time you need. You do not want to be feeling a need to
leave or rush back for any obligation whatsoever.

Write a checklist of things you will need for your day with God. Then, a week before, begin gathering them together.

Nutritional Needs: Plan your nutritional needs for the entire day. Prepare all your food and water ahead of time so you do not need to spend time preparing anything on your day off. Include:

- plenty of pure, fresh water
- naturally healthy, whole foods with no preservatives or additives
- a simple treat, like a favorite cookie or candy from childhood

Clothing: Consider the temperature of the space you will be in. Plan to bring comfortable warm and cool clothing you can layer if necessary: the old sweatpants and sweatshirt you love so much, your favorite T-shirt with the hole in it, that old cotton dress you have worn 50 times but is just so special you cannot give it away, that sweater in your closet you just do not want to throw away because it is your favorite—if you want to wear it, wear it. On the other hand, a piece of new clothing you have just bought and want to wear for this special occasion would also be perfect—a new sweater, or a comfortable pair of pants. Wear what you feel good in.

Seating: Plan to have something comfortable to sit on. Consider a blanket if you will be sitting outside, or if you think it could be cold.

Money: The cost of the day should be minimal, if anything. Bring only the amount of money you will need for the day.

Medications: bring any medication you will need during the day.

Supplies: below are suggestions for supplies you might want to bring with you:

- blank paper, pencil, pen, and a new pack of crayons so you can write down or draw out your thoughts as new insights appear during your day (no cassette recorder or recording devices)
- facial tissues
- a candle and matches if you like
- anything else to help you be as comfortable and focused as possible

Communication and Responsibilities: Inform only the people who really need to know that you are taking the day off and will not be available for the designated amount of time. Designate a contact person whom you can reach should you need to, such as a friend, spouse, minister, or other support person with whom you feel comfortable. Make arrangements for any necessary activities to continue in your absence.

Experience Your Day with God

The day has arrived. Today is your day with God. Waking up and getting started is part of this special day.

If possible, wake before daylight so you can watch the day begin. Dawn can be a magical time. Try to wake up on your own, without an alarm clock. Be present in thought to this special day as soon as you open your eyes. Realize that today is your day with God. Get out of bed when you feel you are ready.

Consider a morning prayer or meditation for the day. Take care of the daily hygiene routine for your body. If you had planned to drink and eat now, do so while taking time to thank God for this nourishment. Check to be sure you do not forget anything before you proceed to your destination, whether at home or away.

Think of your day as having no schedule. You are just going to be with yourself and God. When you arrive at your special place, get comfortable and warm. Have all your writing and drawing materials around you.

You may want to light a candle. This is to be a day of relaxation and vision. Most of the time, stress can stop you from seeing what you're supposed to see in your life, so take some deep breaths to help you relax. Better yet, try the wonderful breathing technique from earlier in the chapter.

Once you have done this relaxation breathing, you will be in a very comfortable state of mind. Allow your day to unfold as it comes. If you feel you are not connected, ask why. You will know when you need to take a break for food, but be sure not to overeat. If you don't feel like eating, that's okay. If you have ideas coming to you and need to write them down or draw them, do so. Go with whatever comes to you. Any thoughts that come to mind should be the ones you follow. Have a fun, magical, happy experience!

As your day with God—or whatever God is to you—comes to a close, take some time to write down your experience, any insights you gained, and how you are going to use the information you learned. For the next few nights, pay attention to what comes to you. Write down your dreams and thoughts.

Continue to be connected with God or whomever you believe your creator to be, so the journey you have chosen will be a happy and productive one.

Chapter Seventeen

PLANNING AND SUPPORTING YOUR NUTRITIONAL CHANGE

Factors that will support you in making the desired nutritional changes include:

- making changes in a mindful and organized manner
- avoiding to make too many changes at one time
- education—knowing why you need to change your diet
- knowing how to accomplish nutritional changes related to taste

Let's now look in more detail at this final point.

The Sense of Taste and Nutritional Change

Taste is one of our most powerful senses, providing a direct chemical connection between the outside world and our nervous system. Many of us were taught that there are four basic tastes: salt, sour, bitter, and sweet. However, there are two more: umami, which is described as a sort of robust or "meaty" taste, and fat, which researchers are beginning to discover has a taste of its own, although it hasn't yet been well described. Each taste category produces its own chemical response on the tongue, and is delivered to the brain via our taste receptor cells, called papillae. These papillae are found on the surface of the tongue and in the olfactory (smell) system. A host of chemical changes occur in this process, and the different tastes result from the brain receiving different signals from the various foods.

Our taste system has a direct connection to the brain, and alters brain chemistry. When a food is eaten frequently, the brain and nervous system get used to a certain level of taste, because of the chemistry that taste experience produces. When a taste experience changes very quickly, the nervous system responds by producing a different chemical experience. It can be difficult for the nervous system to adapt to sudden taste changes. This is why it's best to make changes slowly—the slower, the better.

When you make taste changes, give your nervous system time to adjust to the new chemistry that is produced, or the shock on the nervous system will insist that you go back to the old taste. Bottom line: make changes to your diet slowly.

A Patient's Story: Janet

When Janet first came to see me, she was taking eight medications every day. She had chronic body pain, some joint pain, deep fatigue, migraines, and diarrhea 12 to 14 times a day. Her cholesterol was also dangerously high. During the past few years, she had seen many doctors and undergone extensive testing to find a diagnosis, yet no one could provide a definitive reason for her condition. Eventually, she was given a diagnosis of suspected fibromyalgia with arthritic tendencies and chronic diarrhea. She was prescribed eight different drugs, and even though she hated taking any drugs at all, found that she needed them just to function each day.

Janet's gastroenterologist had worked with me on several other cases and suggested that Janet see me. He thought I could help with her cholesterol problem as well as her diet, to determine whether making some dietary changes would reduce or relieve her chronic illnesses. Believing she had nothing to lose, Janet made an appointment with me.

I did a full physical and an extensive medical history, plus a full blood-chemistry evaluation, and recommended an Apo E gene test. Her total cholesterol was 304, her LDL was 214, and her Apo E genotype was 4/4.

I asked Janet to begin keeping a diet log. This revealed that she often fasted for an unhealthy 12 to 16 hours at a time, and that the foods she did eat were extremely inflammatory—the standard American diet, or SAD, loaded with animal fat, trans fat, and too many simple carbohydrates. Janet said she loved eating "good, hearty, American food," but with an Apo E of 4/4, which cannot tolerate a high-fat diet or long periods of time without adequate food, it was producing the high levels of inflammation in her body that were responsible for her debilitating symptoms.

We discussed all the findings and together developed a plan so Janet could begin slowly, making dietary changes. Despite its dangers, she loved her current diet and had been eating it for years, so it was best she make small changes each week. This way, her system would not be shocked by the changes, and her taste system would adjust slowly so she would be more likely to continue with the new plan designed around her Apo E 4/4.

Janet's dietary changes went very well from the start. After just two weeks, her diarrhea decreased from 12 to 6 times daily; after four weeks, it was cut in half again. Her migraines had decreased, and her chronic pain was reduced to only three areas in her body instead of all over. She was thrilled with such rapid results—but they were only the beginning.

Once she underwent cardiovascular screening and was cleared to begin an exercise program, Janet started a low-intensity aerobic-exercise program. She soon felt so good, she began working out at a higher intensity, but immediately her pain level increased. She couldn't understand why this should happen when she had been improving so well.

I explained that when we exercise for a long time or at high intensity, we burn up fat stores—long-term fuel—in the body, which are built over time from the foods we eat. Janet's body was still storing old inflammatory fuel from her former poor eating habits, so when she bumped up her exercise intensity, those inflammatory fats were released from storage, causing her pain to return as they circulated through her body. I told her that when she had cleared these poor-quality fat stores from her body, she would no longer feel the inflammatory response when she performed higher-intensity exercise. I recommended that she drop her exercise intensity to the original levels prescribed for her and begin taking a ginger supplement, which would help reduce inflammation. Once again, Janet felt much better.

Even though she still had a long way to go, Janet was sufficiently motivated by her positive results to continue slowly making dietary changes, and exercising at the appropriate levels for her. She now understood that it just takes time, and was happy that she had finally found a way back to health.

Personal Nutritional Change Process

There are myriad ways to implement changes in your usual routine. In an earlier chapter, we looked at several tools for change that you might want to draw on at this point. Perhaps you already have a favored technique that works well for you. If so, this is the best way for you to make a change in your diet. If not, take a minute and think back to a time when you made a lasting change in some area of your life. Think about how you accomplished that change. If you have never been able to sustain a change over a reasonable period, speak to others who have. When you have some ideas, you may want to fill out your own Nutritional Change Plan Form, shown on the next page. Remember, this is for you, not for anyone else. No one does things quite like you, so stay focused on you. Family and friends love to give advice, and while you may want to carefully review their advice, accept only what feels right to you, and let the rest go. The only person who can make the right change and choice for you—is you.

17.1 Sample Nutritional Change Plan Form						
	Old Behavior	New Behavior	Food Change	Carbo-hydrates	Fat	Protein
Week 1 Breakfast	2 cups of coffee with 2 spoons of sugar and cream	2 cups of coffee with 1 spoon of sugar and milk	Gradual changes of sugar & cream	Decreased (sugar)	Decreased	No Change

17.2 Nutritional Change Plan Form					
	Old Behavior	New Behavior	Food Change	Carbo-hydrates	Fat	Protein
Week 1 Breakfast						
Week 2 Breakfast						
Week 3 Morning Snack						
Week 4 Morning Snack						
Week 5 Lunch						
Week 6 Lunch						
Week 7 Afternoon Snack						
Week 8 Afternoon Snack						
Week 9 Dinner						
Week 10 Dinner						
Week 11 Evening Snack						
Week 12 Evening Snack						

Making Nutritional Changes

The following recommendations will help you more successfully implement nutritional changes:

- Focus on what you want, such as a healthier diet or more energy.

- Start with "The Big Progressive Cleanout" of kitchen cabinets, the pantry, and the refrigerator. Clear out all those inflammatory and disease-causing foods you have been eating, especially the processed ones.

- Fill out a Personalized Nutritional Change Plan Form (see page 235).

- Look up your Suggested Menus by Genotype and Caloric Level beginning on page 264.

- Make a list of all the healthy foods you are going to eat in the future.

- See the Food Exchange List (pages 256–260) for protein choices, carbohydrates, starches, fruits and vegetables, and good fats.

- Replenish your kitchen with a supply of healthier foods.

- As you begin to incorporate new foods into your diet, go slowly— see the following section on how to make changes week by week.

- Keep a log of your current daily food intake.

My advice is to get help from an Integrative Medicine practitioner trained in nutrition, exercise, stress reduction, and behavioral change, or some other support person.

Supporting Nutritional Changes

When making nutritional changes, most people get excited and want to make changes rapidly. Don't. If your personality is fast and furious, take a deep breath and ask yourself to slow down so you can make this change last a lifetime. Remember, it is best to make changes slowly. As noted above, the human body does not like hasty changes—especially with respect to nutrition and food. Your body is currently used to one level of taste, and it can become physically shocked with too rapid a change, just like it can be shocked with a big psychological change. It also needs time to adapt to any emotional changes that may go along with the new diet.

You need to give your body time to get used to the changes. So go slowly and gently.

For example, if your body is accustomed to consuming four sodas every day, and you suddenly don't drink those sodas, the body will respond to the subsequent chemistry change immediately. Blood-glucose, insulin, and cortisol levels all shift, as do the nervous system and blood vessels, from the drop in the caffeine, sugar, and fluid. To suddenly stop drinking sodas can seem like a good thing to do, but the big shift it causes in body chemistry can generate a negative reaction for the body. It is much better to make changes over a period of time. I would suggest moving, week by week, from four sodas a day to three, then two, then one; and in the meantime, try other drinks in their place. This is the kinder way of doing things.

An important point about this change process can be to understand why you drank four sodas a day in the first place. Many people love soda. It is a fun drink, but it is not a good beverage for a healthy body. So identify the reason why you were drinking it in the first place. Was it because soda was all that was available, or was it purchased by the person in your family who does the grocery shopping? Was it because you had access to free sodas at work, or do you just love the bubbles in soda? For me, I can tell you it's the bubbles—I love drinks with bubbles in them. If sodas weren't so detrimental to my health, I would drink it a lot more. However, I switched to soda water with a little fresh-squeezed lime or lemon juice—this still gives me the bubbles plus some extra vitamin C. Take the time to understand what you eat and drink, and why. It will help you sustain your changes.

Making Nutritional Change

You can start with any meal in the day. However, most people do best if they start with breakfast and slowly work the diet change into other meals throughout the day.

Separate your food intake into six meals. This alone is a lot of change to accomplish all at once, but it's how I have seen change work most effectively with my patients:

Meal 1 Breakfast
Meal 2 Morning snack
Meal 3 Lunch
Meal 4 Afternoon snack
Meal 5 Dinner
Meal 6 Evening snack

Week 1: Make a change in your breakfast meals only. Stop skipping breakfast (if you did). Identify one to two new breakfast meals from your Perfect Gene Diet suggested meal plan and add them to your food intake. Begin eating a correct serving size for breakfast. Possibly, try a new cereal or milk. Try soy, almond, or rice milk rather than dairy.
Reading: Review information on food safety and how to read a food label, at **www.vm.cfsan.fda.gov/~dms/foodlab.html** (this information is constantly being updated).
Journal: Log changes in your Journal.

Week 2: Continue changing the breakfast foods by trying another cereal, fruit, milk, or soymilk.
Reading: Begin to practice reading a food label in the store while you are shopping.
Journal: Log changes in your Journal.

Week 3: Continue with these changes to breakfast, and add one or two morning snacks from your Suggested Diets by genotype and caloric level (see pages 264–332 Begin eating a small morning snack from your suggested menus. This may be a new behavior for you—keep to the recommended serving sizes in your menu. Skipping a morning snack can reduce important calories that your body needs.
Journal: Log changes in your Journal.

Week 4: Continue changing the morning snack by adding one or two additional morning snacks from your suggested menus. Try another morning snack from your menu plan. Consider snacks that taste good and are convenient to prepare and eat in your work setting. Stay with recommended serving sizes.
Reading: Review the benefits of green tea (see page 174), and consider the value of flowers in your day. Next time you are doing your shopping, stop and smell the flowers. Most supermarkets have a flower section.
Journal: Log changes in your Journal.

Week 5: Focus on lunch by adding one or two changes from your lunch food suggestions. Add to last week's successes by making another change to your diet. Try a fruit you have never tried before. Pick from your suggested menus.
Reading: Review sections on smart foods, sodium, and micronutrients (see pages 181–186).
Journal: Log changes in your Journal.

Week 6: Continue changing your lunch intake by adding one or two replacement foods from your suggested menus. For example, instead of white bread choose a whole-grain bread.
Reading: Review section on nutrients (see page 181).
Journal: Log changes in your Journal.

Week 7: Focus on afternoon snacks by adding one or two items from your suggested menus. Consider snacks that taste good and are convenient for your lifestyle. If you are a businessperson and are often in long meetings, it is reasonable to request afternoon refreshments. You will be surprised by how most people welcome the snack break. Make sure you order healthy snacks that will benefit your meeting by providing high-quality foods. Good nutrition makes for good thinking.
Reading: Review section on fats (see page 109). Continue and refine the content of your diet by adding "good fats" into your diet. Try a different fat you have never tried before from your suggested menus.
Journal: Log changes in your Journal.

Week 8: Continue changes by adding one or two different afternoon snacks from your suggested menus. Consider snacks that taste good and are convenient. Continue to refine the content of your diet. Try a protein you have never tried before. Pick from your suggested menus.
Reading: Review section on protein (see page 87).
Journal: Log changes in your Journal.

Week 9: Focus on dinner by adding one or two dinner foods from your suggested menus to your evening meal.
Reading: Review Chapter 14 "Shopping and Dining Tips for Health." Read the section on water (see page 169). Continue to refine the content of your diet. Add improved fluids to your diet. Review the amount of fluids you are drinking and your water source. Evaluate the caffeine content of your diet. Review your alcohol intake—pros, cons. Different teas—pros, cons.
Journal: Log changes in your Journal.

Week 10: Continue changing the dinner meal by adding one or two more dinner foods from your suggested menus. Begin by making a change of a food type. If you have been used to eating excess portions, decrease portion sizes to those recommended. If you are eating in a restaurant, try to order the foods you have on your suggested menu plan. Example: If you want to eat fresh fish, ask for it to be grilled or broiled with olive oil.

Reading: Review section on restaurants (see page 191). Also consider reading the section on glycemic load and glycemic index (see page 84).

Journal: Log changes in your Journal.

Week 11: Continue changing dinner by cutting back on the amount you eat, adding one or two evening snack foods from your suggested menus.

Grocery-store assignment: Ask your supermarket if they sell organic or genetically modified foods. If they don't sell organic, ask them to. They won't until enough people—like you—request this. Similarly, if they sell genetically modified foods, express your concern. Look at the convenience foods, such as frozen dinners, natural packaged food, organic convenience foods, and preservative-free foods. Check your recommended diet plan to see whether these foods are right for you.

Journal: Log changes in your Journal.

Week 12: Focus on evening snack by adding snack foods from your suggested menus. Most of us feel that the evening snack is a meal to skip. However, these calories and nutrients are important to carry you through the night, so be sure not to skip your evening snack (but eat at least 1 hour before you go to bed).

Add to last week's successes by making another change: identify three restaurants that will make changes for you with respect to a specific menu item. Have the sauce on the side. With a salad, get the dressing on the side. Identify a restaurant that serves fresh fish and vegetables. Identify restaurants willing to share and discuss food ingredients on the menu, such as the fats they use in the preparation of food. Find restaurants that have a wide selection on the menu.

Now that you have really begun to make changes, let's focus on *when* you eat. Adjust the time when you eat so you are able to get enough food in at the right time.

Reading: Review section on water (see page 169).

Journal: Log changes in your Journal.

Weeks 13–20: Continue changing by adding new foods to all meals. Make changes with meals eaten in restaurants and take-out foods.

Journal: Log changes in your Journal.

Keep in mind that eating needs to fit in with your lifestyle. Consider what to eat in the following situations:

- Getting up in the morning
- During commute time
- Arriving at work or school
- Morning workload (Do you need to make time to eat during the morning?)
- Morning breaks
- Lunchtime (How convenient is preparing, buying, or bringing your lunch?)
- Afternoon workload
- Return commute time
- Evening

Diet Change Plan Summary

The following list summarizes the things to include in your plans for making dietary changes:

- Read about protein foods and what you can consider for your Apo E genotype.
- Learn about carbohydrate foods you can consider for your Apo E genotype.
- Learn about the right amount and type of fat you can eat for your Apo E genotype.
- Focus on your own dietary recommendations, suggested menus by genotype and caloric level, and learn how to transition to the new food recommendations.
- Understand your diet and why it has been prescribed. This is important, so review the details for your Apo E genotype.
- See individual dietary guidelines.
- Begin nutritional changes by slowly adding in new items to your current eating plan—focusing on making changes to breakfast during the first few weeks.
- Then while continuing the changes made to breakfast, add a morning snack for about 1–2 weeks, and so on.
- Continue your dietary changes.
- Focus on making changes to your lunch for 1–2 weeks.

- Focus on making changes to your afternoon tea/snack for 1–2 weeks.
- Focus on making changes to your dinner for 1–2 weeks.
- Focus on making changes to your evening snack for 1–2 weeks.

Go slowly! Enjoy experimenting with your new foods and recipes. This way you will learn how to eat well for life. To be able to help you make these changes, I encourage you to enlist the aid of a partner or a support person for this process. I have added a support person checklist and process—see support-person section (see page 77).

Chapter Eighteen

STEPS TO DETERMINING YOUR DIET BASED ON THE APO E GENE

Now that you have a bag of tools to support you in making the changes you want to make, let's look at the specifics for determining your recommended nutritional plan. We will discuss the diet in detail. Remember, this is *based on a comprehensive system of caloric calculation and includes nutritional recommendations based on a person's Apo E genotype. This means that this chapter is only of direct relevance to you when you have identified your Apo E genotype.* The recommendations are part of a comprehensive prevention program, and only you and your medical practitioner can properly evaluate how they apply to you.

Caution: Do not use any of these nutritional recommendations unless you know your Apo E genotype. Only then will you know what plan is right for you. Example: If you are an Apo E 2/3 and you follow an Apo E 4/3 diet, this can cause imbalance within your body. If this is taken to an extreme and you eat the wrong diet for a long period of time, it can lead to diseases and illness.

The Apo E Gene-Supportive Environment—Evaluation Levels

In order to gain an optimal gene-supportive environment for an individual Apo E genotype, these evaluation levels are recommended in addition to actually testing for your Apo E genotype.

Basic Evaluation (Level 1)
- height
- weight
- hydration status
- BMI
- individual daily caloric requirements
- body composition: lean mass and fat mass

Health Status Evaluation (Level 2)
- Current health status 1–10
  (1 = high levels of disease; 10 = free of disease)
- Ambulatory level status 1–10
  (1 = bedridden; 10 = no walking limitations)
- Respiratory status 1–10
  (1 = poor respiration status;
  10 = excellent respiration status)
- Vascular/circulatory status 1–10
  (1 = poor vascular status; 10 = excellent vascular status)
- Psychological status 1–10
  (1 = poor psychological status;
  10 = excellent psychological status)
- Family history 1–10
  (1 = extensive family history of disease;
  10 = no current family history of disease)

Advanced Evaluation (Level 3)
- Complete cholesterol screening panel—advanced cholesterol subfraction Apo B particle
- homocysteine level, including an MTHFR gene evaluation TSH, thyroid evaluation
- inflammatory markers—fibrinogen, CRP, Lp-PLA2
- insulin level, fasting glucose, HA1c

A Diet Plan That's Right for You, Based on Your Apo E Gene

Once you know your Apo E genotype, there are three steps to determining the diet plan that's right for you.

- Step 1: determine the calories required for daily activities.
- Step 2: determine your body composition.
- Step 3: identify the Perfect Gene Diet nutritional recommendations for your genotype.

Let's look at these in greater detail.

Step 1: Determine the Calories Required for Daily Activities

I introduced calories in Chapter 3, but now we get into the specific calculations, which are based on two components:

- The calories your body requires to sustain your typical functions— such as digesting food, maintaining your circulation, breathing, plus those required by your general daily level of activity.
- The additional calories required for an exercise program or athletic activity—calories used over and above those of your normal activities, such as 30 minutes of running, 40 minutes of walking, or 60 minutes of biking.

Below are two methods of determining approximately how much energy— how many calories—your body needs from food each day. The first is a manual method that illustrates the principles behind the calculations. The second is the much more practical automated way it is usually done.

Manual Calculation

This method requires no equipment. You simply add together the two caloric requirements mentioned above. This provides you with the approximate number of calories your body requires each day, based on your height and weight as shown in the table below. Keep in mind these are approximate calorie counts.

Male Daily Baseline Calorie Requirements

To compute your baseline number of calories, use this formula:

66 + (6.2 x weight in pounds) + (12.7 x height in inches) - (6.8 x age in years)

For example, a 35-year-old, 5'10" (70"), 150-lb. man yields:

66 + (6.2 x 150) + (12.7 x 70) - (6.8 x 35) = 1,647 kcals per day

Female Daily Baseline Calorie Requirements

To compute your baseline number of calories, use this formula:

655 + (4.35 x weight in pounds) + (4.7 x height in inches) - (4.7 x age in years)

For example, a 35-year-old, 5'6" (66"), 120-lb. woman yields:

655 + (4.35 x 120) + (4.7 x 66) - (4.7 x 35) = 1,323 kcals per day

Additional Daily Calorie Requirements Based on Activity

Now, to allow for the additional calories needed for your daily activities, choose the level below that most closely fits. Then multiply the factor associated with it times the calories you computed above.

Sedentary—little or no exercise: 1.2

Light exercise/sports 1–3 days per week: 1.4

Moderate exercise/sports 3–5 days per week: 1.6

Heavy exercise/sports 6–7 days per week: 1.7

Very heavy exercise/sports & physical job or twice-a-day training: 1.9

For example, the 120-lb. woman above, who is moderately active, needs: 1,323 x 1.6 = 2,116 kcals

Bio-Impedance Test

This is one of the most practical methods of determining caloric needs, but it requires taking a bio-impedance test in a clinical setting. The instrument measures your basal metabolic rate, giving you your daily caloric requirements immediately.

What is your basal metabolic rate (BMR)? Your BMR is the amount of energy you require to maintain basic bodily functions. Approximately three-quarters of the body's energy is needed to support the metabolic cellular function, which includes activities such as that of the cardiopulmonary systems and maintaining body temperature. The rest is the usual amount needed for discretionary movement and thinking.

A bio-impedance test (see page 248) is not only one of the most practical and reproducible methods of determining your daily caloric requirement, it also evaluates your body composition—the second important factor in determining the right diet plan for you.

Step 2: Determine Your Body Composition— the Bathroom Scale and Beyond

Everybody is familiar with the most common of human body surveying tools— the bathroom scale. Few, however, realize that daily "scale jumping" can be hazardous to your health! You jump on the scale and say, "Yes! I lost five pounds yesterday! I am healthier today." This assumption may be true, but most likely it is not. Whether a weight loss is healthy or not depends on what kind of body component you lost: fat, muscle, or water. A bathroom scale detects only your total body weight, and for this reason is a very poor health-evaluation tool.

Body Mass Index

Your *body mass index (BMI, not to be confused with BMR above)* is a measure of your body mass related to your height and weight—specifically your weight (in kilograms) divided by your height (in meters) squared. The BMI is a reliable indicator of total body mass, which can help in identifying health risks. The score applies to both men and women. There are limitations to this index in that:

- It may overestimate body mass in athletes and others who have a muscular build.

- It may underestimate body mass in older people and others who have lost excess muscle mass.

The BMI classifications are:
- underweight = less than 18.5
- normal weight = 18.5–24.9
- overweight = 25–29.9
- obese = 30 or more

Body Composition

We've seen that the bathroom scale gives a very gross idea of your body composition, telling only how many pounds you weigh. Your body-mass index gives a more refined picture of your body composition. Determining caloric needs with a body-composition measurement using a bio-impedance meter gives the most accurate assessment of body composition. It's a simple, painless, noninvasive test that many medical providers and exercise physiologists offer.

A body's composition can be defined as lean mass, fat mass, and fluids where:

- lean mass = muscles, bones, tendons, ligaments, skin, etc.

- fat mass = the body's stored fat

- fluids = water, blood, and a host of other fluids like saliva, bile, and cerebrospinal fluid

Two people who weigh 150 lbs. may have a completely different body makeup. One might have too much fat, and the other could have more muscle and almost no fat. If you eat a balanced diet for your genotype and exercise regularly, chances are you have a normal body composition. If you don't eat a gene supportive-diet, chances are you will have an unhealthy body composition.

The body-composition test is a comprehensive way of assessing health, as it allows us to see the body mass by category. Only when you know the percentage of lean mass, fat mass, and fluids can you determine whether or not you have the correct body composition.

Bio-Impedance—Body-Composition Test

A body-composition test works on the theory that muscles contain more water than fat. A great little device called a bio-impedance body-composition testing machine measures how much water you have in your body, based on the bioelectrical impedance of your tissues—fat and muscle conduct an electric current differently, depending on their water content. By using this machine you can find out the fat mass, lean mass, and water content of your body and thereby determine the ideal calorie intake for you.

Finding Out If Your Body Composition Is Gene Supportive

Here we use BMI and other data, along with your body composition (measured by your provider or at a fitness center), to determine how your body is reflecting the gene supportiveness or unsupportiveness of your environment.

Men should have no more than 16 percent body fat. Women should have no more than 22 percent body fat. A high percentage of body fat indicates you are overfeeding your body for the amount of exercise you are getting. This promotes disease.

Exercise: Finding Your Ideal Body Composition

1. Find and record your body mass index _____
   (from Table 18.2 Body Mass Index, pages 250–251)

2. Is your BMI within the normal range of 18.5–24.9? ___Yes ___No
   If no, is it higher or lower? ____Higher ____Lower

3. Find and record your lean mass range _____
   (from Table 18.1 Lean Mass Recommendation for Males and Females).

4. Determine your current lean mass percentage _____
   (from a body-composition test by your medical provider or
   exercise physiologist).

5. Is your lean mass percentage within the range in step 3?
   _____Yes   _____No
   If no, is it higher or lower?   _____Higher   _____Lower

6. Record your fat mass percentage goal _____
   (Men: 16% or less; Women: 22% or less).

7. Determine your current fat percentage: _____
   (from a body-composition test by your medical provider or
   exercise physiologist).

8. Is your lean mass percentage under the goal in step 6?
   _____Yes   _____No.

This information is valuable in developing your personalized program for minimizing your risk of disease.

18.1 Lean Mass Recommendation for Males and Females[a]

Pounds of Lean Body Mass for Men

5'5"	5'6"	5'7"	5'8"	5'9"	5'10"	5'11"	6'0"	6'1"	6'2"	6'3"
108–120	110–125	112–129	118–132	122–137	127–145	133–153	137–163	140–168	143–176	145–183

Pounds of Lean Body Mass for Women

5'0"	5'1"	5'2"	5'3"	5'4"	5'5"	5'6"	5'7"	5'8"	5'9"	5'10"
70–86	73–89	75–91	78–93	81–96	83–99	86–102	95–105	93–109	95–112	98–119

Recommended Fat Percentage for Males and Females

Male	Less than 16% body fat
Female	Less than 22% body fat

Recommended BMI for Males and Females

Male	BMI less than 25
Female	BMI less than 25

a. Based on research by Covert Bailey.

18.2 Body Mass Index (BMI)

BMI	19	20	21	22	23	24	25	26	27	28	29	30	31	32	33	34	35
Height (inches)							Body Weight (pounds)										
58	91	96	100	105	110	115	119	124	129	134	138	143	148	153	158	162	167
59	94	99	104	109	114	119	124	128	133	138	143	148	153	158	163	168	173
60	97	102	107	112	118	123	128	133	138	143	148	153	158	163	168	174	179
61	100	106	111	116	122	127	132	137	143	148	153	158	164	169	174	180	185
62	104	109	115	120	126	131	136	142	147	153	158	164	169	175	180	186	191
63	107	113	118	124	130	135	141	146	152	158	163	169	175	180	186	191	197
64	110	116	122	128	134	140	145	151	157	163	169	174	180	186	192	197	204
65	114	120	126	132	138	144	150	156	162	168	174	180	186	192	198	204	210
66	118	124	130	136	142	148	155	161	167	173	179	186	192	198	204	210	216
67	121	127	134	140	146	153	159	166	172	178	185	191	198	204	211	217	223
68	125	131	138	144	151	158	164	171	177	184	190	197	203	210	216	223	230
69	128	135	142	149	155	162	169	176	182	189	196	203	209	216	223	230	236
70	132	139	146	153	160	167	174	181	188	195	202	209	216	222	229	236	243
71	136	143	150	157	165	172	179	186	193	200	208	215	222	229	236	243	250
72	140	147	154	162	169	177	184	191	199	206	213	221	228	235	242	250	258
73	144	151	159	166	174	182	189	197	204	212	219	227	235	242	250	257	265
74	148	155	163	171	179	186	194	202	210	218	225	233	241	249	256	264	272
75	152	160	168	176	184	192	200	208	216	224	232	240	248	256	264	272	279
76	156	164	172	180	189	197	205	213	221	230	238	246	254	263	271	279	287

To find your BMI, select your height in the left-hand column. Move across the line to find your weight. The number at the top of that column is your BMI.

18.2 (cont'd.) Body Mass Index (BMI)

BMI	36	37	38	39	40	41	42	43	44	45	46	47	48	49	50	51	52	53	54
Height (inches)	Body Weight (pounds)																		
58	172	177	181	186	191	196	201	205	210	215	220	224	229	234	239	244	248	253	258
59	178	183	188	193	198	203	208	212	217	222	227	232	237	242	247	252	257	262	267
60	184	189	194	199	204	209	215	220	225	230	235	240	245	250	255	261	266	271	276
61	190	195	201	206	211	217	222	227	232	238	243	248	254	259	264	269	275	280	285
62	196	202	207	213	218	224	229	235	240	246	251	256	262	267	273	278	284	289	295
63	203	208	214	220	225	231	237	242	248	254	259	265	270	278	282	287	293	299	304
64	209	215	221	227	232	238	244	250	256	262	267	273	279	285	291	296	302	308	314
65	216	222	228	234	240	246	252	258	264	270	276	282	288	294	300	306	312	318	324
66	223	229	235	241	247	253	260	266	272	278	284	291	297	303	309	315	322	328	334
67	230	236	242	249	255	261	268	274	280	287	293	299	306	312	319	325	331	338	344
68	236	243	249	256	262	269	276	282	289	295	302	308	315	322	328	335	341	348	354
69	243	250	257	263	270	277	284	291	297	304	311	318	324	331	338	345	351	358	365
70	250	257	264	271	278	285	292	299	306	313	320	327	334	341	348	355	362	369	376
71	257	265	272	279	286	293	301	308	315	322	329	338	343	351	358	365	372	379	386
72	265	272	279	287	294	302	309	316	324	331	338	346	353	361	368	375	383	390	397
73	272	280	288	295	302	310	318	325	333	340	348	355	363	371	378	386	393	401	408
74	280	287	295	303	311	319	326	334	342	350	358	365	373	381	389	396	404	412	420
75	287	295	303	311	319	327	335	343	351	359	367	375	383	391	399	407	415	423	431
76	295	304	312	320	328	336	344	353	361	369	377	385	394	402	410	418	426	435	443

National Institutes of Health
National Heart, Lung, and Blood Institute, Bethesda, MD

Step 3: Identify the Perfect Gene Diet Nutritional Recommendations for Your Genotype

Once you know your Apo E genotype, you can use the information in this section to find the specific recommendations for you.

Detailed Perfect Gene Diet Nutritional Recommendations
Building on my overview of the best nutritional recommendations for each genotype in Chapter 11, here I offer more specific information about the Big Three needs of each genotype—starting with the 4/4s so as not to play favorites. Note there are different ratios suggested for higher-calorie diets.

Apo E 4/4 Nutritional Recommendations
For diets less than 2,400 kcal: fat 20%, protein 25%, carbohydrate 55%
For diets greater than 2,400 kcal: fat 20%, protein 20%, carbohydrate 60%

Carbohydrate: From carbohydrates with low glycemic load, regulated by high-fiber content.[1] It is most crucial for this genotype to avoid all refined carbohydrates.

Protein: From plant sources as much as possible.

Fat: Lowest fat content requirement of all genotypes. Obtain fat from monounsaturated and polyunsaturated sources only, avoiding animal saturated fat sources in favor of plant sources and avoiding all trans fats.

Food intake timing: For optimal fuel delivery, eat every three hours while awake to ensure an adequate blood-glucose level at all times.

Apo E 4/3 Nutritional Recommendations
For diets less than 2,400 kcal: fat 20%, protein 25%, carbohydrate 55%
For diets greater than 2,400 kcal: fat 20%, protein 20%, carbohydrate 60%

Carbohydrate: From carbohydrates with low glycemic load, regulated by a high fiber content.[1]

Protein: Mainly from plant protein sources, with some additional protein sources, preferably from an omega-3 fish source, allowing adequate clearance time (24–48 hours) between consuming fish or other animal proteins containing saturated fat.

Fat: Second-lowest fat content requirement of all genotypes. Obtain fat from

---

1   Glycemic load is described in Chapter 8. The high-fiber content in this diet helps slow down glucose release into the bloodstream, and if coupled with a small amount of monounsaturated fat from a plant source, stomach emptying is delayed and blood glucose is prolonged and stabilized. Food intake timing: for optimal fuel delivery, eat every three hours while awake to ensure an adequate blood-glucose level at all times.

monounsaturated and polyunsaturated sources, avoiding most all animal saturated fats and staying with plant sources of saturated fat and avoiding all trans fats.

Apo E 4/2 Nutritional Recommendations
Fat 25%, protein 20%, carbohydrate 55%

Carbohydrate: From carbohydrates with low glycemic load, regulated by a high fiber content.[1]

Protein: Mainly from plant sources, with some additional protein sources, preferably omega-3 fish, allowing adequate clearance time (24–48 hours) between consuming fish or other animal proteins containing saturated fat.

Fat: Needs moderate dietary fat. Obtain fat from a combination of monounsaturated and polyunsaturated sources. No trans fat.

Food intake timing: For optimal fuel delivery, eat every three hours while awake to ensure an adequate blood-glucose level at all times.

Apo E 3/3 Nutritional Recommendations
Fat 25%, protein 20%, carbohydrate 55%

Carbohydrate: From carbohydrates with low glycemic load, regulated by a high fiber content.[1]

Protein: Mainly from plant sources, with some additional sources, preferably omega-3 fish, allowing adequate clearance time (24–48 hours) between consuming fish or other animal proteins containing saturated fat.

Fat: Need moderate dietary fat. Obtain fat mainly from monounsaturated, polyunsaturated sources with limited saturated fat intake. No trans fat.

Food intake timing: For optimal fuel delivery, eat every three hours while awake to ensure an adequate blood-glucose level at all times.

---

1   Glycemic load is described in Chapter 8. The high-fiber content in this diet helps slow down glucose release into the bloodstream, and if coupled with a small amount of monounsaturated fat from a plant source, stomach emptying is delayed and blood glucose is prolonged and stabilized. Food intake timing: for optimal fuel delivery, eat every three hours while awake to ensure an adequate blood-glucose level at all times.

Apo E 2/3 Nutritional Recommendations
Fat 30%, protein 15%, carbohydrate 55%

Carbohydrate: From carbohydrates with low glycemic load, regulated by a high fiber content.[1]

Protein: From a combination of plant and animal protein sources, allowing adequate clearance time (24–48 hours) between consuming fish or other animal protein containing saturated fat.

Fat: Needs more dietary fat than the above genotypes. Obtain mainly from monounsaturated and polyunsaturated sources with limited saturated and trans fats.

Food intake timing: For optimal fuel delivery, eat every three hours while awake to ensure an adequate blood-glucose level at all times.

Apo E 2/2 Nutritional Recommendations
Fat 35%, protein 15%, carbohydrate 50%

Carbohydrate: Greatest need of all genotypes for high-quality carbohydrates with low glycemic load, regulated by a high fiber content.[1]

Protein: From a combination of protein sources, mostly plant sources, but with some additional protein from omega-3 fish, allowing adequate clearance time (24–48 hours) between consuming fish or other animal protein containing saturated fat.

Fat: Needs the most dietary fats of all genotypes. Obtain from monounsaturated and polyunsaturated sources, with limited saturated and trans fats.

Food intake timing: For optimal fuel delivery, eat every three hours while awake to ensure an adequate blood-glucose level at all times.

---

1   Glycemic load is described in Chapter 8. The high-fiber content in this diet helps slow down glucose release into the bloodstream, and if coupled with a small amount of monounsaturated fat from a plant source, stomach emptying is delayed and blood glucose is prolonged and stabilized. Food intake timing: For optimal fuel delivery, eat every three hours while awake to ensure an adequate blood-glucose level at all times.

Apo E Menu Suggestion Plans for Each Genotype and Different Caloric Levels

Chapter 19 contains sample diet meal plans, which include suggestions for breakfast, lunch, and dinner meals, as well as a morning and afternoon snack. When you know your Apo E genotype, you can use the sample meal plans to design your personal meal plans. For example, if you are an Apo E 4/3 with a daily calorie requirement of 1,800, review the Menu Suggestion Plan for Apo E 4/3—1,800 calories.

If you would prefer different food choices for any of the meals listed in the sample meal plans, you can use the Food Exchange List (see pages 256–260) and find a replacement food.

About the Food Exchange List

This exchange list is based on a single serving size within each food category. Remember to stay within your serving recommendations for the day. When selecting a protein food, the serving size can change depending on the food type. For instance, 1 oz. of cooked fish is equal to one serving. You may have 10 servings of protein a day, so be mindful of serving sizes—learn what a serving looks like. With milk-type products (such as skim milk and soy), the serving size changes depending on the type of product.

Keep in mind the following, to ensure that you design appropriate meals:

- Carbohydrates come from grain, starch, fruit, and vegetable sources.
- Fats come from both plant and animal sources.
- Proteins come from both plant and animal sources.
- Always exchange the same food type so your diet will remain balanced.
  - carbohydrate for carbohydrate
  - fat for fat
  - protein for protein
- When substituting a food, be mindful of the serving size.
- When possible, choose organic and avoid all processed and genetically modified foods (GMO).
- Avoid all foods coming from unhealthy farming practices. Consider buying your food locally; farmers' markets can be a great source of good, fresh produce.

Food Exchange List

Carbohydrates

Carbohydrates are the number one energy food source for the body. The single servings listed below are selected because they provide a good variety of shorter-term fuel with low glycemic load (see page 84). With low glycemic load foods, the glucose delivery is lower and slower to the body. It is also regulated by its high fiber content because the fiber slows down the digestion so the food is not absorbed too rapidly and therefore doesn't raise blood sugar as rapidly.

Carbohydrates: Fruits
1 cup or 18 grapes
1 cup or 15 cherries
4 fresh apricots or 7 halves, dried
1 fresh apple or 4 rings, dried
1 medium orange or 2 mandarins/tangerines
½ cup kiwi
¾ cup blueberries
1 cup papaya/mango/guava/pineapple
¾ cup raspberries
1 medium peach/nectarine
1 medium plum or pear or ½ large pear
1¼ cups melon (watermelon, honeydew, cantaloupe)
¾ cup strawberries
¾ cup loganberries
2 tbsp. dried cranberries or raisins
3 medium prunes
½ banana
1½ figs
¾ cup blackberries

Carbohydrates: Vegetables
½ cup cooked, 1 cup raw:
    turnips
    bok choy/leeks
    broccoli/broccolini/cauliflower

    carrots/celery
    onions/scallions
    summer squash
    green beans
    asparagus
    artichoke
    brussel sprouts
    radishes
    turnips/rutabaga/parsnips/beets
    eggplant
    English peapods
    cabbage, red and white—kohlrabi
    peppers—red, yellow, green/tomatoes
    mushrooms, cooked

1 cup leafy greens such as:
    spinach/mustard greens
    kale
    romaine lettuce
    mixed salad greens

Carbohydrates: Grains/Starches
¾ cup plain high-fiber dry cereal
½ cup cooked cereals: oat bran, whole oatmeal
¼ cup low-fat granola
½ small whole-grain bagel
1 slice whole-grain bread
½ whole-grain bun
6-inch whole-wheat tortilla
6-inch corn tortilla
½ whole-wheat pita
¾ oz. whole-wheat pretzels
½ cup whole-wheat pasta
⅓ cup brown rice
½ cup corn, lima beans, peas
3 oz. baked potato (w/skin), waxy type

⅓ cup sweet potato, yam, pumpkin
3 cups plain dry popcorn, no seasonings
7 whole-grain crackers (rounds)
3 ginger biscuits/cookies (1 serving of recipe)
1 slice angel food cake ($1/12$ of a 10" diameter pan)
½ cup beans, non-GMO (black, kidney, red, lima, navy, white)[2]

Fats

These suggested servings of fats provide longer-term fuel. Fat is much more complex than carbohydrates. It still contains carbon, hydrogen, and oxygen, but the atoms are linked together with different chemical bonds that cause it to take longer to digest. Fats come as saturated and unsaturated, depending on the type of chemical bonds. This makes a big difference in how they interact with our bodies. Also, some fat sources have a greater percentage of fat in them than others. This translates into different amounts per serving size.

1 oz. avocado
1 tsp. canola, olive, peanut oil (small amounts only—non-GMO)
8 olives
6 almonds
10 peanuts
4 cashews
4 halves pecans
4 halves walnuts
1 tbsp. sesame seeds
2 tsp. nut butter (peanut, almond, cashew, sesame)
1 tbsp. pumpkin, sunflower seeds
¼ cup purslane
2 tsp. linseed
2 tbsp. flaxseed (ground)
1 tbsp. light mayonnaise

Protein

Different protein foods have different concentrations of protein in them. Also, protein has something that carbohydrates and fat don't

---

2   Also counts as 1 protein

have—nitrogen from the amino acids. When these are digested and used as fuel in the bloodstream, it is hard on the body because of the nitrogen. They break down to produce a waste product in the liver, called urea, which then has to be cleared by the kidneys.

Protein: Plant Legume
½ cup beans, non-GMO (black, kidney, red, lima, navy, white)[3]
½ cup soybeans
½ cup legumes—split peas, lentils
1 garden or veggie burger = 2 protein servings
4 oz. tofu/tempeh (non-GMO)

Protein: Egg
¼ cup egg substitute
2 medium egg whites
1 organic whole egg

Protein: Fish
1 oz. of cooked fish/seafood:
  black cod
  crab
  halibut
  lobster
  oysters (6)
  salmon
  sardines
  scallops
  sea bass
  shrimp
  trout
  tuna
  herring
  mackerel
  smaller plant-eating wild fish and seafoods

Protein: Poultry
1 oz. white meat, no skin cooked
1 oz. organic chicken, turkey, Cornish game hen, wild; no skin, cooked
1 oz. organic, nonprocessed sliced meat; cooked

---

3   Also counts as 1 grain

Protein: Dairy & Soy

1 cup nonfat milk (from organic source, nonpregnant cows)

1 cup soymilk—(carrageenan free)

½ cup evaporated nonfat milk

⅓ cup dry nonfat milk

1 cup nonfat buttermilk

1 cup nonfat yogurt

1 cup almond milk

1 cup hemp milk

1 cup soy yogurt

1 oz. nonfat cheese

1 oz. low-fat soy cheese

1 oz. soy cream cheese

¼ cup nonfat cottage cheese

¼ cup nonfat ricotta cheese

¼ cup nonfat soy cottage cheese

¼ cup nonfat soy ricotta cheese

* If you presently consume products made from cow's milk, or are thinking about doing so, consider those that are organic and come from animals that are grass fed only and not treated with antibiotics or the genetically engineered hormones rbST and rbGH.

Chapter Nineteen

SAMPLE MEAL PLANS BY GENOTYPE AND CALORIE ALLOWANCE

As you plan your daily menus, keep in mind that most foods are a combination of the Big Three food categories—carbohydrate, protein, and fat. It is very rare that a food contains only one of these components. Foods typically break down into the following components:

- fruit contains mostly carbohydrate (with plant fiber)
- beans contain a mixture of protein and carbohydrate
- dairy foods contain mostly protein, fat, and some carbohydrate
- animal protein (meat and eggs) contains protein and animal fat
- most plant protein (beans, nuts, rice, seeds, and soy) contains a more diluted protein and good anti-inflammatory fat

If your suggested food plan calls for a food that you don't like or don't want to eat, see the food exchange list on page 256. Here you can look up any particular food and exchange it for another that you prefer; e.g., if your Apo E 4/4 plan calls for a serving of halibut and you don't like halibut, look at the list of fish on page 259 and select one you prefer.

Important Points to Remember

Use local, organic ingredients wherever available: organic foods are grown without the use of pesticides, synthetic fertilizers, sewage sludge, genetically modified organisms, or radiation. Organically raised animals that produce meat, poultry, eggs, and dairy products are not given antibiotics or growth hormones. Organic foods are produced by farmers who emphasize the use of renewable resources and the conservation of soil and water to enhance environmental quality for future generations. The closer it is grown to where you live, the more likely it is to be fresher as well as tree- or vine-ripened, with more nutrients present. Local production also reduces energy costs for transport.

Other important points:

- Honey: It is especially important to use local, organic honey if a person has seasonal allergies. Local honey can reduce allergy symptoms because the bees go the local plants that a person is allergic to and this actually helps reduce local allergies.

- Beverages: In addition to the beverages listed in the Sample Meal Plans below, most people will have water with meals. You may dress it up with ice, lemon, cucumber, or use sparkling waters for special occasions—and don't forget to use a special crystal glass (or bone china with your hot tea) for a treat.

- Lettuce: Choose romaine lettuce whenever possible. It has the highest nutritional value of any of the lettuce family.

- Eggs: Choose free-range, antibiotic free, organically fed, omega-3 fortified eggs. Eggs may be poached, boiled, or scrambled. When poaching or boiling, remove the yolks after cooking. When scrambling, use only the egg whites. When scrambling eggs, cook in a little olive oil over a low heat to minimize the production of free radicals. If you use a nonstick pan, also make sure the heat is very low, as toxic products can be released from the coating.

- Yogurt and soy products: Choose soy cheeses that do *not* contain soy isolate. Be sure yogurt and soymilk are carrageenan free and are organic—not the common genetically modified soy.

- You can make your own soy yogurt from the recipe section or choose a GMO-free brand such as Wildwood, Nancy's, or Trader Joe's.

- Angel food cake: A serving of angel food cake is $^1/_{12}$ of a 10" diameter pan.

Access to some of the less well-known foods (marked in "Suggested Diets" with a †, starting on page 264) are:

- Matcha tea: at Whole Foods Markets and
  www.teance.com/Wako_Matcha_Made_from_Shade_Grown_ Gyokuro_Teance_p/matchacan.htm
  Jasmine tea: **www.teance.com/Immortal_Peach_Hand_Tied_ Jasmine_Green_Teance_p/tea121.htm**

- Organic sardines, black cod, or sablefish: **vitalchoice.com**

- Soy yogurt and frozen yogurt: **wholesoyco.com**

- Veggie burgers: Amy's Texas Burgers at **amyskitchen.com**

- Oat bran bread or bran flax bread: **vitalvittles.com**

- Olive oil mayonaise and ground flaxseed (Spectrum Brand): at Whole Foods Market or Trader Joe's or **spectrumorganics.com** (click on "Products" and then use left menu).

- Sweet potato fries: **alexiafoods.com**

- Vegetable broth: **www.imaginefoods.com/content/organic -vegetable-broth**

- Gluten-free flour: **www.kingarthurflour.com**

In the following pages you will find detailed custom diets for your individual Apo E genotype. These suggestions provide you with a personalized dietary plan, taking into account your optimal caloric needs and dietary fat, protein, and carbohydrate requirements. We have further simplified your diet by providing you with the correct serving amounts for each food group broken down into fat, protein, and carbohydrate.

By providing you with the number of servings for a specific calorie level, it makes it very simple to get the calorie level and recommended carbohydrate, fat, and protein percentages needed for that day. These custom diets are further supported by the recipes found in the recommended diets based on your Apo E gene.

In addition to these specific diets, we have provided additional calorie levels located in Appendix B, beginning on page 417. These are based on broader recommendations once your initial diet has been perfected. It allows more freedom to choose various food options that fit into your new eating pattern. All of our calorie level tables take into consideration your specific individual Apo E genotype.

Although our data was produced by professionals with extensive training in nutritional science and research, we recognize that your individual circumstances may create exceptions. Please contact us if you think your situation has not been fully addressed and we will do our best to tailor a plan that is best for you.

Suggested Diets

* = See recipe by same name in next chapter.

† = Indicates that the product (usually a tea) can be found in the product listings above.

The following sample meal plans are organized by genotype with the highest numbers first, i.e., Apo E 4/4, followed by 4/3, etc. Using the gray "tabs" printed on the edge of the pages, locate your genotype and caloric level as determined by the formula for your gender on pages 245–246. Each section offers four days of meal plans for the most common caloric levels: 1,600–2,400 kcal.

APO E GENE
4/4 1,600 KCAL, DAY 1
Serving considerations per day:
   (be mindful of serving sizes)

Carbohydrates
6 servings grain/starch
7 servings fruit/vegetable

Protein
10 servings plant protein or fish

Fat
4.5 servings anti-inflammatory fat

Breakfast
1 slice whole-grain toast
1 tbsp. nut butter
1 medium orange
1 cup nonfat Almond Milk*
Japanese Matcha Tea†
Apo E Diet Multivitamins™

Morning Snack
¼ cup whole-grain granola
½ cup Soy Yogurt*
Ginger Green Tea*

Lunch
Sandwich:
2 slices whole-grain bread
3 oz. baby shrimp
Romaine lettuce (1 leaf)
¼ cup sliced tomato
⅛ cup onions
1 oz. avocado
1 tbsp. olive or canola oil mayonnaise†

Sparkling Lemon Juice Iced Water*

Afternoon Snack
¼ cup Original Hummus*
½ cup carrots
½ cup cherry tomatoes
White Tea*

Dinner
3 oz. Grilled or Baked Fish (halibut)*
Pam's Baked Potato*
2 tbsp. Tomato Salsa Cream* (¼ serving)
1 tbsp. chives
1 cup steamed broccoli
1 slice whole-grain bread
1 oz. avocado
Chamomile Peach Tea*

Supper (evening snack)
Scottish Fruit Pottage*
½ cup nonfat soy ice cream
Chamomile Hibiscus Tea*

APO E GENE
4/4 1,600 KCAL, DAY 2
Serving considerations per day:

Carbohydrates
5 servings grain/starch
8.5 servings fruit/vegetable

Protein
7 servings plant protein or fish

Fat
2 servings anti-inflammatory fat

Breakfast
½ cup nonfat Soy Yogurt*
½ banana
½ whole-grain bagel
½ tbsp. honey
Green Tea*
Apo E Diet Multivitamins™

Morning Snack
½ medium apple
½ tbsp. nut butter

White Tea with Cranberries*

Lunch
Sandwich:
1 whole-grain pita bread
2 oz. fresh crab
1 oz. low-fat soy cheese, shredded
Romaine lettuce (1 leaf)
¼ cup sliced tomato
⅛ cup onions
2 tbsp. nonfat Caesar dressing

Sparkling Orange Juice Iced Water*

Afternoon Snack
Carrot and Cucumber Yogurt Salad*
4 whole-grain crackers
Peach Herbal Tea*

Dinner
Shiitake Mushroom and Spinach Lasagna*
(¾ serving)
1 tbsp. Parmesan cheese
1 cup steamed spinach

1 slice whole-grain bread
Sparkling Orange Juice Iced Water *
  and Rosehip Green Tea*

Supper (evening snack)
3 Raspberry Ginger Biscuits (cookies)*
1 cup nonfat milk

APO E GENE
4/4 1,600 KCAL, DAY 3
Serving considerations per day:

Carbohydrates
9.5 servings grain/starch
4 servings fruit/vegetable

Protein
9.5 servings plant protein or fish

Fat
6 servings anti-inflammatory fat

Breakfast
Eggs (½–¾ cup egg whites or substitute)
1 slice whole-grain oat flax toast†
1 oz. avocado
1½ oz. fat-free soy cheese
½ cup Tomato Salsa Cream*
Ginger Green Tea*
Apo E Diet Multivitamins™

Morning Snack
½ cup nonfat Almond Milk*
½ cup blueberries
Ginger Green Tea*

Lunch
Tofu Salad* (¾ serving)
¾ cup grapes
¾ cup nonfat milk
Black Currant, Ginger, and Turmeric Tea*

Afternoon Snack
Trail mix:
⅛ cup almonds
⅛ cup cranberries or raisins
½ cup low-fat granola
Matcha Tea†

Dinner
3 oz. grilled tuna with 1 serving
  Teriyaki Sauce*
⅓ cup black beans
Salad: 1 cup spinach
⅓ cup cherry tomatoes
⅓ cup cabbage
⅓ cup shredded carrots
Fat Free Salad Dressing* with 1 tsp.
  of olive oil added
Sparkling Lime Juice Iced Water* and
  White Mint Tea*

Supper (evening snack)
¾ cup strawberries
Angel food cake
Chamomile Peach Tea*

**APO E GENE
4/4 1,600 KCAL, DAY 4**
Serving considerations per day:

Carbohydrates
6 servings grain/starch
10.5 servings fruit/vegetable

Protein
8 servings plant protein or fish

Fat
4 servings anti-inflammatory fat

Breakfast
Scottish Oatmeal*
1 cup nonfat milk
Green Tea*
Apo E Diet Multivitamins™

Morning Snack
¼ cup whole-grain granola
1 cup nonfat Soy Yogurt*
Peach Hibiscus Tea*

Lunch
Sandwich:
1 whole-grain pita bread
3 oz. water-packed tuna

Romaine lettuce (1 leaf)
¼ cup sliced tomato
⅛ cup onions
1 tbsp. fat-free ranch dressing

Sparkling Hibiscus Iced Water*

Afternoon Snack
1½ oz. low-fat soy cream cheese
1 whole-grain Wasa Cracker†
½ cup grapes
Ginger Green Tea*

Dinner
Vegetable Spaghetti or Pasta* (¾ serving)
1 tbsp. soy cheese
Green Salad*
Hibiscus Elder Tea*

Supper (evening snack)
3 Lemon Ginger Biscuits (cookies)*
Chamomile Peach Tea*

APO E GENE
4/4 1,800 KCAL, DAY 1
Serving considerations per day:
(be mindful of serving sizes)

Carbohydrates
11.5 servings grain/starch
5.5 servings fruit/vegetable

Protein
10 servings plant protein or fish

Fat
2.5 servings anti-inflammatory fat

Breakfast
1 slice whole-grain oat flax toast[†]
½ tbsp. honey
½ cup blueberries
½ cup Almond Milk*
Matcha Tea[†]
Apo E Diet Multivitamins™

Morning Snack
½ cup cherries
¾ cup Soy Yogurt*
Green Ginger Tea*

Lunch
Vegetable and Bean Tacos*
½ cup Tomato Salsa Cream*
1 cup low-fat soymilk
Iced Green Tea* with lemon slice

Afternoon Snack
Sultana, Carrot, Ginger Coleslaw*
4 oz. whole-wheat pretzels
½ cup cherry tomatoes
The Green and Red Tea*

Dinner
3 oz. Grilled or Baked Fish (wild halibut)*
Pam's Baked Potato*
3 tbsp. plain yogurt
1 tbsp. chives
1 cup steamed broccoli
½ slice whole-grain bread
1 oz. avocado
Classic English Tea with Milk*

Supper (evening snack)
Scottish Fruit Pottage*
½ cup frozen yogurt
Chamomile Peach Tea*

APO E GENE
4/4 1,800 KCAL, DAY 2
Serving considerations per day:

Carbohydrates
3.5 servings grain/starch
12.5 servings fruit/vegetable

Protein
11 servings plant protein or fish

Fat
2 servings anti-inflammatory fat

Breakfast
Eggs (½–¾ cup egg whites or substitute)
¼ cup Tomato Salsa Cream* (½ serving)
1 slice whole-grain toast or
whole-wheat tortilla
½ tbsp. honey
Ginger Green Tea*
Apo E Diet Multivitamins™

Morning Snack
Sultana, Carrot, Ginger Coleslaw*
1½ oz. soy cheese
Black Currant, Ginger, and Turmeric Tea*

Lunch
Tofu Salad*
1 medium apple
1 cup nonfat milk
Sparkling Orange Juice Iced Water*

Afternoon Snack
Carrot and Cucumber Yogurt Salad*
5 whole-wheat crackers
White Mint Tea*

Dinner
3 oz. Grilled or Baked Fish (trout)*
with Soy Ginger Sauce*

APO E 4/4 1,800 KCAL

Pam's Baked Potato*
Mevagissey Ratatouille*
Hibiscus Elder Tea*

Supper (evening snack)
Pear and Blueberry Crumble* (½ serving)
English Vanilla Custard*
Peach Tea*

**APO E GENE
4/4 1,800 KCAL, DAY 3**
Serving considerations per day:

Carbohydrates
9.5 servings grain/starch
10.5 servings fruit/vegetable

Protein
12 servings plant protein or fish

Fat
4 servings anti-inflammatory fat

Breakfast
2 six-inch corn tortillas
¼ cup egg substitute
1½ oz. fat-free soy cheese
½ cup Tomato Salsa Cream* (½ serving)
Ginger Green Tea*
Apo E Diet Multivitamins™

Morning Snack
1 cup blueberries
1 cup nonfat Almond Milk*
The Green and Red Tea*

Lunch
Sandwich:
2 slices whole-grain bread
3 oz. shrimp or crab
Romaine lettuce (1 leaf)
¼ cup sliced tomato
⅛ cup onions
1 tbsp. low-fat canola or olive
    oil mayonnaise†

Sparkling Lemon Juice Iced Water* and
    fresh mint (consider using a crystal glass)

Afternoon Snack
Trail mix:
⅛ cup almonds
⅛ cup cranberries or raisins
½ cup low-fat granola

Matcha Tea†

Dinner
3 oz. Baked Fish (sea bass)* with squeeze
    of lime and ½ cup Tomato Salsa Cream*
½ cup black beans
Green Salad*
1 slice multigrain bread
Lemon Lime Tea with Wild Mint* and
    Rosehip Green Tea*

Supper (evening snack)
1 cup strawberries
Angel food cake
Chamomile Peach Tea*

**APO E GENE
4/4 1,800 KCAL, DAY 4**
Serving considerations per day:

Carbohydrates
7 servings grain/starch
12 servings fruit/vegetable

Protein
11 servings plant protein or fish

Fat
3 servings anti-inflammatory fat

Breakfast
Scottish Oatmeal*
1 cup nonfat soymilk
Lemon Ginger Green Tea*
Apo E Diet Multivitamins™

Morning Snack
¼ cup whole-grain granola
1 cup nonfat yogurt with ½ cup berries
White Mint Tea*

Lunch
Sandwich:
1 whole-grain pita bread
4 oz. water-packed tuna
1 tbsp. fat-free ranch dressing
Romaine lettuce (1 leaf)
¼ cup sliced tomato
⅛ cup spring onions

Cornish Pixie Rose-Lemon Green Tea*

Afternoon Snack
1 oz. soy cheese
1 whole-grain Wasa Cracker†
½ cup grapes
Ginger Green Tea*

Dinner
Vegetable Spaghetti*
1 tbsp. grated soy cheese
Green Salad*
Sparkling Orange Juice Iced Water*
  and Peach Tea*

Supper (evening snack)
3 Ginger Biscuits (cookies)*
White Mint Tea*

APO E GENE
4/4 2,000 KCAL, DAY 1
Serving considerations per day:
  (be mindful of serving sizes)

Carbohydrates
5.5 servings grain/starch
9 servings fruit/vegetable

Protein
10 servings plant protein or fish

Fat
5 servings anti-inflammatory fat

Breakfast
Scottish Oatmeal*
⅛ cup raisins or cranberries
1 cup Soy or Almond Milk*
Matcha Tea†
Apo E Diet Multivitamins™

Morning Snack
Granola mix:
¼ cup low-fat granola
⅛ cup chopped walnuts
⅛ cup dried apricots
¾ cup nonfat yogurt

Classic English Tea with Milk*

Lunch
Vegetable and Bean Tacos* (1.5 servings)
½ cup Tomato Salsa Cream*
½ medium apple
1 cup nonfat milk

Green Tea*

Afternoon Snack
Simple Vegetarian Black Bean Soup*
  (½ serving)
¼ cup cherry tomatoes
Hibiscus Elder Tea*

Dinner
4 oz. Baked Trout*
Pam's Baked Potato*
1½ oz. nonfat cheese
1 tbsp. chives
Mevagissey Ratatouille*
Peach Tea*

Supper (evening snack)
½ cup low-fat chocolate frozen yogurt
Chamomile Hibiscus Tea*

APO E 4/4 2,000 KCAL

APO E GENE
4/4 2,000 KCAL, DAY 2
Serving considerations per day:

Carbohydrates
8.5 servings grain/starch
7.5 servings fruit/vegetable

Protein
13 servings plant protein or fish

Fat
2 servings anti-inflammatory fat

Breakfast
1 whole-grain bagel
Eggs (½–¾ cup egg whites or substitute)
½ banana
½ tbsp. honey
Classic English Tea with Milk*
Apo E Diet Multivitamins™

Morning Snack
½ cup cherries or cherry tomatoes
1 oz. sliced soy cheese
8 whole-grain crackers
Green Tea*

Lunch
Sandwich:
1 veggie burger
1½ oz. low-fat soy cheese
1 slice whole-grain bread
Romaine lettuce (1 leaf)
¼ cup sliced tomato
⅛ cup onions
4 green or black olives
1 oz. avocado
1 tbsp. low-fat canola or olive
   oil mayonnaise†

1 cup nonfat milk
Sparkling Orange Juice Iced Water*
   (consider a crystal glass)

Afternoon Snack
Quick Fresh Fruit Shake-to-Go*
   (¾ serving)

Dinner
4 oz. Grilled or Baked Fish (ahi tuna*)
½ cup black beans
Mevagissey Ratatouille*
1 slice whole-grain bread or roll
Iced or hot Peach Herbal Tea*

Supper (evening snack)
3 Ginger Biscuits (cookies)*
1 cup nonfat Almond Milk*

APO E GENE
4/4 2,000 KCAL, DAY 3
Serving considerations per day:

Carbohydrates
7.5 servings grain/starch
11 servings fruit/vegetable

Protein
14.5 servings plant protein or fish

Fat
4 servings anti-inflammatory fat

Breakfast
1 six-inch corn tortilla
½ cup egg substitute
1½ oz. fat-free cheese
¼ cup Tomato Salsa Cream* (½ serving)
½ cup melon
Ginger and Turmeric Tea*
Apo E Diet Multivitamins™

Morning Snack
1 medium apple
½ tbsp. nut butter
White Mint Tea*

Lunch
Open-faced sandwich:
1 slice whole-grain bread
4 oz. tofu
Romaine lettuce (1 leaf)
¼ cup sliced tomato
⅛ cup onions

1 tbsp. low-fat canola or olive
  oil mayonnaise†

1 cup nonfat or soymilk

Afternoon Snack
Trail mix:
⅛ cup almonds
⅛ cup cranberries or raisins
½ cup low-fat granola
⅛ cup nuts

Matcha Tea†

Dinner
Vegetable Spaghetti or Pasta*
  (¾ recipe serving)
1 tbsp. Parmesan cheese
Green Salad*
1 slice whole-grain bread
Sparkling Lime Juice Iced Water*
  and The Green and Red Tea*

Supper (evening snack)
1 cup blackberries
Vanilla angel food cake
1 cup nonfat Almond Milk*

APO E GENE
4/4 2,000 KCAL, DAY 4
Serving considerations per day:

Carbohydrates
8.5 servings grain/starch
10 servings fruit/vegetable

Protein
13.5 servings plant protein or fish

Fat
3 servings anti-inflammatory fat

Breakfast
1 cup whole-grain dry cereal
½ banana
1 cup Almond Milk*
Ginger Green Tea*
Apo E Diet Multivitamins™

Morning Snack
Snack break mix:
½ cup low-fat granola
⅛ cup of your favorite dried fruit, such as
  dried apricots
½ cup nonfat vanilla soy yogurt

Lemon Lime Tea with Wild Mint*

Lunch
Pam's Baked Potato*
1 cup Cornish Chili*
1½ oz. fat-free soy cheese, shredded
1 cup cooked broccoli
Romaine lettuce (1 leaf)
¼ cup sliced tomato
⅛ cup onions
Sparkling Hibiscus Iced Water*

Afternoon Snack
Carrot and Cucumber Yogurt Salad*
Lemon Ginger Green Tea*

Dinner
4 oz. Grilled or Baked Fish (wild salmon)*
Pam's Baked Potato* (½ serving)
Wok-steamed kale (½ cup raw), with
  onion (¼ cup), one medium tomato,
  corn (¼ cup), and garlic
1 tbsp. Parmesan cheese
Sparkling Lemon Juice Iced Water*
  and Hibiscus Elder Tea*

Supper (evening snack)
Peach and Blackberry Crumble*
  (½ serving)
1 cup nonfat milk or soymilk

APO E 4/4 2,000 KCAL

APO E GENE
4/4 2,400 KCAL, DAY 1
Serving considerations per day:
(be mindful of serving sizes)

Carbohydrates
6.5 servings grain/starch
9.5 servings fruit/vegetable

Protein
14.5 servings plant protein or fish

Fat
2.5 servings anti-inflammatory fat

Breakfast
Orange Shake-to-Go* (½ serving)
½ whole-grain bagel
½ tbsp. honey
⅛ cup raisins or cranberries
1 cup nonfat or Almond Milk*
Jasmine Green Tea†
Apo E Diet Multivitamins™

Morning Snack
Granola mix:
¼ cup low-fat granola
⅛ cup chopped walnuts
⅛ cup dried apricots

½ cup Soy Yogurt*

Lunch
Vegetable and Bean Tacos*
¼ cup Tomato Salsa Cream* (½ serving)
⅓ cup black beans
½ medium apple
1 cup Almond Milk*
Cornish Pixie Rose-Lemon Green Tea*

Afternoon Snack
Cornish Chili* (¾ serving)
4 whole-grain crackers
Iced or hot Peach Herbal Tea*

Dinner
5 oz. Grilled or Baked Fish (wild halibut)*
with Soy Ginger Sauce*
Pam's Baked Potato*

1½ oz. nonfat Almond Cheese*
1 tbsp. chives
½ cup grilled yellow squash
6–8 asparagus spears
Sparkling Orange Juice Iced Water*

Supper (evening snack)
1 cup strawberries
Angel food cake
¾ cup nonfat warm vanilla yogurt
Chamomile Peach Tea*

APO E GENE
4/4 2,400 KCAL, DAY 2
Serving considerations per day:

Carbohydrates
4.5 servings grain/starch
15.5 servings fruit/vegetable

Protein
12.5 servings plant protein or fish

Fat
3 servings anti-inflammatory fat

Breakfast
Scottish Oatmeal*
⅛ cup raisins
½ tbsp. honey
1 cup nonfat milk
Black Currant, Ginger, and Turmeric Tea*
Apo E Diet Multivitamins™

Morning Snack
1 slice whole-grain oat flax bread
1½ tbsp. raisins
½ cup nonfat cottage cheese
Rosehip Green Tea*

Lunch
Open-faced sandwich:
½ whole-grain bun or 1 slice bread
Tofu Salad* (¾ serving)

½ medium apple
1 cup nonfat milk
Sparkling Orange Juice Iced Water*

Afternoon Snack
Carrot and Cucumber Yogurt Salad*
  (1½ servings)
½ cup carrots or jicama slices
1 slice multigrain bread
The Green and Red Tea*

Dinner
4 oz. Grilled or Baked Fish (mackerel)*
  with rosemary, olive oil, and orange juice
Green Salad*
Olive Oil Potato Wedgewood Fries*
  (½ serving)
Peach Tea*

Supper (evening snack)
Kelly's Fore Street Dessert* (½ serving)
White Tea with Cranberries*

**APO E GENE
4/4 2,400 KCAL, DAY 3**
Serving considerations per day:

Carbohydrates
8 servings grain/starch
16.5 servings fruit/vegetable

Protein
16.5 servings plant protein or fish

Fat
8.5 servings anti-inflammatory fat

Breakfast
2 six-inch corn tortillas
¾ cup egg white, or substitute
¼ cup Fresh Tomato Salsa*
3 oz. fat-free cheese
¼ cup baked beans
1 oz. avocado
½ cup melon
Lemon Ginger Green Tea*
Apo E Diet Multivitamins™

Morning Snack
1 medium apple
½ tbsp. natural nut butter

½ cup Almond Cheese*
White Mint Tea*

Lunch
Fish Salad*
1 whole-grain pita bread
1 cup nonfat milk
Sparkling Lemon or Lime Juice Iced Water*
  (don't forget a pretty glass)

Afternoon Snack
Fruit Shake-to-Go* (¾ serving)

Dinner
Vegetable Spaghetti or Pasta*
1 tbsp. Parmesan cheese
Green Salad*
1 slice whole-grain bread
1 cup nonfat milk
Rosehip Green Tea*

Supper (evening snack)
½ cup frozen soy yogurt
Scottish Fruit Pottage* (2 servings)
Chamomile Peach Tea*

**APO E GENE
4/4 2,400 KCAL, DAY 4**
Serving considerations per day:

Carbohydrates
9.5 servings grain/starch
15 servings fruit/vegetable

Protein
15 servings plant protein or fish

Fat
4.5 servings anti-inflammatory fat

Breakfast
Blueberry Oat Muffin*
Baked Apples* (½ serving)
Eggs (½–¾ cup egg whites or substitute)
1 medium orange
1 cup Almond Milk*
Jasmine Green Tea†
Apo E Diet Multivitamins™

Morning Snack
⅓ cup low-fat whole-grain granola
¾ cup nonfat Soy Yogurt*
1 cup fresh strawberries
Sparkling Lime Juice Iced Water*

Lunch
Rustic Tuscany Pizza*
Green Salad*
Sparkling Hibiscus Iced Water*

Afternoon Snack
Carrot and Cucumber Yogurt Salad*
1 cup Almond Milk*
Lemon Ginger Green Tea*

Dinner
5 oz. Grilled or Baked Fish (tuna steak)*
    with ¼ cup Teriyaki Sauce*
Pam's Baked Potato* (½ serving)
Mevagissey Ratatouille*
1 tbsp. Parmesan cheese
1 slice whole-grain bread
1 tsp. avocado
Sparkling Lemon Juice Iced Water*
    and Hibiscus Elder Tea*

Supper (evening snack)
½ cup Apple Blueberry Crumble*
¾ cup nonfat warm vanilla yogurt
Peach Tea*

APO E 4/4 2,400 KCAL

APO E GENE
4/3 1,600 KCAL, DAY 1

Serving considerations per day:
(be mindful of serving sizes)

Carbohydrates
6 servings grain/starch
7 servings fruit/vegetable

Protein
9 servings plant protein or fish

Fat
4.5 servings anti-inflammatory fat

Breakfast
1 slice whole-grain toast
1 tbsp. nut butter
1 medium orange
1 cup nonfat soymilk
Matcha Tea†
Apo E Diet Multivitamins™

Morning Snack
¼ cup whole-grain granola
½ cup yogurt
Black Currant, Ginger, and Turmeric Tea*

Lunch
Sandwich:
2 slices whole-grain bread
1 tbsp. olive oil mayonnaise†
3 oz. crabmeat
Romaine lettuce (1 leaf)
¼ cup sliced tomato
⅛ cup onions
1 oz. avocado

Sparkling Lemon Juice Iced Water*

Afternoon Snack
¼ cup nonfat yogurt
½ cup carrots
½ cup cherry tomatoes
Rosehip Green Tea*

Dinner
3 oz. Grilled or Baked Fish (wild black cod)*
Pam's Baked Potato*
2 tbsp. Tomato Salsa Cream* (¼ serving)

1 tbsp. chives
1 cup steamed broccoli
1 slice whole-grain bread
1 oz. avocado
White Mint Tea*

Supper (evening snack)
Scottish Fruit Pottage*
½ cup nonfat frozen yogurt
Chamomile Peach Tea*

APO E GENE
4/3 1,600 KCAL, DAY 2

Serving considerations per day:

Carbohydrates
5 servings grain/starch
8.5 servings fruit/vegetable

Protein
7 servings plant protein or fish

Fat
2 servings anti-inflammatory fat

Breakfast
½ whole-grain bagel
½ banana
½ tbsp. honey
½ cup nonfat Almond Milk*
White Mint Tea*
Apo E Diet Multivitamins™

Morning Snack
½ medium apple
½ tbsp. nut butter
Lemon Lime Tea with Wild Mint*

Lunch
Sandwich:
1 whole-grain pita bread
2 oz. fresh crab
1 oz. low-fat soy cheese, grated
Romaine lettuce (1 leaf)
¼ cup sliced tomato
⅛ cup onions
2 tbsp. nonfat Caesar dressing

Sparkling Orange Juice Iced Water*

Afternoon Snack
Carrot and Cucumber Yogurt Salad*
4 whole-grain crackers
Lemon Ginger Green Tea*

Dinner
Shiitake Mushroom and Spinach Lasagna*
  (¾ serving)
1 tbsp. Parmesan cheese
1 cup steamed spinach
1 slice whole-grain bread
Sparkling Orange Juice Iced Water* and
  White Tea with Cranberries*

Supper (evening snack)
3 Raspberry Ginger Biscuits (cookies)*
1 cup nonfat milk

**APO E GENE
4/3 1,600 KCAL, DAY 3**
Serving considerations per day:

Carbohydrates
9.5 servings grain/starch
4 servings fruit/vegetable

Protein
9.5 servings plant protein or fish

Fat
6 servings anti-inflammatory fat

Breakfast
Eggs (½–¾ cup egg whites or substitute)
1 slice whole-grain oat flax toast†
1 oz. avocado
1½ oz. fat-free cheese
½ cup Tomato Salsa Cream*
Ginger Green Tea*
Apo E Diet Multivitamins™

Morning Snack
¼ cup vanilla soy yogurt
½ cup blueberries
White Mint Tea

Lunch
Tofu Salad* (¾ serving)
¾ cup grapes
¾ cup nonfat Almond Milk*
Rosehip Green Tea*

Afternoon Snack
Trail mix:
⅛ cup almonds
⅛ cup cranberries or raisins
½ cup low-fat granola

Matcha Tea†

Dinner
3 oz. Grilled or Baked Fish (sea bass)*
  with Teriyaki Sauce*
⅓ cup black beans
Salad: 1 cup spinach, ⅓ cup cherry tomatoes,
  ⅓ cup cabbage, ⅓ cup shredded carrots
Simple Salad Dressing*
Sparkling Lime Juice Iced Water*
Chamomile Peach Tea*

Supper (evening snack)
¾ cup raspberries
Angel food cake
Classic English Tea with Milk*

**APO E GENE
4/3 1,600 KCAL, DAY 4**
Serving considerations per day:

Carbohydrates
6 servings grain/starch
10.5 servings fruit/vegetable

Protein
8 servings plant protein or fish

Fat
4 servings anti-inflammatory fat

Breakfast
Scottish Oatmeal*
1 cup nonfat milk
Green Tea*
Apo E Diet Multivitamins™

Morning Snack
¼ cup whole-grain granola
1 cup nonfat Soy Yogurt*
Iced Ginger and Turmeric Tea*

Lunch
Sandwich:
1 whole-grain pita bread
3 oz. water-packed tuna
Romaine lettuce (1 leaf)
¼ cup sliced tomato
⅛ cup onions
1 tbsp. fat-free ranch dressing

Sparkling Hibiscus Iced Water*

Afternoon Snack
1½ oz. low-fat cheese
½ cup grapes
Ginger Green Tea*

Dinner
Vegetable Spaghetti or Pasta* (¾ serving)
1 tbsp. soy cheese, grated
Green Salad*
Cornish Pixie Rose-Lemon Green Tea*

Supper (evening snack)
3 Lemon Ginger Biscuits (cookies)*
Chamomile Peach Tea*

APO E GENE
4/3 1,800 KCAL, DAY 1
Serving considerations per day:
　(be mindful of serving sizes)

Carbohydrates
11.5 servings grain/starch
5.5 servings fruit/vegetable

Protein
10 servings plant protein or fish

Fat
2.5 servings anti-inflammatory fat

Breakfast
1 slice whole-grain oat flax toast†
½ tbsp. honey
½ cup blueberries
½ cup soymilk
Jasmine Green Tea†
Apo E Diet Multivitamins™

Morning Snack
½ cup cherries
¾ cup cottage cheese or yogurt
Classic English Tea with Milk*

Lunch
Vegetable and Bean Tacos*
½ cup Tomato Salsa Cream*
1 cup low-fat soymilk
Ginger Green Tea*

Afternoon Snack
Sultana, Carrot, Ginger Coleslaw*
4 oz. whole-wheat pretzels
½ cup cherry tomatoes
The Green and Red Tea*

Dinner
3 oz. Grilled or Baked Fish (wild sea bass)*
Pam's Baked Potato*
3 tbsp. plain yogurt
1 tbsp. chives
1 cup steamed broccoli
½ slice whole-grain bread
1 oz. avocado
Peach Tea*

APO E 4/3 1,800 KCAL

Supper (evening snack)
Scottish Fruit Pottage*
½ cup frozen yogurt
Chamomile Hibiscus Tea*

APO E GENE
4/3 1,800 KCAL, DAY 2
Serving considerations per day:

Carbohydrates
3.5 servings grain/starch
12.5 servings fruit/vegetable

Protein
11 servings plant protein or fish

Fat
2 servings anti-inflammatory fat

Breakfast
Eggs (½–¾ cup egg whites or substitute)
¼ cup Tomato Salsa Cream* (½ serving)
1 slice whole-grain toast or
   whole-wheat tortilla
½ tbsp. honey
Ginger Green Tea*
Apo E Diet Multivitamins™

Morning Snack
Sultana, Carrot, Ginger Coleslaw*
1½ oz. soy cheese
Hibiscus Elder Tea*

Lunch
Tofu Salad*
1 medium apple
1 cup nonfat milk
Sparkling Orange Juice Iced Water*

Afternoon Snack
Carrot and Cucumber Yogurt Salad*
5 whole-wheat crackers
Lemon Lime Tea with Wild Mint*

Dinner
3 oz. Grilled or Baked Fish (trout)* with
   Soy Ginger Sauce*

Olive Oil Potato Wedgewood Fries*
Mevagissey Ratatouille* (2 servings)
Ginger and Turmeric Tea*

Supper (evening snack)
Apple and Blueberry Crumble*
   (½ serving)
English Vanilla Custard*
Peach Tea*

APO E GENE
4/3 1,800 KCAL, DAY 3
Serving considerations per day:

Carbohydrates
9.5 servings grain/starch
10.5 servings fruit/vegetable

Protein
12 servings plant protein or fish

Fat
4 servings anti-inflammatory fat

Breakfast
2 six-inch corn tortillas
2 egg whites or ¼ cup egg substitute
1½ oz. fat-free Almond Cheese*
½ cup Tomato Salsa Cream* (½ serving)
Jasmine Green Tea†
Apo E Diet Multivitamins™

Morning Snack
½ cup vanilla yogurt
1 cup blueberries
White Mint Tea*

Lunch
Sandwich:
2 slices whole-grain bread
3 oz. rock shrimp or crab
Tomato, lettuce, and onions
1 tbsp. low-fat canola or olive oil
   mayonnaise†

Sparkling Lemon Juice Iced Water*
   (consider using a crystal glass)

Afternoon Snack

Trail mix:

¼ cup almonds

¼ cup cranberries or raisins

½ cup low-fat granola

Matcha Tea†

Dinner

3 oz. Grilled or Baked Fish (sea bass)*

½ cup Tomato Salsa Cream*

½ cup black beans

Green Salad*

1 slice multigrain bread

Sparkling Lime Juice Iced Water*

Chamomile Peach Tea*

Supper (evening snack)

1 cup raspberries

Angel food cake

Chamomile Peach Tea*

APO E GENE

4/3 1,800 KCAL, DAY 4

Serving considerations per day:

Carbohydrates

7 servings grain/starch

12 servings fruit/vegetable

Protein

11 servings plant protein or fish

Fat

3 servings anti-inflammatory fat

Breakfast

Scottish Oatmeal*

1 cup nonfat milk

Ginger Green Tea*

Apo E Diet Multivitamins™

Morning Snack

¼ cup whole-grain granola

1 cup nonfat yogurt

½ cup berries

White Mint Tea*

Lunch

Sandwich:

1 whole-grain pita bread

4 oz. water-packed tuna

Romaine lettuce (1 leaf)

¼ cup sliced tomato

⅛ cup onions

1 tbsp. fat-free ranch dressing

Sparkling Hibiscus Iced Water*

Afternoon Snack

1 oz. soy cheese

½ cup grapes

Ginger Green Tea*

Dinner

Vegetable Spaghetti or Pasta*

1 tbsp. grated soy cheese

Green Salad*

Matcha Tea†

Supper (evening snack)

3 Raspberry Ginger Biscuits (cookies)*

Peach Tea*

APO E GENE
4/3 2,000 KCAL, DAY 1

Serving considerations per day:
  (be mindful of serving sizes)

Carbohydrates
5.5 servings grain/starch
9 servings fruit/vegetable

Protein
10 servings plant protein or fish

Fat
3 servings anti-inflammatory fat

Breakfast
Scottish Oatmeal*
⅛ cup raisins or cranberries
1 cup nonfat milk or soymilk
Matcha Tea†
Apo E Diet Multivitamins™

Morning Snack
Granola mix:
¼ cup low-fat granola
⅛ cup chopped walnuts
⅛ cup dried apricots
¾ cup nonfat yogurt

Lemon Ginger Green Tea*

Lunch
Vegetable and Bean Tacos* (1½ servings)
½ cup Tomato Salsa Cream*
½ medium apple
1 cup nonfat milk
Rosehip Green Tea*

Afternoon Snack
Simple Vegetarian Black Bean Soup*
  (½ serving)
¼ cup cherry tomatoes
Hibiscus Elder Tea*

Dinner
4 oz. Pam's Lime Rosemary
  Baked Chicken*
Pam's Baked Potato*
1½ oz. nonfat Almond Cheese*
1 tbsp. chives
Mevagissey Ratatouille*
Elder Hibiscus Tea*

Supper (evening snack)
½ cup low-fat chocolate frozen yogurt
Chamomile Hibiscus Tea*

APO E GENE
4/3 2,000 KCAL, DAY 2

Serving considerations per day:

Carbohydrates
8.5 servings grain/starch
7.5 servings fruit/vegetable

Protein
13 servings plant protein or fish

Fat
2 servings anti-inflammatory fat

Breakfast
1 whole-grain bagel
Eggs (½–¾ cup egg whites or substitute)
½ banana
½ tbsp. honey
Classic English Tea with Milk*
Apo E Diet Multivitamins™

Morning Snack
½ cup cherries or cherry tomatoes
½ cup nonfat cottage cheese
8 whole-grain crackers
Green Tea* (don't forget to consider a
  bone china cup)

Lunch
1 veggie burger
1½ oz. low-fat soy cheese
1 slice whole-grain bread
Romaine lettuce (1 leaf)
¼ cup sliced tomato
⅛ cup onions
4 green or black olives
1 oz. avocado
1 tbsp. low-fat canola or olive oil
  mayonnaise†
1 cup nonfat milk
Sparkling Orange Juice Iced Water*
  (consider a crystal glass)

Afternoon Snack
Quick Fresh Fruit Shake-to-Go*
(¾ serving)
Lemon Ginger Green Tea*

Dinner
4 oz. Grilled or Baked Fish (ahi tuna)*
½ cup black beans
1 slice whole-grain bread or oat flax
roll or bread
Mevagissey Ratatouille*
½ cup broccolini
Black Currant, Ginger, and Turmeric Tea*

Supper (evening snack)
3 small Lemon Ginger Biscuits (cookies)*
1 cup nonfat milk

APO E GENE
4/3 2,000 KCAL, DAY 3
Serving considerations per day:

Carbohydrates
7.5 servings grain/starch
11 servings fruit/vegetable

Protein
14.5 servings plant protein or fish

Fat
4 servings anti-Inflammatory fat

Breakfast
1 six-inch corn tortilla
½ cup egg substitute
1½ oz. fat-free cheese
¼ cup Tomato Salsa Cream* (½ serving)
½ cup melon
Ginger Green Tea*
Apo E Diet Multivitamins™

Morning Snack
1 medium apple
½ tbsp. natural nut butter
White Mint Tea*

Lunch
Sandwich:
1 slice whole-grain bread
4 oz. tofu
Romaine lettuce (1 leaf)
¼ cup sliced tomato
⅛ cup onions
1 tbsp. low-fat canola or olive oil
mayonnaise†

1 cup nonfat or soymilk

Afternoon Snack
Trail mix:
⅛ cup almonds
¼ cup cranberries or raisins
½ cup low-fat granola
⅔ cup nonfat Soy Yogurt*

Matcha Tea†

Dinner
Vegetable Spaghetti or Pasta* (¾ serving)
1 tbsp. Parmesan cheese
Green Salad
1 slice whole-grain bread
Sparkling Lime Juice Iced Water* and
Chamomile Peach Tea*

Supper (evening snack)
1 cup blackberries
Vanilla angel food cake
1 cup nonfat milk

APO E GENE
4/3 2,000 KCAL, DAY 4
Serving considerations per day:

Carbohydrates
8.5 servings grain/starch
10 servings fruit/vegetable

Protein
13.5 servings plant protein or fish

Fat
3 servings anti-inflammatory fat

Breakfast
1 cup whole-grain dry cereal
½ banana
1 cup soymilk or nonfat milk
Ginger Green Tea*
Apo E Diet Multivitamins™

Morning Snack
Snack break mix:
½ cup low-fat granola
⅛ cup of your favorite dried fruit,
    such as dried apricots
½ cup nonfat cottage cheese

The Red and Green Tea*

Lunch
Olive Oil Potato Wedgewood Fries*
1 cup Cornish Chili*
1½. oz. fat-free soy cheese, shredded
1 cup cooked broccoli
Lettuce, tomatoes, and onions (1–2 cups)

Sparkling Hibiscus Iced Water*

Afternoon Snack
Carrot and Cucumber Yogurt Salad*
Lemon Ginger Green Tea*

Dinner
4 oz. Grilled or Baked Fish (wild salmon)*
Pam's Baked Potato (½ serving)
Wok-steamed: ½ cup raw kale, garlic, ¼
    chopped onion, ¼ cup corn, and 1
    tomato.
1 tbsp. Parmesan cheese
Sparkling Lemon Juice Iced Water*

Supper (evening snack)
Pear and Black Currant Crumble*
    (½ serving)
Chamomile Peach Tea*

APO E GENE
4/3 2,400 KCAL, DAY 1
Serving considerations per day:
(be mindful of serving sizes)

Carbohydrates
6.5 servings grain/starch
9.5 servings fruit/vegetable

Protein
14.5 servings plant protein or fish

Fat
2.5 servings anti-inflammatory fat

Breakfast
Orange Shake-to-Go* (½ serving)
½ whole-grain bagel
½ tbsp. honey
⅛ cup raisins or cranberries
1 cup nonfat milk or soymilk and
   Ginger Green Tea*
Apo E Diet Multivitamins™

Morning Snack
Granola mix:
¼ cup low-fat granola
⅛ cup chopped walnuts
⅛ cup dried apricots
¾ cup Almond Milk*

Peach Tea*

Lunch
Vegetable and Bean Tacos*
¼ cup Tomato Salsa Cream* (½ serving)
⅓ cup black beans
½ medium apple
1 cup nonfat or soymilk
Cornish Pixie Rose-Lemon Green Tea*

Afternoon Snack
Cornish Chili* (¾ serving)
4 whole-grain crackers
Iced or hot Hibiscus Elder Tea*

Dinner
5 oz. Grilled or Baked Fish (halibut)* with
   Soy Ginger Sauce*

Pam's Baked Potato*
1½ oz. nonfat cheese
1 tbsp. chives
Grilled vegetables: ½ cup yellow squash
   and 6–8 asparagus spears
Iced Classic English Tea with Milk*

Supper (evening snack)
1 cup blueberries
Angel food cake
¾ cup nonfat warm vanilla yogurt
Iced Chamomile Peach Tea*

APO E GENE
4/3 2,400 KCAL, DAY 2
Serving considerations per day:

Carbohydrates
4.5 servings grain/starch
15.5 servings fruit/vegetable

Protein
12.5 servings plant protein or fish

Fat
3 servings anti-inflammatory fat

Breakfast
Scottish Oatmeal™
⅛ cup raisins
½ tbsp. honey
1 cup nonfat milk
Black Currant, Ginger, and Turmeric Tea*
Apo E Diet Multivitamins™

Morning Snack
1 slice whole-grain oat flax bread
1½ tbsp. raisins
½ cup nonfat yogurt
Iced or hot Ginger Green Tea*

Lunch
Open-faced sandwich:
½ whole-grain bun or 1 slice bread
Tofu Salad* (¾ serving)

½ medium apple

1 cup nonfat milk
Sparkling Orange Juice Iced Water*

Afternoon Snack
Carrot and Cucumber Yogurt Salad*
   (1½ servings)
½ cup carrots or jicama slices
1 slice multigrain bread
Sparkling Orange Juice Iced Water*

Dinner
4 oz. Baked Fish (Flounder)*
Green Salad*
Olive Oil Potato Wedgewood Fries*
   (½ serving)
Iced Rosehip Green Tea*

Supper (evening snack)
Kelly's Fore Street Dessert* (½ serving)
White Tea with Cranberries*

**APO E GENE
4/3 2,400 KCAL, DAY 3**
Serving considerations per day:

Carbohydrates
8 servings grain/starch
16.5 servings fruit/vegetable

Protein
16.5 servings plant protein or fish

Fat
8.5 servings anti-inflammatory fat

Breakfast
2 six-inch corn tortillas
Eggs (½–¾ cup egg whites or substitute)
3 oz. fat-free cheese
¼ cup baked beans
1 oz. avocado
¼ cup Fresh Tomato Salsa*
½ cup melon
Green Tea*
Apo E Diet Multivitamins™

Morning Snack
1 medium apple
½ tbsp. natural nut butter
½ cup nonfat Almond Cheese*
White Mint Tea*

Lunch
Fish Salad*
1 whole-grain pita bread
1 cup Almond Milk*
Sparkling Lemon or Lime Juice Iced Juice
Water*
   (don't forget a pretty glass)

Afternoon Snack
Quick Fresh Fruit Shake-to-Go*
   (¾ serving)
Ginger Green Tea*

Dinner
Vegetable Pasta*
1 tbsp. Parmesan cheese
Green Salad*
1 slice whole-grain bread
1 cup nonfat soymilk
Chamomile Peach Tea*

Supper (evening snack)
½ cup orange frozen yogurt
Scottish Fruit Pottage* (2 servings)
Hibiscus Elder Tea*

**APO E GENE
4/3 2,400 KCAL, DAY 4**
Serving considerations per day:

Carbohydrates
9.5 servings grain/starch
15 servings fruit/vegetable

Protein
15 servings plant protein or fish

Fat
4.5 servings anti-inflammatory fat

Breakfast
Blueberry Oat Muffin*
Baked Apples* (½ serving)
Eggs (½–¾ cup egg whites or substitute)
1 medium orange
1 cup nonfat milk
Jasmine Green Tea†
Apo E Diet Multivitamins™

Morning Snack
⅓ cup low-fat whole-grain granola
¾ cup nonfat Soy Yogurt*
1 cup fresh strawberries
White Mint Tea*

Lunch
Rustic Tuscany Pizza*
Green Salad*
Chamomile Hibiscus Tea*

Afternoon Snack
Carrot and Cucumber Yogurt Salad*
¾ cup nonfat cottage cheese
Lemon Ginger Green Tea*

Dinner
5 oz. Grilled or Baked Salmon
   with Teriyaki Shiitake Mushroom Sauce*
Pam's Baked Potato* (½ serving)
Mevagissey Ratatouille*
1 tbsp. Parmesan cheese
1 slice whole-grain bread
1 tsp. avocado
Sparkling Orange Juice Iced Water* and
   Elder Hibiscus Tea*

Supper (evening snack)
½ cup Peach and Blackberry Crumble*
¾ cup nonfat warm vanilla yogurt
Ginger Green Tea*

APO E 4/3 2,400 KCAL

APO E GENE
4/2 1,600 KCAL, DAY 1
Serving considerations per day:
(be mindful of serving sizes)

Carbohydrates
6 servings grain/starch
13.5 servings fruit/vegetable

Protein
7 servings protein

Fat
5 servings anti-inflammatory fat

Breakfast
1 slice whole-grain toast
½ tbsp. nut butter
½ banana
1 tbsp. honey
Classic English Tea with Milk*
Apo E Diet Multivitamins™

Morning Snack
1½ cups jicama, radish, and carrot sticks
2 tbsp. Original Hummus*
Sparkling Lime Juice Iced Water*

Lunch
Sandwich:
2 slices whole-grain bread
3 oz. sliced tuna steak
Romaine lettuce (1 leaf)
¼ cup sliced tomato
¼ cup sliced cucumber
⅛ cup red onion
1 oz. avocado

Sparkling Lemon Juice Iced Water*

Afternoon Snack
½ medium apple, sliced
1 oz. soy cheese
Lemon Ginger Green Tea*

Dinner
Vegetable Spaghetti or Pasta* (¾ serving)
1 tbsp. soy Parmesan cheese
Green Salad*
Chamomile Peach Tea*

Supper (evening snack)
Black Currant and Rhubarb Crumble*
(½ serving)
1 cup nonfat milk

APO E GENE
4/2 1,600 KCAL, DAY 2
Serving considerations per day:

Carbohydrates
6.5 servings grain/starch
10 servings fruit/vegetable

Protein
8.5 servings protein

Fat
3 servings anti-inflammatory fat

Breakfast
Blueberry Sultana Oat Bread* (¾ serving)
1 tbsp. honey
Green Tea*
Apo E Diet Multivitamins™

Morning Snack
1 cup Soy Yogurt*
¼ cup low-fat granola
1 cup grapes or cherries
White Mint Tea*

Lunch
Sandwich:
½ whole-grain pita bread
2 oz. fresh crab
Romaine lettuce (1 leaf)
¼ cup sliced tomato
⅛ cup red onion
1 oz. avocado
1 tbsp. low-fat ranch dressing (olive or
canola oil)
1 oz. low-fat soy cheese

Sparkling Orange Juice Iced Water*

Afternoon Snack
Carrot and Cucumber Yogurt Salad*
5 whole-grain crackers
Ginger Green Tea*

Dinner
4 oz. Grilled or Baked Fish (wild salmon)*
Green Salad*
1 slice whole-grain bread
½ cup steamed spinach
1 cup soymilk
Rosehip Green Tea*

Supper (evening snack)
Orange angel food cake
1 cup nonfat milk
Chamomile Peach Tea*

APO E GENE
4/2 1,600 KCAL, DAY 3
Serving considerations per day:

Carbohydrates
5.5 servings grain/starch
10 servings fruit/vegetable

Protein
8 servings protein

Fat
8 servings anti-inflammatory fat

Breakfast
Omelet* (¾ serving)
½ cup mixed berries
1 cup Tomato Salsa Cream* (2 servings)
Classic English Tea with Milk *
Apo E Diet Multivitamins™

Morning Snack
1 medium apple, sliced
½ tbsp. nut butter
White Mint Tea*

Lunch
Open-faced sandwich:
1 slice whole-grain bread
2 oz. herring or tuna

1 tbsp. low-fat canola or olive oil
    mayonnaise†
1 cup romaine lettuce
¼ cup chopped cabbage
½ cup broccoli
1 oz. avocado

1 cup nonfat milk
Ginger Green Tea*

Afternoon Snack
Carrot and Cucumber Yogurt Salad*
¾ oz. pretzels
Matcha Tea†

Dinner
Salad: spinach, cherry tomatoes, cabbage,
    broccoli, carrots (1½ cups)
2 oz. Roast Rosemary Turkey*
½ cup cooked basmati rice
Simple Salad Dressing*
Sparkling Lime Juice Iced Water* and
    Green Tea*

Supper (evening snack)
3 Ginger Biscuits (cookies)*
1 cup nonfat milk

APO E GENE
4/2 1,600 KCAL, DAY 4
Serving considerations per day:

Carbohydrates
4.75 servings grain/starch
15 servings fruit/vegetable

Protein
4.75 servings protein

Fat
5.5 servings anti-inflammatory fat

Breakfast
Scottish Oatmeal*
½ cup nonfat milk
Green Tea* with orange slices
Apo E Diet Multivitamins™

Morning Snack
½ banana
Golf Snack Mix* (½ serving)
½ cup nonfat milk

Lunch
1 veggie burger
2 slices whole-grain toast
1 oz. low-fat soy cheese
Romaine lettuce (1 leaf)
¼ cup sliced tomato
⅛ cup red onion
1 oz. avocado

Small cooked red potato
1 tbsp. nonfat dressing
Sparkling Hibiscus Iced Water*

Afternoon Snack
Carrot and Cucumber Yogurt Salad*
    (¾ serving)
Ginger Green Tea*

Dinner
Shiitake Mushroom and Spinach Lasagna*
    (½ serving)
1 tbsp. grated low-fat cheese
Green Salad* (1½ servings)
1 slice multigrain bread
Sparkling Orange Juice Iced Water* and
    Hibiscus Elder Tea*

Supper (evening snack)
½ cup plain nonfat yogurt
½ cup fresh strawberries
Peach Tea*

APO E GENE
4/2 1,800 KCAL, DAY 1
Serving considerations per day:
(be mindful of serving sizes)

Carbohydrates
7.5 servings grain/starch
11.5 servings fruit/vegetable

Protein
7 servings protein

Fat
5 servings anti-inflammatory fat

Breakfast
1 slice whole-grain toast
½ tbsp. nut butter
1 banana
Green Tea*
Apo E Diet Multivitamins™

Morning Snack
1 cup nonfat Soy Yogurt*
Snack mix (½ cup low-fat granola, and
⅛ cup apricots)
Jasmine Green Tea†

Lunch
Sandwich:
2 slices whole-grain bread
3 oz. fresh wild baby shrimp
Romaine lettuce (1 leaf)
¼ cup sliced tomato
¼ cup sliced cucumber
⅛ cup red onion

Classic English Tea with Milk*

Afternoon Snack
1 medium apple, sliced
1 oz. soy cheese
Lemon Ginger Green Tea*

Dinner
Vegetable Spaghetti or Pasta* (¾ serving)
1 tbsp. soy Parmesan cheese
Green Salad*
1 slice whole-grain bread
1 oz. avocado

Matcha Tea†

Supper (evening snack)
½ cup strawberry low-fat soy frozen yogurt
Chamomile Peach Tea*

APO E GENE
4/2 1,800 KCAL, DAY 2
Serving considerations per day:

Carbohydrates
8.5 servings grain/starch
8 servings fruit/vegetable

Protein
9.5 servings protein

Fat
4 servings anti-inflammatory fat

Breakfast
Raspberry Oat Bread (¾ serving)
1 tbsp. honey
Green Tea*
Apo E Diet Multivitamins™

Morning Snack
1 cup Soy Yogurt*(2 servings)
¼ cup low-fat granola
½ cup grapes or cherries
White Mint Tea*

Lunch
Sandwich:
1 whole-grain pita bread
3 oz. sardines†
Romaine lettuce (1 leaf)
¼ cup sliced tomato
¼ cup sliced cucumber
⅛ cup red onion
1 oz. avocado
8 olives

Sparkling Orange Juice Iced Water *

Afternoon Snack
Carrot and Cucumber Yogurt Salad*
4 whole-grain crackers
Matcha Tea†

APO E 4/2 1,800 KCAL

Dinner
3 oz. Baked Fish (wild halibut)*
½ cup steamed broccolini
½ cup steamed spinach
¾ cup cooked wild rice
¼ cup white beans
2 tbsp. Salsa Cream*
1 tbsp. chives
Chamomile Tea* with rosehips and lemon

Supper (evening snack)
½ cup red grapes
3 Orange Ginger Biscuits (cookies)
1 cup soymilk

APO E GENE
4/2 1,800 KCAL, DAY 3
Serving considerations per day:

Carbohydrates
8 servings grain/starch
6.5 servings fruit/vegetable

Protein
10 servings protein

Fat
5.5 servings anti-inflammatory fat

Breakfast
1 cup bran cereal
1 cup soymilk
½ cup blueberries
1 tbsp. honey
Black Currant, Ginger, and Turmeric Tea*
Apo E Diet Multivitamins™

Morning Snack
Banana Almond Shake-to-Go* (¾ serving)
White Mint Tea*

Lunch
1 veggie burger
2 slices whole-grain bread
Romaine lettuce (1 leaf)
¼ cup sliced tomato
⅛ cup red onion

1 oz. avocado
Ginger Green Tea*

Afternoon Snack
Carrot and Cucumber Yogurt Salad*
Rosehip Green Tea*

Dinner
12-inch corn tortilla or four 6-inch tortillas
3 oz. Pam's Lime Rosemary Baked Chicken*
   (¾ serving)
1½ oz. low-fat soy cheese
Romaine lettuce (1 leaf)
¼ cup sliced tomato
⅛ cup red onion
1 oz. avocado
2 tbsp. Tomato Salsa Cream* (¼ serving)
Sparkling Lime Juice Iced Water* and
   Peach Tea*

Supper (evening snack)
½ cup fresh sliced strawberries
5 Raspberry Ginger Biscuits (cookies)*
   (1½ servings)
Rosehip Green Tea*

APO E GENE
4/2 1,800 KCAL, DAY 4
Serving considerations per day:

Carbohydrates
5.5 servings grain/starch
11.5 servings fruit/vegetable

Protein
7 servings protein

Fat
4 servings anti-inflammatory fat

Breakfast
Scottish Oatmeal*
½ tbsp. honey
⅛ cup sultanas
½ cup nonfat milk
Ginger Green Tea*
Apo E Diet Multivitamins™

Morning Snack
¾ oz. whole-wheat pretzels
½ cup raspberry nonfat yogurt
Jasmine Green Tea[†]

Lunch
Sandwich:
½ whole-grain pita bread
Romaine lettuce (1 leaf)
¼ cup sliced tomato
¼ cup celery
⅛ cup red onion
1 oz. avocado
3 oz. Grilled or Baked Fish (black cod)*

Lemon Lime Tea with Wild Mint*

Afternoon Snack
Carrot and Cucumber Yogurt Salad*
4 whole-grain crackers
White Tea with Cranberries*

Dinner
Shiitake Mushroom and Spinach Lasagna*
  (¾ serving)
1 tbsp. Parmesan cheese
Green Salad*
½ slice whole-grain bread
4 steamed asparagus spears with lemon
Iced Hibiscus Elder Tea*

Supper (evening snack)
3 Ginger Biscuits (cookies)*
1 cup ice-cold nonfat milk

APO E 4/2 1,800 KCAL

APO E GENE
4/2 2,000 KCAL, DAY 1
Serving considerations per day:
   (be mindful of serving sizes)

Carbohydrates
6 servings grain/starch
7 servings fruit/vegetable

Protein
7 servings protein

Fat
5 servings anti-inflammatory fat

Breakfast
1 cup oatmeal
½ tbsp. honey
1 tbsp. ground flaxseed[†]
⅛ cup sultanas
1 cup soymilk
The Green and Red Tea*
Apo E Diet Multivitamins™

Morning Snack
1 medium apple
2 dates
½ tbsp. nut butter
Rosehip Green Tea*

Lunch
Mevagissey Fish Tacos* (¾ serving)
2 tbsp. Nonfat Papaya Salsa Cream*
   (¼ serving)
Sparkling Lemon Juice Iced Water*

Afternoon Snack
Sultana, Carrot, Ginger Coleslaw*
   (½ serving)
1 cup nonfat milk
Lemon Ginger Green Tea*

Dinner
3 oz. Grilled or Baked Fish (halibut)* with
   Teriyaki Sauce*
6 steamed asparagus spears
Pam's Baked Potato* (½ serving)
½ slice whole-grain bread

1 oz. avocado
Hibiscus Elder Tea*

Supper (evening snack)
Peach and Blackberry Crumble*
   (¾ serving)
½ cup frozen yogurt
Chamomile Peach Tea*

APO E GENE
4/2 2,000 KCAL, DAY 2
Serving considerations per day:

Carbohydrates
10 servings grain/starch
11 servings fruit/vegetable

Protein
9 servings protein

Fat
5 servings anti-inflammatory fat

Breakfast
2 slices whole-grain bread
1 tbsp. nut butter
1 banana
½ tbsp. honey
Matcha Tea[†]
Apo E Diet Multivitamins™

Morning Snack
½ cup low-fat granola
1 cup nonfat Soy Yogurt*
Black Currant, Ginger, and Turmeric Tea*

Lunch
1 veggie burger
2 slices whole-grain bread
Romaine lettuce (1 leaf)
¼ cup sliced tomato
1 tbsp. low-fat canola or olive oil
   mayonnaise[†]
Sparkling Orange Juice Iced Water*

Afternoon Snack
Sultana, Carrot, Ginger Coleslaw*
   (½ serving)

1 slice multigrain bread
White Tea with Cranberries*

Dinner
4 oz. Grilled or Baked Fish (tuna steak)*
    with Teriyaki Sauce*
½ cup broccoli or broccolini
¼ cup cooked white beans
Green Salad*
½ cup steamed spinach
½ slice whole-grain bread
1 cup nonfat milk
Chamomile Peach Tea*

Supper (evening snack)
Scottish Fruit Pottage*
½ cup low-fat frozen soy yogurt
Rosehip Green Tea*

APO E GENE
4/2 2,000 KCAL, DAY 3
Serving considerations per day:

Carbohydrates
10.5 servings grain/starch
10 servings fruit/vegetable

Protein
12 servings protein

Fat
5 servings anti-inflammatory fat

Breakfast
Eggs (½–¾ cup egg whites or substitute)
½ cup baked beans
¼ cup Fresh Tomato Salsa*
1 oz. avocado
½ whole-grain bagel, toasted
½ cup fresh cut melon
The Green and Red Tea*
Apo E Diet Multivitamins™

Morning Snack
Golf Snack Mix*
1 medium peach
White Mint Tea*

Lunch
Prawn salad sandwich:
1 whole-wheat pita bread
3 oz. grilled prawns
Romaine lettuce (1 leaf)
¼ cup sliced tomato
⅛ cup red onion
4 Mediterranean olives

1 cup nonfat milk
Ginger Green Tea*

Afternoon Snack
1 cup Pam's Vegetable Soup*
7 whole-grain crackers
Matcha Tea†

Dinner
3 oz. Roast Rosemary Chicken*
    (¾ serving)
Olive Oil Potato Wedgewood Fries*
Green Salad*
1 slice whole-grain bread
Sparkling Lime Juice Iced Water*
Peach Tea*

Supper (evening snack)
3 Ginger Biscuits (cookies)*
1 cup nonfat milk

APO E GENE
4/2 2,000 KCAL, DAY 4
Serving considerations per day:

Carbohydrates
10 servings grain/starch
9 servings fruit/vegetable

Protein
10.5 servings protein

Fat
4.5 servings anti-inflammatory fat

Breakfast
1 orange
Blueberry Sultana Oat Bread* (¾ serving)
Eggs (½–¾ cup egg whites or substitute)

1 tbsp. honey
White Tea with Cranberries*
Apo E Diet Multivitamins™

Morning Snack
1 medium apple
1 cup Soy Yogurt*
⅓ cup low-fat granola
Sparkling Orange Juice Iced Water*

Lunch
Sandwich:
1 whole-grain pita bread
3 oz. Grilled or Baked Fish (sea bass)*
1 tbsp. fat-free ranch dressing
Romaine lettuce (1 leaf)
¼ cup sliced tomato
¼ cup celery
⅛ cup red onion
1 oz. avocado

Iced Black Currant, Ginger, and
    Turmeric Tea*

Afternoon Snack
⅓ cup Original Hummus*
7 whole-grain crackers
White Tea with Cranberries*

Dinner
3 oz. Grilled or Baked Fish (wild salmon)*
1 tbsp. chopped almonds
Green Salad*
2 slices whole-grain bread
6 steamed asparagus spears with lemon
1 cup nonfat milk
Peach Tea*

Supper (evening snack)
¾ cup sliced strawberries and blueberries
Chocolate angel food cake
Chamomile Hibiscus Tea*

APO E GENE
4/2 2,400 KCAL, DAY 1
Serving considerations per day:
   (be mindful of serving sizes)

Carbohydrates
10 servings grain/starch
11.5 servings fruit/vegetable

Protein
12.5 servings protein

Fat
6 servings anti-inflammatory fat

Breakfast
Eggs (½–¾ cup egg whites or substitute)
2 slices toasted oat bran bread
1 tbsp. nut butter
½ cup fresh mixed berries
Jasmine Green Tea†
Apo E Diet Multivitamins™

Morning Snack
Golf Snack Mix*
½ cup nonfat soy cottage cheese
Ginger and Turmeric Tea*

Lunch
Sandwich:
1 whole-grain pita bread
1 cup mixed shredded lettuce
   and chopped onions
2 oz. Grilled or Baked Fish (mackerel)*
1 oz. avocado

1 cup fresh papaya slices
Sparkling Lemon Juice Iced Water*

Afternoon Snack
2 tbsp. almonds
1 cup Pam's Vegetable Soup*
2 mandarin oranges
Lemon Ginger Green Tea*

Dinner
3 oz. grilled Cornish game hen breast
1 cup whole-wheat spaghetti
1 tbsp. Parmesan cheese

1 cup steamed broccoli
½ cup steamed carrots
1 cup nonfat milk
Hibiscus Elder Tea*

Supper (evening snack)
Peach and Blackberry Crumble*
   (¾ serving)
½ cup low-fat vanilla soy ice cream
Chamomile Hibiscus Tea*

APO E GENE
4/2 2,400 KCAL, DAY 2
Serving considerations per day:

Carbohydrates
11 servings grain/starch
8.5 servings fruit/vegetable

Protein
14 servings protein

Fat
8 servings anti-inflammatory fat

Breakfast
2 six-inch corn tortillas
¼ cup egg substitute
¼ avocado
1½ oz. low-fat soy cheese
¼ cup Fresh Tomato Salsa*
½ cup melon
White Mint Tea* with lemon
Apo E Diet Multivitamins™

Morning Snack
1 whole-grain bagel, toasted
1 tbsp. nut butter
1 cup soymilk
Ginger Green Tea*

Lunch
1 veggie burger
Blueberry Sultana Oat Bread*
Romaine lettuce (1 leaf)
¼ cup sliced tomato
⅛ cup red onion

1 tbsp. low-fat canola or olive oil mayonnaise[†]
1 oz. avocado

Sparkling Orange Juice Iced Water*

Afternoon Snack
Sultana, Carrot, Ginger Coleslaw (½ serving)
4 whole-grain crackers
Matcha Tea[†]

Dinner
6 oz. Grilled Shrimp with Teriyaki Sauce*
9 steamed asparagus spears
½ cup cooked basmati rice
Sliced tomato with balsamic vinegar
Pam's Baked Potato*
2 tbsp. Nonfat Papaya Salsa Cream*
   (¼ serving)
1 tbsp. fresh chopped chives
Sparkling Lemon Juice Iced Water* and
   Chamomile Tea*

Supper (evening snack)
1 cup Mixed Berry Crumble*
½ cup low-fat frozen soy yogurt
Peach Tea*

**APO E GENE
4/2 2,400 KCAL, DAY 3**
Serving considerations per day:

Carbohydrates
9 servings grain/starch
12.5 servings fruit/vegetable

Protein
11 servings protein

Fat
5.5 servings anti-inflammatory fat

Breakfast
1 cup oat bran flakes
¼ cup sultanas
½ banana
1 cup soymilk
Ginger Green Tea*
Apo E Diet Multivitamins™

Morning Snack
1 tbsp. nut butter
1 slice whole-grain bread, toasted
1 medium apple, sliced
White Mint Tea*

Lunch
Rustic Tuscany Pizza*
Green Salad*
Iced lemon Green Tea*
Afternoon Snack
Sultana, Carrot, Ginger Coleslaw*
   (½ serving)
8 whole-grain crackers
Matcha Tea[†]

Dinner
5 oz. Grilled or Baked Fish (halibut)*
¼ cup Mango Salsa Cream*
6 steamed asparagus spears
1 slice whole-grain bread
1 cup soymilk
Hibiscus Elder Tea*

Supper (evening snack)
Kelly's Fore Street Dessert* (½ serving)
1 cup nonfat milk

**APO E GENE
4/2 2,400 KCAL, DAY 4**
Serving considerations per day:

Carbohydrates
9.5 servings grain/starch
7.5 servings fruit/vegetable

Protein
11 servings protein

Fat
6 servings anti-inflammatory fat

Breakfast
Blueberry Sultana Oat Bread*
1 cup nonfat strawberry yogurt
Green Tea*
Apo E Diet Multivitamins™

Morning Snack
Banana Almond Shake-to-Go* (¾ serving)
Peach Tea*

Lunch
Sandwich:
1 veggie burger
1½ oz. slice low-fat soy cheese
2 slices whole-grain bread
Romaine lettuce (1 leaf)
¼ cup sliced tomato
⅛ cup red onion
1 tbsp. low-fat canola or olive oil
    mayonnaise†

Ginger and Turmeric Tea* and Lemon
    Lime Tea with Wild Mint*

Afternoon Snack
2 fresh dates
1 medium orange or apple
White Tea with Cranberries *

Dinner
Pam's Lime Rosemary Baked Chicken*
1 medium baked red potato (2.5" by 4.5")
Mcvagissey Ratatouille*
1 slice whole-grain bread
Sparkling Orange Juice Iced Water* and
    Chamomile Peach Tea*

Supper (evening snack)
Peach and Blackberry Crumble*
½ cup low-fat soy ice cream
Lemon Ginger Green Tea*

APO E 4/2 2,400 KCAL

APO E GENE
3/3 1,600 KCAL, DAY 1

Serving considerations per day:
(be mindful of serving sizes)

Carbohydrates
6 servings grain/starch
13.5 servings fruit/vegetable

Protein
7 servings protein

Fat
5 servings anti-inflammatory fat

Breakfast
1 slice whole-grain toast
½ tbsp. nut butter
½ banana
1 tbsp. honey
White Mint Tea*
Apo E Diet Multivitamins™

Morning Snack
1½ cups jicama, radish, and carrot sticks
2 tbsp. Original Hummus*
Cornish Pixie Rose-Lemon Green Tea*

Lunch
Sandwich:
2 slices whole-grain bread
3 oz. sliced chicken breast
Romaine lettuce (1 leaf)
¼ cup sliced tomato
¼ cup sliced cucumber
⅛ cup red onion
1 oz. avocado

Sparkling Lemon Juice Iced Water*

Afternoon Snack
½ medium apple, sliced
1 oz. soy cheese
Lemon Ginger Green Tea*

Dinner
Vegetable Spaghetti or Pasta* (¾ serving)
1 tbsp. soy Parmesan cheese
Green Salad*
Classic English Tea with Milk*

Supper (evening snack)
Black Currant and Rhubarb Crumble*
(½ serving)
1 cup nonfat milk
Chamomile Hibiscus Tea*

APO E GENE
3/3 1,600 KCAL, DAY 2

Serving considerations per day:

Carbohydrates
6.5 servings grain/starch
10 servings fruit/vegetable

Protein
8.5 servings protein

Fat
3 servings anti-inflammatory fat

Breakfast
Blueberry Sultana Oat Bread* (¾ serving)
1 tbsp. honey
Green Tea*
Apo E Diet Multivitamins™

Morning Snack
Soy Yogurt*
¼ cup low-fat granola
1 cup grapes or cherries
White Tea with Cranberries*

Lunch
Sandwich:
½ whole-grain pita bread
Lettuce, cucumber, onion, and tomato
(1–2 cups)
2 oz. sliced chicken
1 oz. avocado
1 tbsp. low-fat ranch dressing (olive or
canola oil)
1 oz. low-fat soy cheese

Sparkling Orange Juice Iced Water*

Afternoon Snack
Carrot and Cucumber Yogurt Salad*
5 whole-grain crackers
Green Tea*

Dinner
4 oz. Grilled or Baked Fish (wild salmon)*
½ cup steamed spinach
Green Salad*
1 slice whole-grain bread
1 cup soymilk
Chamomile Hibiscus Tea*

Supper (evening snack)
Orange angel food cake
1 cup nonfat milk
Rosehip Green Tea*

**APO E GENE
3/3 1,600 KCAL, DAY 3**
Serving considerations per day:

Carbohydrates
5.5 servings grain/starch
10 servings fruit/vegetable

Protein
8 servings protein

Fat
8 servings anti-inflammatory fat

Breakfast
Omelet* (¾ serving)
½ cup mixed berries
1 cup Tomato Salsa Cream* (2 servings)
White Mint Tea*
Apo E Diet Multivitamins™

Morning Snack
1 medium apple, sliced
½ tbsp. nut butter
Ginger Green Tea*

Lunch
Open-faced sandwich:
1 slice whole-grain bread
2 oz. herring or tuna
1 tbsp. olive or canola oil mayonnaise†
Romaine lettuce, chopped onions,
cabbage, broccoli, and carrots (1–2 cups)
1 oz. avocado

1 cup nonfat milk
Ginger Green Tea*

Afternoon Snack
Carrot and Cucumber Yogurt Salad*
¾ oz. pretzels
Matcha Tea†

Dinner
Salad: spinach, cherry tomatoes, cabbage,
  broccoli, carrots (1½ cups)
2 oz. Roast Rosemary Turkey*
½ cup cooked basmati rice
Simple Salad Dressing*
Sparkling Lime Juice Iced Water*
Peach Tea*

Supper (evening snack)
3 Lemon Ginger Biscuits (cookies)*
1 cup nonfat milk

**APO E GENE
3/3 1,600 KCAL, DAY 4**
Serving considerations per day:

Carbohydrates
4.75 servings grain/starch
15 servings fruit/vegetable

Protein
4.75 servings protein

Fat
5.5 servings anti-inflammatory fat

Breakfast
Scottish Oatmeal*
½ cup nonfat milk
Green Tea* with orange slices
Apo E Diet Multivitamins™

Morning Snack
½ banana
Golf Snack Mix* (½ serving)
½ cup nonfat milk

Lunch
Sandwich:
1 veggie burger
2 slices whole-grain toast
1½ oz. slice low-fat soy cheese

1 oz. avocado
1 tbsp. nonfat dressing

Sparkling Orange Juice Iced Water*

Afternoon Snack
Carrot and Cucumber Yogurt Salad*
    (¾ serving)
Ginger Green Tea*

Dinner
Shiitake Mushroom and Spinach Lasagna*
    (½ serving)
1 tbsp. grated low-fat cheese
Green Salad* (1½ serving)
1 slice multigrain bread
Sparkling Orange Juice Iced Water* and
    White Tea with Cranberries*

Supper (evening snack)
½ cup plain nonfat yogurt
½ cup fresh strawberries
Chamomile Hibiscus Tea*

APO E GENE
3/3 1,800 KCAL, DAY 1
Serving considerations per day:
  (be mindful of serving sizes)

Carbohydrates
7.5 servings grain/starch
11.5 servings fruit/vegetable

Protein
7 servings protein

Fat
5 servings anti-inflammatory fat

Breakfast
1 slice whole-grain toast
½ tbsp. nut butter
1 banana
Black Currant, Ginger, and Turmeric Tea*
Apo E Diet Multivitamins™

Morning Snack
1 cup nonfat yogurt
Snack mix (½ cup low-fat granola and
  ⅛ cup apricots)
White Mint Tea*

Lunch
Sandwich:
2 slices whole-grain bread
3 oz. sliced chicken breast
1½ oz. slice low-fat soy cheese
1 oz. avocado

Sparkling Lemon Juice Iced Water*

Afternoon Snack
1 medium apple, sliced
1 oz. whole soy cheese
Lemon Ginger Green Tea*

Dinner
Vegetable Spaghetti or Pasta* (¾ serving)
1 tbsp. soy Parmesan cheese
Green Salad*
1 slice whole-grain bread
1 oz. avocado
Hibiscus Elder Tea*

Supper (evening snack)
½ cup strawberry low-fat soy frozen yogurt
Chamomile Peach Tea*

APO E GENE
3/3 1,800 KCAL, DAY 2
Serving considerations per day:

Carbohydrates
8.5 servings grain/starch
8 servings fruit/vegetable

Protein
9.5 servings protein

Fat
4 servings anti-inflammatory fat

Breakfast
Blueberry Sultana Oat Bread*
  (¾ serving)
1 tbsp. honey
Green Tea* with fresh squeezed juice of
  ½ lemon
Apo E Diet Multivitamins™

Morning Snack
1 cup Soy Yogurt* (2 servings)
¼ cup low-fat granola
½ cup grapes or cherries
Black Currant, Ginger, and Turmeric Tea*

Lunch
Sandwich:
1 whole-grain pita bread
3 oz. sardines
Romaine lettuce (1 leaf)
¼ cup sliced tomato
¼ cup sliced cucumber
⅛ cup red onion
1 oz. avocado
8 olives

Sparkling Orange Juice Iced Water*

Afternoon Snack
1 cup sliced carrot and cucumber
¼ cup Original Hummus*

4 whole-grain crackers
Matcha Tea†

Dinner
3 oz. Grilled or Baked Fish (halibut)*
½ cup steamed broccolini
½ cup steamed spinach
¾ cup cooked wild rice
¼ cup white beans
2 tbsp. Hawaiian Mango Salsa*
1 tbsp. chives
Chamomile Tea* with rosehips and lemon

Supper (evening snack)
½ cup red grapes
3 Lemon Ginger Biscuits (cookies)*
1 cup soymilk
Rosehip Green Tea*

**APO E GENE
3/3 1,800 KCAL, DAY 3**
Serving considerations per day:

Carbohydrates
8 servings grain/starch
6.5 servings fruit/vegetable

Protein
10 servings protein

Fat
5.5 servings anti-inflammatory fat

Breakfast
1 cup bran cereal
1 cup soymilk
½ cup blueberries
1 tbsp. honey
Peach Tea*
Apo E Diet Multivitamins™

Morning Snack
Banana Almond Shake-to-Go* (¾ serving)
White Mint Tea*

Lunch
Sandwich:
1 veggie burger

2 slices whole-grain bread
Romaine lettuce (1 leaf)
¼ cup sliced tomato
⅛ cup onion
1 oz. avocado

½ cup black beans
Iced Lemon Ginger Green Tea*

Afternoon Snack
Carrot and Cucumber Yogurt Salad*
Matcha Tea†

Dinner
12-inch corn tortilla or four 6-inch tortillas
Pam's Lime Rosemary Baked Chicken*
   (¾ serving)
2 tbsp. Tomato Salsa Cream* (¼ serving)
Chopped romaine lettuce, tomatoes, and
   onions (1–2 cups)
1½ oz. low-fat soy cheese
1 oz. avocado
Sparkling Lime Juice Iced Water* and
   Chamomile Peach Tea*

Supper (evening snack)
½ cup fresh sliced strawberries
5 Lemon Ginger Biscuits (cookies)*
   (1.5 servings)
Jasmine Green Tea†

**APO E GENE
3/3 1,800 KCAL, DAY 4**
Serving considerations per day:

Carbohydrates
5.5 servings grain/starch
11.5 servings fruit/vegetable

Protein
7 servings protein

Fat
4 servings anti-inflammatory fat

Breakfast
Scottish Oatmeal*
½ tbsp. honey

⅛ cup sultanas
1 cup nonfat milk
Ginger Green Tea*
Apo E Diet Multivitamins™

Morning Snack
¾ oz. whole-wheat pretzels
½ cup raspberry nonfat yogurt
Ginger and Turmeric Tea*

Lunch
Sandwich:
½ whole-grain pita bread
3 oz. Grilled or Baked Fish (black cod*)
Romaine lettuce (1 leaf)
¼ cup sliced tomato
¼ cup celery
⅛ cup red onion
1 oz. avocado

Lemon Lime Tea with Wild Mint*

Afternoon Snack
Carrot and Cucumber Yogurt Salad*
4 whole-grain crackers
Classic English Tea with Milk*

Dinner
Shiitake Mushroom and Spinach Lasagna*
1 tbsp. Parmesan cheese
4 steamed asparagus spears with lemon
Green Salad*
½ slice whole-grain bread
Sparkling Orange Juice Iced Water* and
   Green Tea*

Supper (evening snack)
3 Raspberry Ginger Biscuits (cookies)*
1 cup ice-cold nonfat milk
Chamomile Peach Tea* with rosehips

APO E GENE
3/3 2,000 KCAL, DAY 1

Serving considerations per day:
(be mindful of serving sizes)

Carbohydrates
6 servings grain/starch
7 servings fruit/vegetable

Protein
7 servings protein

Fat
5 servings anti-inflammatory fat

Breakfast
1 cup oatmeal
1 cup soymilk
½ tbsp. honey
1 tbsp. ground flaxseed†
⅛ cup sultanas
White Mint Tea*
Apo E Diet Multivitamins™

Morning Snack
1 medium apple
2 dates
½ tbsp. nut butter
The Green and Red Tea*

Lunch
Mevagissey Fish Tacos* (¾ serving)
2 tbsp. Papaya Salsa Cream* (¼ serving)
Sparkling Lemon Juice Iced Water*
and Ginger and Turmeric Tea*

Afternoon Snack
Sultana, Carrot, Ginger Coleslaw*
(½ serving)
1 cup nonfat milk
Lemon Ginger Green Tea*

Dinner
3 oz. Grilled or Baked Fish (halibut)* with
Teriyaki Sauce*
6 steamed asparagus spears
Pam's Baked Potato* (½ serving)
½ slice whole-grain bread
1 oz. avocado
Peach Tea*

Supper (evening snack)
Peach and Blackberry Crumble*
(¾ serving)
½ cup frozen yogurt
Chamomile Hibiscus Tea*

APO E GENE
3/3 2,000 KCAL, DAY 2

Serving considerations per day:

Carbohydrates
10 servings grain/starch
11 servings fruit/vegetable

Protein
9 servings protein

Fat
5 servings anti-inflammatory fat

Breakfast
2 slices whole-grain bread
1 tbsp. nut butter
1 banana
½ tbsp. honey
Matcha Tea†
Apo E Diet Multivitamins™

Morning Snack
½ cup low-fat granola
1 cup nonfat Soy Yogurt*
The Green and Red Tea*

Lunch
Sandwich:
1 veggie burger
2 slices whole-grain bread
1 leaf romaine lettuce
¼ tomato
1 tbsp. low-fat canola or olive oil
mayonnaise†

Sparkling Orange Juice Iced Water*

Afternoon Snack
Sultana, Carrot, Ginger Coleslaw* (½ serving)
1 slice multigrain bread
Jasmine Green Tea†

Dinner
4 oz. Grilled or Baked Fish (tuna steak)*
    with Teriyaki Sauce*
½ cup broccoli or broccolini
½ cup steamed spinach
¼ cup cooked white beans
Green Salad*
½ slice whole-grain bread
1 cup nonfat milk
Chamomile Peach Tea* with rosehips

Supper (evening snack)
Scottish Fruit Pottage*
½ cup low-fat frozen soy yogurt
Hibiscus Elder Tea*

**APO E GENE
3/3 2,000 KCAL, DAY 3**
Serving considerations per day:

Carbohydrates
10.5 servings grain/starch
10 servings fruit/vegetable

Protein
12 servings protein

Fat
5 servings anti-inflammatory fat

Breakfast
Eggs (½–¾ cup egg whites or substitute)
½ cup baked beans
2 tbsp. Tomato Salsa Cream* (¼ serving)
½ whole-grain bagel, toasted
1 oz. avocado
½ cup fresh cut melon
Ginger Green Tea*
Apo E Diet Multivitamins™

Morning Snack
Golf Snack Mix*
1 medium peach
White Mint Tea*

Lunch
Prawn salad sandwich:

1 whole-wheat pita bread
3 oz. grilled prawns
Romaine lettuce (1 leaf)
¼ cup sliced tomato
⅛ cup onion
4 Mediterranean olives
1 tbsp. low-fat canola or olive oil
    mayonnaise†

1 cup nonfat milk
Black Currant, Ginger, and Turmeric Tea*

Afternoon Snack
1 cup Pam's Vegetable Soup*
7 whole-grain crackers
Matcha Tea†

Dinner
Pam's Lime Rosemary Baked Chicken*
    (¾ serving)
Pam's Baked Potato*
Green Salad*
1 small slice whole-grain bread
Sparkling Lime Juice Iced Water* and
    Green Tea*

Supper (evening snack)
3 Raspberry Ginger Biscuits (cookies)*
1 cup nonfat milk
Chamomile Hibiscus Tea*

**APO E GENE
3/3 2,000 KCAL, DAY 4**
Serving considerations per day:

Carbohydrates
10 servings grain/starch
9 servings fruit/vegetable

Protein
10.5 servings protein

Fat
4.5 servings anti-inflammatory fat

APO E 3/3 2,000 KCAL

Breakfast
Blueberry Sultana Oat Bread* (¾ serving)
Eggs (½–¾ cup egg whites or substitute)
1 tbsp. honey
1 orange
Classic English Tea with Milk*
Apo E Diet Multivitamins™

Morning Snack
1 medium apple
1 cup Soy Yogurt*
⅓ cup low-fat granola
Cornish Pixie Rose-Lemon Green Tea*

Lunch
Sandwich:
1 whole-grain pita bread
3 oz. Grilled or Baked Fish (sea bass)*
Romaine lettuce (1 leaf)
¼ cup sliced tomato
¼ cup celery
⅛ cup red onion
1 oz. avocado
1 tbsp. fat-free ranch dressing

Black Currant, Ginger, and Turmeric Tea*

Afternoon Snack
⅓ cup Original Hummus*
7 whole-grain crackers
White Mint Tea*

Dinner
3 oz. Grilled or Baked Fish (wild salmon)*
6 steamed asparagus spears with lemon
1 tbsp. almonds
Green Salad*
2 slices whole-grain bread
1 cup nonfat milk
The Green and Red Tea*

Supper (evening snack)
¾ cup sliced strawberries and blueberries
Chocolate angel food cake
Chamomile Peach Tea*

½ cup steamed carrots
1 cup nonfat milk
Hibiscus Elder Tea*

Supper (evening snack)
Peach and Blackberry Crumble*
  (¾ serving)
½ cup low-fat vanilla soy ice cream
Chamomile Peach Tea*

APO E GENE
3/3 2,400 KCAL, DAY 2
Serving considerations per day:

Carbohydrates
11 servings grain/starch
8.5 servings fruit/vegetable

Protein
14 servings protein

Fat
8 servings anti-inflammatory fat

Breakfast
2 six-inch corn tortillas
¼ cup egg substitute
¼ avocado
1½ oz. low-fat soy cheese
¼ cup Fresh Tomato Salsa*
½ cup melon
White Mint Tea*
Apo E Diet Multivitamins™

Morning Snack
1 toasted whole-grain bagel
1 tbsp. nut butter
1 cup soymilk
Ginger Green Tea*

Lunch
1 veggie burger
Blueberry Sultana Oat Bread*
Romaine lettuce and tomatoes (1–2 cups)
1 tbsp. low-fat canola or olive oil mayonnaise†
1 oz. avocado
Sparkling Orange Juice Iced Water*

APO E GENE
3/3 2,400 KCAL, DAY 1
Serving considerations per day:
  (be mindful of serving sizes)

Carbohydrates
10 servings grain/starch
11.5 servings fruit/vegetable

Protein
12.5 servings protein

Fat
6 servings anti-inflammatory fat

Breakfast
Eggs (½–¾ cup egg whites or substitute)
2 slices toasted oat bran bread
1 tbsp. nut butter
½ cup fresh mixed berries
Jasmine Green Tea†
Apo E Diet Multivitamins™

Morning Snack
Golf Snack Mix*
½ cup nonfat soy cottage cheese
Lemon Ginger Green Tea*

Lunch
Sandwich:
1 whole-grain pita bread
2 oz. Grilled or Baked Fish (mackerel)*
Shredded lettuce and chopped onions
1 oz. avocado

1 cup fresh papaya slices
Sparkling Lemon Juice Iced Water*

Afternoon Snack
2 tbsp. almonds
1 cup Pam's Vegetable Soup*
2 mandarin oranges
Lemon Ginger Green Tea*

Dinner
3 oz. grilled chicken breast
1 cup whole-wheat spaghetti
1 tbsp. Parmesan cheese
1 cup steamed broccoli

Afternoon Snack
Sultana, Carrot, Ginger Coleslaw*
   (½ serving)
4 whole-grain crackers
Matcha Tea†

Dinner
6 oz. grilled shrimp with Teriyaki Sauce*
   to taste
9 steamed asparagus spears
½ cup cooked basmati rice
1 medium sliced tomato with balsamic
   vinegar
Pam's Baked Potato*
2 tbsp. Nonfat Papaya Salsa Cream*
   (¼ serving)
1 tbsp. fresh chopped chives
Chamomile Peach Tea *

Supper (evening snack)
Peach and Blackberry Crumble*
   (2 servings)
½ cup low-fat frozen soy yogurt
Rosehip Green Tea*

**APO E GENE
3/3 2,400 KCAL, DAY 3**
Serving considerations per day:

Carbohydrates
9 servings grain/starch
12.5 servings fruit/vegetable

Protein
11 servings protein

Fat
5.5 servings anti-inflammatory fat

Breakfast
1 cup oat bran flakes
¼ cup sultanas
½ banana
1 cup soymilk
Ginger Green Tea*
Apo E Diet Multivitamins™

Morning Snack
1 tbsp. nut butter
1 slice whole-grain toast
1 medium apple, sliced
White Mint Tea*

Lunch
Rustic Tuscany Pizza*
Green Salad*
Ginger and Turmeric Tea*

Afternoon Snack
Sultana, Carrot, Ginger Coleslaw*
   (½ serving)
8 whole-grain crackers
Matcha Tea†

Dinner
5 oz. Grilled or Baked Fish (halibut)*
   with Hawaiian Mango Salsa*
   (½ serving)
6 steamed asparagus spears
2 slices whole-grain bread
1 cup soymilk
Sparkling Lime Juice Iced Water* and
Chamomile Peach Tea*

Supper (evening snack)
1 cup nonfat milk
Kelly's Fore Street Dessert* (½ serving)
Jasmine Green Tea† with rosehips

**APO E GENE
3/3 2,400 KCAL, DAY 4**
Serving considerations per day:

Carbohydrates
9.5 servings grain/starch
7.5 servings fruit/vegetable

Protein
11 servings protein

Fat
6 servings anti-inflammatory fat

APO E 3/3 2,400 KCAL

Breakfast
Blueberry Sultana Oat Bread
1 cup nonfat strawberry yogurt
Green Tea* with mint
Apo E Diet Multivitamins™

Morning Snack
Banana Shake-to-Go* (¾ serving)
The Green and Red Tea*

Lunch
Sandwich:
1 veggie burger
1½-oz. slice low-fat soy cheese
2 slices whole-grain bread
Romaine lettuce (1 leaf)
½ cup sliced tomato
⅛ cup onion
1 tbsp. low-fat canola or olive oil
    mayonnaise†

White Tea with Cranberries*

Afternoon Snack
2 fresh dates
Medium orange or apple
Ginger Green Tea*

Dinner
Pam's Lime Rosemary Baked Chicken*
Pam's Baked Potato*
Mevagissey Ratatouille*
1 slice whole-grain bread
Iced Hibiscus Elder Tea*

Supper (evening snack)
Peach and Blackberry Crumble*
½ cup low-fat soy ice cream
Lemon Ginger Green Tea*

APO E 3/3 2,400 KCAL

APO E GENE
2/3 1,600 KCAL, DAY 1
Serving considerations per day:
  (be mindful of serving sizes)

Carbohydrate
4 servings grain/starch
9.5 servings fruit/vegetable

Protein
8.5 servings protein

Fat
4.5 servings anti-inflammatory fat

Breakfast
Quick Fresh Fruit Shake-to-Go*
  (¾ serving)
Jasmine Green Tea†
Apo E Diet Multivitamins™

Morning Snack
1 cup Soy Yogurt*
¼ cup dried apricots
White Mint Tea*

Lunch
Open-faced sandwich:
1 slice whole-grain bread
2 oz. sliced chicken breast
1 tbsp. low-fat olive oil or canola oil
  mayonnaise†
Romaine lettuce (1 leaf)
½ cup sliced tomato
⅛ cup onion
1 oz. avocado

1 cup nonfat milk
Sparkling Lemon Juice Iced Water*

Afternoon Snack
Sultana, Carrot, Ginger Coleslaw*
  (½ serving)
7 whole-grain crackers
Lemon Ginger Green Tea*

Dinner
3 oz. Grilled or Baked Fish (wild salmon)*
¼ cup white beans

2 tbsp. Hawaiian Mango Salsa*
  (¼ serving)
Green Salad*
Lemon Lime Tea with Wild Mint* and
  Hibiscus Elder Tea*

Supper (evening snack)
3 Orange Ginger Biscuits (cookies)*
Chamomile Peach Tea*

APO E GENE
2/3 1,600 KCAL, DAY 2
Serving considerations per day:

Carbohydrates
4.5 servings grain/starch
7.5 servings fruit/vegetable

Protein
8.5 servings protein

Fat
6 servings anti-inflammatory fat

Breakfast
1 slice whole-grain bread
1 tbsp. nut butter
½ banana
1 tsp. honey
Green Tea*
Apo E Diet Multivitamins™

Morning Snack
Golf Snack Mix* (½ serving)
1 oz. soy cheese
½ cup grapes or cherries
Sparkling Lemon Juice Iced Water*

Lunch
Sandwich:
1 whole-grain pita bread
3 oz. sliced chicken
1 oz. soy cheese
Romaine lettuce (1 leaf)
½ cup sliced tomato
⅛ cup onion
1 oz. avocado

1 tbsp. low-fat ranch dressing (olive or
canola oil)

Ginger and Turmeric Tea*

Afternoon Snack
Sultana, Carrot, Ginger Coleslaw*
(½ serving)
1 cup soymilk
White Mint Tea*

Dinner
1 cup whole-wheat pasta
½ cup fresh marinara sauce
½ cup shiitake mushrooms
1 tsp. olive oil
½ cup steamed spinach
1 oz. soy cheese
1 oz. avocado
Sparkling Orange Juice Iced Water* and
Chamomile Peach Tea*

Supper (evening snack)
½ cup low-fat frozen yogurt or soy ice cream
Green Rosehip Tea*

**APO E GENE
2/3 1,600 KCAL, DAY 3**
Serving considerations per day:

Carbohydrates
5.5 servings grain/starch
7.5 servings fruit/vegetable

Protein
4.5 servings protein

Fat
10 servings anti-inflammatory fat

Breakfast
Blueberry Sultana Oat Bread*
Ginger Green Tea*
Apo E Diet Multivitamins™

Morning Snack
1 medium apple, sliced

1 tbsp. nut butter
White Mint Tea* with squeeze of lemon

Lunch
Open-faced sandwich:
1 slice whole-grain bread
3 oz. Grilled or Baked Fish (tuna steak)*
with Teriyaki Sauce*
1 tbsp. olive or canola oil mayonnaise†
Romaine lettuce (1 leaf)
¼ cup sliced tomato
¼ cup celery
⅛ cup red onion
1 oz. avocado

Jasmine Green Tea†

Afternoon Snack
Golf Snack Mix* (½ serving)
1 cup nonfat yogurt
Matcha Tea†

Dinner
Shiitake Mushroom and Spinach Lasagna*
(¾ serving)
Salad: 1 cup spinach and ½ cup of
veggies such as cherry tomatoes,
cucumber, or carrots
Simple Salad Dressing*
1 slice whole-grain bread
1 oz. avocado
Sparkling Lime Juice Iced Water*
Peach Tea*

Supper (evening snack)
½ cup fresh mixed berries
Lemon angel food cake
Chamomile Hibiscus Tea*

APO E GENE
2/3 1,600 KCAL, DAY 4

Serving considerations per day:

Carbohydrates
5 servings grain/starch
5 servings fruit/vegetable

Protein
9 servings protein

Fat
7 servings anti-inflammatory fat

Breakfast
Scottish Oatmeal*
1 cup nonfat milk
White Mint Tea*
Apo E Diet Multivitamins™

Morning Snack
⅛ cup almonds
1 oz. soy cheese
Sparkling Orange Juice Iced Water*

Lunch
1 veggie burger
1 slice whole-grain bread
Salad: 1 cup lettuce with ½ cup tomato,
    onion, peppers, and grated carrot
1½ oz. low-fat soy cheese
2 tbsp. Tomato Salsa Cream* (¼ serving)
Iced Green and Red Tea*

Afternoon Snack
1 tbsp. nut butter
½ cup carrot slices
Ginger Green Tea*

Dinner
1 six-inch tortilla
Shredded lettuce and diced tomato
    (1–2 cups)
1½ oz. low-fat soy cheese
¼ cup black beans
2 tbsp. Tomato Salsa Cream* (¼ serving)
1 oz. avocado
Sparkling Lemon Juice Iced Water* and
    White Tea with Cranberries*

Supper (evening snack)
Apple and Peach Crumble* (¾ serving)
English Vanilla Custard*
Peach Tea*

APO E GENE
2/3 1,800 KCAL, DAY 1
Serving considerations per day:
  (be mindful of serving sizes)

Carbohydrates
5.5 servings grain/starch
9 servings fruit/vegetable

Protein
9 servings protein

Fat
5 servings anti-inflammatory fat

Breakfast
Orange Shake-to-Go* (¾ serving)
Jasmine Green Tea†
Apo E Diet Multivitamins™

Morning Snack
Blueberry Sultana Oat Bread* (¾ serving)
1 cup soymilk
Ginger and Turmeric Tea*

Lunch
Rustic Tuscany Pizza* (¾ serving)
Green Salad*
Sparkling Lemon Juice Iced Water*

Afternoon Snack
Golf Snack Mix*
Lemon Ginger Green Tea*

Dinner
4 oz. roasted chicken
Mevagissey Ratatouille*
1½ oz. low-fat soy cheese
Pam's Baked Potato* (½ serving)
2 tbsp. Tomato Salsa Cream* (¼ serving)
Hibiscus Elder Tea*

Supper (evening snack)
Pear and Currant Crumble* (½ serving)
½ cup low-fat soy ice cream
Chamomile Peach Tea*

APO E GENE
2/3 1,800 KCAL, DAY 2
Serving considerations per day:

Carbohydrates
4.5 servings grain/starch
12.5 servings fruit/vegetable

Protein
7 servings protein

Fat
6 servings anti-inflammatory fat

Breakfast
Eggs (½–¾ cup egg whites or substitute)
2 slices whole-grain oat flax toast†
1 oz. avocado
1 medium orange, sliced
The Green and Red Tea*
Apo E Diet Multivitamins™

Morning Snack
1 tbsp. nut butter
1 medium apple, sliced
1 cup nonfat milk
Cornish Pixie Rose-Lemon Green Tea*

Lunch
Tofu and Bean Tacos* (¾ serving)
2 tbsp. Tomato Salsa Cream* (¼ serving)
Sparkling Orange Juice Iced Water*
Lemon Ginger Green Tea*

Afternoon Snack
Sultana, Carrot, Ginger Coleslaw*
4 whole-grain crackers
White Mint Tea*

Dinner
Vegetable Spaghetti or Pasta* (¾ serving)
½ cup steamed spinach
Green Salad*
Chamomile Peach Tea* with rosehips
  and lemon

Supper (evening snack)
3 Raspberry Ginger Biscuits (cookies)*
1 cup nonfat milk
Hibiscus Elder Tea*

APO E 2/3 1,800 KCAL

APO E GENE
2/3 1,800 KCAL, DAY 3
Serving considerations per day:

Carbohydrates
7.5 servings grain/starch
3 servings fruit/vegetable

Protein
10 servings protein

Fat
6.5 servings anti-inflammatory fat

Breakfast
1 tbsp. almond butter
1 slice multigrain toast
1 cup soymilk
Lemon Ginger Green Tea*
Apo E Diet Multivitamins™

Morning Snack
1 cup nonfat yogurt
¼ cup low-fat granola
White Mint Tea* with a squeeze of lemon

Lunch
Sandwich:
1 veggie burger
2 slices whole-grain bread
Romaine lettuce (1 leaf)
¼ cup sliced tomato
¼ cup celery
⅛ cup red onion
1½ oz. low-fat soy cheese
1 tbsp. light canola mayonnaise†
1 oz. avocado

Iced Black Currant, Ginger, and
    Turmeric Tea*

Afternoon Snack
Wheat Pasta Salad* (½ serving)
10 green olives
Matcha Tea†

Dinner
3 oz. Grilled or Baked Fish (wild salmon)*
    with Thai Hazelnut Sauce*
1 cup basmati rice

8 steamed asparagus spears
Sparkling Lime Juice Iced Water* and
    Chamomile Peach Tea*

Supper (evening snack)
Peach and Blackberry Crumble* (¾
serving)
1 cup English Vanilla Custard (½ serving)
Green Tea* with a squeeze of orange

APO E GENE
2/3 1,800 KCAL, DAY 4
Serving considerations per day:

Carbohydrates
5 servings grain/starch
12.5 servings fruit/vegetable

Protein
2.5 servings protein

Fat
8 servings anti-inflammatory fat

Breakfast
Scottish Oatmeal with Dates*
Jasmine Green Tea†
Apo E Diet Multivitamins™

Morning Snack
Trail mix:
½ cup oat bran cereal
⅛ cup nuts
¼ cup currants
⅔ cup nonfat cottage cheese

Lemon Lime Tea with Wild Mint*

Lunch
Vegetable and Bean Tacos*
½ cup Fresh Tomato Salsa*
2 tbsp. Soy Yogurt*
Sparkling Hibiscus Iced Water*
Green Tea* with lemon

Afternoon Snack
1 slice whole-grain bread
1 tbsp. nut butter
Ginger Green Tea*

Dinner

Shiitake Mushroom and Spinach Lasagna*
   (¾ serving)
1 tbsp. Parmesan cheese
Green Salad*
2 tbsp. Simple Salad Dressing* (in place
   of the vinaigrette dressing in Green
   Salad recipe)
Sparkling Hibiscus Iced Water*
Peach Tea*

Supper (evening snack)

Lemon angel food cake
¾ cup sliced strawberries
Chamomile Peach Tea*

APO E 2/3 1,800 KCAL

APO E GENE
2/3 2,000 KCAL, DAY 1
Serving considerations per day:
   (be mindful of serving sizes)

Carbohydrates
8 servings grain/starch
6.5 servings fruit/vegetable

Protein
10 servings protein

Fat
7.5 servings anti-inflammatory fat

Breakfast
Eggs (½–¾ cup egg whites or substitute)
1 slice whole-grain toast
1 medium orange
1 tbsp. honey
Jasmine Green Tea[†]
Apo E Diet Multivitamins™

Morning Snack
Blueberry Sultana Oat Bread* (¾ serving)
White Mint Tea*

Lunch
Rustic Tuscany Pizza*
Green Salad*
Cilantro Soy Ginger Dressing* (in place
   of the vinaigrette dressing in Green
   Salad recipe)
½ oz. kalamata olives
Sparkling Lemon Juice Iced Water*

Afternoon Snack
1 medium apple, sliced
1 tbsp. nut butter
1 oz. soy cheese
Ginger Green Tea*

Dinner
Pam's Lime Rosemary Baked Chicken*
Pam's Baked Potato*
2 tbsp. Tomato Salsa Cream* (¼ serving)
1 tbsp fresh chives
1 cup cooked broccoli

1 cup nonfat milk
Hibiscus Elder Tea*

Supper (evening snack)
Pear and Currant Crumble* (½ serving)
½ cup low-fat soy ice cream
Chamomile Peach Tea*

APO E GENE
2/3 2,000 KCAL, DAY 2
Serving considerations per day:

Carbohydrates
5.5 servings grain/starch
5.5 servings fruit/vegetable

Protein
8 servings protein

Fat
6 servings anti-inflammatory fat

Breakfast
Scottish Oatmeal*
¼ cup black currants
1 cup soymilk
Jasmine Green Tea[†]
Apo E Diet Multivitamins™

Morning Snack
1 tbsp. nut butter
1 slice whole-grain bread
White Mint Tea*

Lunch
Simple Vegetarian Black Bean Soup*
   (¾ serving)
1 slice whole-grain bread
Romaine lettuce and tomatoes (1–2 cups)
1½ oz. low-fat soy cheese
1 tbsp. light canola mayonnaise[†]
1 oz. avocado
Sparkling Lemon Juice Iced Water*
Lemon Ginger Green Tea*

Afternoon Snack
Golf Snack Mix* (½ serving)
Matcha Tea[†]

Dinner
Mevagissey Fish Tacos* (¾ serving)
2 tbsp. Tomato Salsa Cream* (¼ serving)
½ cup black beans
Sparkling Lime Juice Iced Water*
Chamomile Peach Tea*

Supper (evening snack)
1 cup chocolate milk

APO E GENE
2/3 2,000 KCAL, DAY 3
Serving considerations per day:

Carbohydrates
7 servings grain/starch
9.5 servings fruit/vegetable

Protein
7.5 servings protein

Fat
9 servings anti-inflammatory fat

Breakfast
Omelet or Burrito*
1 oz. avocado
½ cup sliced potatoes grilled with 1 tsp.
  olive oil
2 tbsp. fresh diced tomato
Classic English Tea with Milk*
Apo E Diet Multivitamins™

Morning Snack
1 tbsp. nut butter
1 slice whole-grain toast
Rosehip Green Tea*

Lunch
Sandwich:
1 veggie burger
2 slices whole-grain bread
1½ oz. low-fat soy cheese
1 tbsp. canola oil mayonnaise†
Romaine lettuce (1 leaf)
¼ cup sliced tomato
¼ cup celery

⅛ cup red onion
1 oz. avocado

Sparkling Orange Juice Iced Water*

Afternoon Snack
1 Blueberry Oat Muffin*
The Green and Red Tea*

Dinner
Shiitake Mushroom and Spinach Lasagna*
Mevagissey Ratatouille*
1 cup romaine lettuce
1 tbsp. fat-free Caesar dressing
Chamomile Peach Tea* with rosehips
  and lemon

Supper (evening snack)
½ cup soy ice cream
Scottish Fruit Pottage*
Rosehip Green Tea*

APO E GENE
2/3 2,000 KCAL, DAY 4
Serving considerations per day:

Carbohydrates
7 servings grain/starch
9.5 servings fruit/vegetable

Protein
8.5 servings protein

Fat
8 servings anti-inflammatory fat

Breakfast
Orange Shake-to-Go* (¾ serving)
Green Tea*
Apo E Diet Multivitamins™

Morning Snack
1 medium peach
8 almonds
White Mint Tea*

Lunch
Sandwich:
2 slices whole-grain bread

3 oz. sliced chicken
¼ avocado
¼ cup sliced tomato
¼ cup sliced Maui onion

½ cup baked sweet potato fries or ½ cup
   sweet potato baked with 1 tsp. olive oil
Sparkling Hibiscus Iced Water*

Afternoon Snack
1 cup carrots
¼ cup Original Hummus*
Ginger Green Tea*

Dinner
3 oz. Grilled or Baked Fish (wild salmon)*
Pam's Baked Potato*
1 tbsp. chopped almonds
1 cup romaine lettuce
1 tbsp. olive oil-based dressing
Cornish Pixie Rose-Lemon Green Tea*
The Green and Red Tea*

Supper (evening snack)
Apple and Peach Crumble* (½ serving)
1 cup fresh sliced strawberries
1 cup nonfat milk
Hibiscus Elder Tea*

APO E 2/3 2,000 KCAL

APO E GENE
2/3, DAY 1
Serving considerations per day:
(be mindful of serving sizes)

Carbohydrates
8.5 servings grain/starch
11.5 servings fruit/vegetable

Protein
14 servings protein

Fat
5.5 servings anti-inflammatory fat

Breakfast
Banana Almond Shake-to-Go* (½ serving)
½ whole-grain bagel
1 tbsp. honey
Jasmine Green Tea†
Apo E Diet Multivitamins™

Morning Snack
⅛ cup raisins
1 tsp. ground flaxseed†
1 peach, sliced
1 cup nonfat Soy Yogurt*
White Tea with Cranberries*

Lunch
Sandwich:
1 whole-grain pita bread
3 oz. grilled chicken breast, sliced
Romaine lettuce (1 leaf)
¼ cup sliced tomato
¼ cup red pepper
⅛ cup Maui onion
1 tbsp. Cilantro Soy Ginger Salad
    Dressing* (¾ serving)
1½ oz. low-fat soy cheese
1 oz. avocado

Sparkling Lemon Juice Iced Water*

Afternoon Snack
Simple Vegetarian Black Bean Soup*
    (¾ serving)
3 tbsp. chopped tomato

3 tbsp. chopped green onion
2 slices whole-grain bread
Ginger Green Tea*

Dinner
5 oz. Grilled or Baked Fish (black cod)*
¼ cup Tomato Salsa Cream* (½ serving)
½ cup pinto beans
1 cup broccoli
Hibiscus Elder Tea*

Supper (evening snack)
3 Raspberry Ginger Biscuits (cookies)*
1 cup soymilk
Chamomile Peach Tea*

APO E GENE
2/3 2,400 KCAL, DAY 2
Serving considerations per day:

Carbohydrates
7 servings grain/starch
10.5 servings fruit/vegetable

Protein
13.5 servings protein

Fat
9 servings anti-inflammatory fat

Breakfast
Eggs (½–¾ cup egg whites or substitute)
1 six-inch whole-wheat tortilla
½ cup Fresh Tomato Salsa*
1 oz. avocado
½ cup mixed chopped melon
1 cup soymilk
Lemon Ginger Green Tea*
Apo E Diet Multivitamins™

Morning Snack
1 medium apple, sliced
1 cup peach yogurt
8 raw almonds
1 tbsp. ground flaxseed†
White Mint Tea* with lemon

Lunch

Sandwich:

1 veggie burger
2 slices whole-grain bread
Romaine lettuce (1 leaf)
¼ cup sliced tomato
¼ cup celery
1 tbsp. light canola mayonnaise[†]
¼ avocado

Iced Black Currant, Ginger, and
    Turmeric Tea*

Afternoon Snack

Simple Vegetarian Black Bean Soup*
    (¾ serving)
Matcha Tea[†]

Dinner

5 oz. Grilled or Baked Fish (wild salmon)*
1 cup steamed broccoli
½ cup cooked white beans
Green Salad* (1½ cups)
2 tbsp. Simple Salad Dressing* (in place
    of the vinaigrette dressing in the Green
    Salad recipe)
1 slice multigrain bread
Sparkling Lime Juice Iced Water*
Peach Tea*

Supper (evening snack)

Pear and Blueberry Crumble*
½ cup low-fat soy frozen yogurt
Green Tea* with squeeze of orange

**APO E GENE
2/3 2,400 KCAL, DAY 3**

Serving considerations per day:

Carbohydrates

6 servings grain/starch
13.5 servings fruit/vegetable

Protein

7.5 servings protein

Fat

9 servings anti-inflammatory fat

Breakfast

Blueberry Oat Muffin*
1 medium pear, sliced
1 tbsp. nut butter
½ cup nonfat cottage cheese
Ginger Green Tea*
Apo E Diet Multivitamins™

Morning Snack

Quick Fresh Fruit Shake-to-Go*
    (¾ serving)

Lunch

Sandwich:

2 slices whole-grain bread
Chicken Salad*
Green Salad* (1–2 cups)

¼ cup mixed melons
Sparkling Orange Juice Iced Water*

Afternoon Snack

Sultana, Carrot, Ginger Coleslaw*
    (½ serving)
⅛ cup almonds
Lemon Lime Tea with Wild Mint*

Dinner

Shiitake Mushroom and Spinach Lasagna*
    (¾ serving)
1 tbsp. Parmesan cheese
Green Salad*
2 tbsp. Fat Free Salad Dressing*
1 slice whole-grain bread
Chamomile Peach Tea* with rosehips

Supper (evening snack)
¾ cup blackberries
½ cup low fat frozen yogurt
Green Tea* with rosehips

APO E GENE
2/3 2,400 KCAL, DAY 4
Serving considerations per day:

Carbohydrates
7.5 servings grain/starch
12.5 servings fruit/vegetable

Protein
13.5 servings protein

Fat
4.5 servings anti-inflammatory fat

Breakfast
Red Pepper Tofu Scramble*
½ cup grilled baby potatoes (slice thinly, boil potatoes for 5-6 minutes, brush with olive oil and grill)
1 medium apple
Classic English Tea with Milk*
Apo E Diet Multivitamins™

Morning Snack
Snack mix: ½ cup oat bran squares and ¼ cup dried cranberries or raisins
2 oz. soy cheese
Lemon Ginger Green Tea*

Lunch
Sandwich:
2 slices whole-grain bread
4 oz. sliced skinless chicken
Romaine lettuce (1 leaf)
¼ cup sliced tomato
¼ cup celery
⅛ cup red onion
1 tbsp. canola mayonnaise†

1 peach, sliced
Sparkling Hibiscus Iced Water*

Afternoon Snack
Vegetable and Bean Tacos*
1 oz. soy cheese
1 oz. avocado
Rosehip Green Tea*

Dinner
5 oz. Grilled or Baked Fish (wild black cod)*
1 medium red skin potato, baked
1 oz. avocado
1 cup steamed broccoli
½ cup cooked carrots
Salad: spinach, red pepper, tomatoes, and corn (1–2 cups)
Cornish Pixie Rose-Lemon Green Tea*

Supper (evening snack)
½ cup low-fat soy ice cream or frozen yogurt
1 cup fresh sliced strawberries
Hibiscus Elder Tea*

APO E GENE
2/2 1,600 KCAL, DAY 1

Serving considerations per day:
(be mindful of serving sizes)

Carbohydrates
4.5 servings grain/starch
14 servings fruit/vegetable

Protein
4.5 servings protein

Fat
7 servings anti-inflammatory fat

Breakfast
Quick Fresh Fruit Shake-to-Go*
(¾ serving)
Jasmine Green Tea†
Apo E Diet Multivitamins™

Morning Snack
1 cup Soy Yogurt
¼ cup dried apricots
The Green and Red Tea*

Lunch
Open-faced sandwich:
1 slice whole-grain bread
2 oz. sliced chicken breast
Lettuce, cucumber, sliced tomato, and
onion (1–2 cups)
1 tbsp. low-fat olive oil or canola oil
mayonnaise†
¼ avocado
1 cup nonfat milk
Sparkling Lemon Juice Iced Water*

Afternoon Snack
1 medium apple
7 whole-grain crackers
Lemon Ginger Green Tea*

Dinner
2 oz. Grilled or Baked Fish (wild salmon)*
2 tbsp. Mango Salsa Cream* (¼ serving)
⅛ cup almonds
Green Salad*

1 slice whole-grain bread
White Tea with Cranberries*

Supper (evening snack)
3 Orange Ginger Biscuits (cookies)*
Chamomile Peach Tea

APO E GENE
2/2 1,600 KCAL, DAY 2

Serving considerations per day:

Carbohydrates
5 servings grain/starch
8.5 servings fruit/vegetable

Protein
7 servings protein

Fat
8 servings anti-inflammatory fat

Breakfast
2 slices whole-grain bread
2 tbsp. nut butter
½ banana
Ginger Green Tea*
Apo E Diet Multivitamins™

Morning Snack
Golf Snack Mix* (½ serving)
1 oz. soy cheese
½ cup grapes or cherries
Sparkling Hibiscus Iced Water*

Lunch
Sandwich:
½ whole-grain pita bread
2 oz. sliced chicken
Romaine lettuce (1 leaf)
½ cup sliced tomato
⅛ cup onion
1 oz. avocado
1 tbsp. Fat-Free Salad Dressing*
1 oz. soy cheese

Sparkling Orange Juice Iced Water*

Afternoon Snack
Sultana, Carrot, Ginger Coleslaw*
  (½ serving)
1 cup soymilk
Lemon Ginger Green Tea*

Dinner
1 cup whole-wheat pasta
½ cup fresh marinara sauce
½ cup shiitake mushrooms
1 tsp. olive oil
½ cup steamed spinach
½ oz. soy cheese
1 oz. avocado
Chamomile Tea* with rosehips and lemon

Supper (evening snack)
½ cup low-fat frozen yogurt or soy
  ice cream
Green Tea* with rosehips

APO E GENE
2/2 1,600 KCAL, DAY 3
Serving considerations per day:

Carbohydrates
5.5 servings grain/starch
9.5 servings fruit/vegetable

Protein
4 servings protein

Fat
9 servings anti-inflammatory fat

Breakfast
Blueberry Sultana Oat Bread* (¾ serving)
Lemon Ginger Green Tea*
Apo E Diet Multivitamins™

Morning Snack
1 apple, sliced
1 tbsp. nut butter
Classic English Tea with Milk*

Lunch
Sandwich:
2 slices whole-grain bread
2 oz. Grilled or Baked Fish (tuna steak)*
  with Teriyaki Sauce*
1 tbsp. olive or canola oil mayonnaise[†]
Chopped romaine lettuce, celery, and
  onion (1–2 cups)
¼ avocado

Iced Lemon Ginger Green Tea*

Afternoon Snack
1 sliced carrot
1 cup nonfat yogurt
Matcha Tea[†]

Dinner
Shiitake Mushroom and Spinach Lasagna*
  (½ serving)
Salad:
1 cup spinach
½ cup cherry tomatoes
½ cup cucumber
¼ cup carrots
1. oz. avocado
Simple Salad Dressing*

Sparkling Lime Juice Iced Water*
Peach Tea*

Supper (evening snack)
½ cup fresh mixed berries
Lemon angel food cake

APO E GENE
2/2 1,600 KCAL, DAY 4
Serving considerations per day:

Carbohydrates
4 servings grain/starch
6.5 servings fruit/vegetable

Protein
6 servings protein

Fat
10 servings anti-inflammatory fat

Breakfast
Scottish Oatmeal with Dates* (½ serving)
1 cup nonfat milk
White Mint Tea*
Apo E Diet Multivitamins™

Morning Snack
⅛ cup plain almonds
1 oz. soy cheese
Hibiscus Tea*

Lunch
1 veggie burger
1 slice whole-grain bread
2 tbsp. Tomato Salsa Cream* (¼ serving)
1 oz. avocado
Lettuce, tomatoes, and onion (1–2 cups)
Sparkling Orange Juice Iced Water*

Afternoon Snack
2 tbsp. nut butter
10 carrot slices
Ginger Green Tea*

Dinner
1 six-inch whole-wheat tortilla
Shredded lettuce and diced tomato
    (1–2 cups)
1½ oz. low-fat soy cheese
¼ cup black beans
2 tbsp. Mango Salsa Cream* (¼ serving)
1 oz. avocado
Black Currant, Ginger, and Turmeric Tea*

Supper (evening snack)
Apple and Peach Crumble* (½ serving)
English Vanilla Custard* (½ serving)

APO E GENE
2/2 1,800 KCAL, DAY 1
Serving considerations per day:
  (be mindful of serving sizes)

Carbohydrates
6.5 servings grain/starch
9.5 servings fruit/vegetable

Protein
6.5 servings protein

Fat
6 servings anti-inflammatory fat

Breakfast
Orange Shake-to-Go* (¾ serving)
Jasmine Green Tea†
Apo E Diet Multivitamins™

Morning Snack
Blueberry Sultana Oat Bread (¾ serving)
1 cup soymilk
The Green and Red Tea*

Lunch
Rustic Tuscany Pizza* (¾ serving)
Green Salad*
8 olives, green
Sparkling Lemon Juice Iced Water*

Afternoon Snack
Golf Snack Mix*
Lemon Ginger Green Tea*

Dinner
2 oz. roasted chicken
Pam's Baked Potato* (½ serving)
2 tbsp. Tomato Salsa Cream* (¼ serving)
Mevagissey Ratatouille*
1 oz. low-fat soy cheese

Supper (evening snack)
Pear and Currant Crumble* (½ cup)
½ cup low-fat soy ice cream
Chamomile Tea*

APO E GENE
2/2 1,800 KCAL, DAY 2
Serving considerations per day:

Carbohydrates
5.5 servings grain/starch
12.5 servings fruit/vegetable

Protein
7 servings protein

Fat
6.5 servings anti-inflammatory fat

Breakfast
Eggs (½–¾ cup egg whites or substitute)
"Green" Toast*
1 orange
Classic English Tea with Milk*
Apo E Diet Multivitamins™

Morning Snack
1 tbsp. nut butter
½ apple, sliced
½ cup nonfat milk

Lunch
Tofu and Bean Tacos*
2 tbsp. Mango Salsa Cream* (¼ serving)
Sparkling Orange Juice Iced Water*

Afternoon Snack
Sultana, Carrot, Ginger Coleslaw*
  (½ serving)
6 whole-grain crackers
The Green and Red Tea*

Dinner
Vegetable Spaghetti or Pasta* (¾ serving)
Green Salad*
½ cup steamed spinach
Chamomile Tea* with rosehips and lemon

Supper (evening snack)
3 Ginger Biscuits (cookies)*
1 cup Soy Yogurt*
Hibiscus Elder Tea*

APO E GENE
2/2 1,800 KCAL, DAY 3
Serving considerations per day:

Carbohydrates
8 servings grain/starch
5 servings fruit/vegetable

Protein
6.5 servings protein

Fat
7 servings anti-inflammatory fat

Breakfast
⅔ cup low-fat granola
¾ cup soymilk
White Mint Tea* with lemon
Apo E Diet Multivitamins™

Morning Snack
1 banana
2 tbsp. almond butter
Lemon Lime Tea with Wild Mint*

Lunch
½ veggie burger
1 slice whole-grain bread
Romaine lettuce, tomatoes, and red onion
  (1–2 cups)
1 tbsp. light canola mayonnaise†
¼ avocado
Iced Ginger and Turmeric Tea* with lemon

Afternoon Snack
Wheat Pasta Salad* (½ serving)
8 ripe, green olives
Matcha Tea†

Dinner
2 oz. Grilled or Baked Fish (wild salmon)*
  with Thai Hazelnut Sauce*
½ cup cooked basmati rice
8 steamed asparagus spears
Sparkling Lime Juice Iced Water*
Rosehip Green Tea*

Supper (evening snack)
Peach and Blackberry Crumble*
English Vanilla Custard (soy)* (½ serving)
Hibiscus Elder Tea*

APO E GENE
2/2 1,800 KCAL, DAY 4
Serving considerations per day:

Carbohydrates
6.5 servings grain/starch
13.5 servings fruit/vegetable

Protein
2.5 servings protein

Fat
8.5 servings anti-inflammatory fat

Breakfast
Scottish Oatmeal*
¾ cup fresh blackberries
Jasmine Green Tea†
Apo E Diet Multivitamins™

Morning Snack
Trail mix:
½ cup oat bran cereal
⅛ cup almonds
¼ cup currants

¼ cup nonfat cottage cheese
Cornish Pixie Rose-Lemon Green Tea*

Lunch
Tofu and Bean Tacos*
2 tbsp. low-fat Soy Yogurt*
½ cup Fresh Tomato Salsa*
8 fresh olives
Sparkling Hibiscus Iced Water*
Green Tea* with lemon

Afternoon Snack
1 slice whole-grain bread
1 tbsp. nut butter
White Tea with Cranberries*

Dinner

Shiitake Mushroom and Spinach Lasagna*
(¾ serving)
Green Salad*

Supper (evening snack)

Lemon angel food cake
¾ cup fresh sliced strawberries
Chamomile Hibiscus Tea*

**APO E GENE
2/2 2,000 KCAL, DAY 1**

Serving considerations per day:
(be mindful of serving sizes)

Carbohydrates

8 servings grain/starch
10.5 servings fruit/vegetable

Protein

9 servings protein

Fat

7.5 servings anti-inflammatory fat

Breakfast

Eggs (½–¾ cup egg whites or substitute)
1 slice whole-grain toast
1 tbsp. almond butter
1 orange
Jasmine Green Tea†
Apo E Diet Multivitamins™

Morning Snack

Blueberry Sultana Oat Bread* (¾ serving)
The Green and Red Tea*

Lunch

Rustic Tuscany Pizza*
Green Salad*
½ oz. kalamata olives
Sparkling Lemon Juice Iced Water*

Afternoon Snack

1 medium apple, sliced
2 tbsp. nut butter
1 oz. soy cheese
Lemon Ginger Green Tea*

Dinner

3 oz. Pam's Lime Rosemary Baked
Chicken* (¾ serving)
Pam's Baked Potato
2 tbsp. Tomato Salsa Cream*
Fresh chives
1 cup cooked broccoli
1 cup nonfat milk
Hibiscus Elder Tea*

Supper (evening snack)
Pear and Currant Crumble* (½ serving)
½ cup low-fat soy ice cream
Chamomile Peach Tea*

Sparkling Lime Juice Iced Water*
Peach Tea*

Supper (evening snack)
1 cup hot chocolate (nonfat milk)

APO E GENE
2/2 2,000 KCAL, DAY 2
Serving considerations per day:

Carbohydrates
5 servings grain/starch
5 servings fruit/vegetable

Protein
5 servings protein

Fat
8 servings anti-inflammatory fat

Breakfast
Scottish Oatmeal*
½ cup black currants
Rosehip Green Tea*
Apo E Diet Multivitamins™

Morning Snack
1 tbsp. nut butter
1 slice whole-grain bread
White Mint Tea*

Lunch
Simple Vegetarian Black Bean Soup*
Romaine lettuce and tomatoes (1–2 cups)
1½ oz. low-fat soy cheese
1 tbsp. light canola mayonnaise†
1 slice whole-grain bread
¼ avocado
Iced Ginger and Turmeric Tea* with lemon

Afternoon Snack
Golf Snack Mix* (¾ serving)
Matcha Tea†

Dinner
Fish Tacos* (¾ serving)
2 tbsp. Tomato Salsa Cream* (¼ serving)
1 cup black beans
10 olives

APO E GENE
2/2 2,000 KCAL, DAY 3
Serving considerations per day:

Carbohydrates
6.5 servings grain/starch
10 servings fruit/vegetable

Protein
6 servings protein

Fat
10.5 servings anti-inflammatory fat

Breakfast
Omelet or Burrito*
1 oz. avocado
2 tbsp. fresh diced tomato
1 orange
White Mint Tea*
Apo E Diet Multivitamins™

Morning Snack
1 slice whole-grain toast
1 tbsp. nut butter
Sparkling Hibiscus Iced Water*

Lunch
Sandwich:
1 veggie burger
2 slices whole-grain bread
1½ oz. low-fat soy cheese
1 tbsp. canola oil mayonnaise†
Romaine lettuce (1 leaf)
¼ cup sliced tomato
¼ cup sliced cucumber
⅛ cup red onion
¼ avocado

Iced Lemon Ginger Green Tea*

Afternoon Snack
1 Blueberry Oat Muffin*
Black Currant, Ginger, and Turmeric Tea*

Dinner
Shiitake Mushroom and Spinach Lasagna*
   (¾ serving)
Mevagissey Ratatouille*
Romaine lettuce (1 cup)
1 tbsp. Fat-Free Salad Dressing*
Chamomile Tea* with rosehips and lemon

Supper (evening snack)
½ cup soy ice cream
Scottish Fruit Pottage*
Hibiscus Elder Tea*

**APO E GENE
2/2 2,000 KCAL, DAY 4**
Serving considerations per day:

Carbohydrates
6 servings grain/starch
8 servings fruit/vegetable

Protein
6 servings protein

Fat
9.5 servings anti-inflammatory fat

Breakfast
Orange Shake-to-Go* (¾ serving)
Green Tea*
Apo E Diet Multivitamins™

Morning Snack
1 peach
8 almonds

Lunch
Sandwich:
2 slices whole-grain bread
2 oz. cooked sliced chicken
2 oz. avocado
1 medium sliced tomato
Maui onion, sliced

½ cup baked sweet potato fries†
Sparkling Hibiscus Iced Water*

Afternoon Snack
1 cup carrots
¼ cup Original Hummus*
Ginger Green Tea*

Dinner
3 oz. Grilled or Baked Fish (wild salmon)*
Olive Oil Potato Wedgewood Fries*
1 tbsp. chopped almonds
1 cup romaine lettuce with Simple
   Salad Dressing*

Supper (evening snack)
Apple and Peach Crumble* (½ serving)
¾ cup sliced strawberries
1 cup nonfat milk

APO E 2/2 2,000 KCAL

APO E GENE
2/2 2,400 KCAL, DAY 1
Serving considerations per day:
  (be mindful of serving sizes)

Carbohydrates
9 servings grain/starch
12 servings fruit/vegetable

Protein
9.5 servings protein

Fat
8.5 servings anti-inflammatory fat

Breakfast
Quick Fresh Fruit Shake-to-Go*
  (¾ serving)
1 slice whole-grain toast
1 tbsp. honey
Jasmine Green Tea†
Apo E Diet Multivitamins™

Morning Snack
1 cup nonfat Soy Yogurt*
1 peach, sliced
1 tbsp. ground flaxseed†
Ginger and Turmeric Tea*

Lunch
Sandwich:
1 whole-grain pita bread
2 oz. grilled chicken breast, sliced
Romaine lettuce (1 leaf)
¼ cup sliced tomato
¼ cup red pepper
⅛ cup Maui onion
1 tbsp. Cilantro Soy Ginger
  Dressing* (½ serving)
¼ avocado
Maui onion and red pepper, sliced
Iced Classic English Tea with Milk*
  with lemon

Afternoon Snack
Simple Vegetarian Black Bean Soup*
  (½ serving)
3 tbsp. chopped tomato

3 tbsp. chopped green onion
1½ slices whole-grain bread
Ginger Green Tea*

Dinner
3 oz. Grilled or Baked Fish
  (wild black cod)*
¼ cup Tomato Salsa Cream* (½ serving)
¼ avocado
½ cup pinto beans
1 cup broccoli
Chamomile Tea*

Supper (evening snack)
3 ginger biscuits (cookies)
1 cup soymilk

APO E GENE
2/2 2,400 KCAL, DAY 2
Serving considerations per day:

Carbohydrates
6.5 servings grain/starch
8.5 servings fruit/vegetable

Protein
10 servings protein

Fat
10 servings anti-inflammatory fat

Breakfast
Eggs (½–¾ cup egg whites or substitute)
1 six-inch whole-wheat tortilla
½ cup Fresh Tomato Salsa*
¼ avocado
½ cup mixed melon
1 cup soymilk
Ginger and Turmeric Tea*
Apo E Diet Multivitamins™

Morning Snack
1 medium apple, sliced
1 cup peach yogurt
8 raw almonds
1 tbsp. ground flaxseed†
White Mint Tea*

Lunch
1 veggie burger
1 slice whole-grain bread
Romaine lettuce and tomatoes (1–2 cups)
1 tbsp. light canola mayonnaise†
½ avocado
Iced Ginger Green Tea* with lemon

Afternoon Snack
Simple Vegetarian Black Bean Soup*
   (½ serving)
1 cup cooked basmati rice
Matcha Tea†

Dinner
3 oz. Grilled or Baked Fish (wild salmon)*
½ cup fresh steamed broccoli
1 cup cooked white beans
Green Salad*
Sparkling Lime Juice Iced Water*
Peach Tea*

Supper (evening snack)
Black Currant and Rhubarb Crumble*
   (¾ serving)
½ cup low-fat soy frozen yogurt
Hibiscus Elder Tea*

APO E GENE
2/2 2,400 KCAL, DAY 3
Serving considerations per day:

Carbohydrates
4 servings grain/starch
15.5 servings fruit/vegetable

Protein
6 servings protein

Fat
13 servings anti-inflammatory fat

Breakfast
1 Blueberry Oat Muffin*
1 pear, sliced
1 tbsp. fruit preserves

1 tbsp. nut butter
1 cup soymilk
Green Tea*
Apo E Diet Multivitamins™

Morning Snack
Quick Fresh Fruit Shake-to-Go*

Lunch
Chicken Salad* (½ serving)
Romaine lettuce, cucumber, tomatoes
   (1–2 cups)
1 slice whole-grain bread
¼ cup mixed melons
Sparkling Orange Juice Iced Water*

Afternoon Snack
Sultana, Carrot, Ginger Coleslaw*
   (½ serving)
¼ cup almonds
White Mint Tea*

Dinner
Shiitake Mushroom and Spinach Lasagna*
(¾ serving)
1 tbsp. Parmesan cheese
Spinach salad (1½ cups)
2 tbsp. Fat-Free Salad Dressing*
Chamomile Tea* with lemon and rosehips

Supper (evening snack)
¾ cup blackberries
1 cup nonfat ice cream
Chamomile Hibiscus Tea*

APO E 2/2 2,400 KCAL

APO E GENE
2/2 2,400 KCAL DAY 4
Serving considerations per day:

Carbohydrates
8 servings grain/starch
11 servings fruit/vegetable

Protein
9.5 servings protein

Fat
8 servings anti-inflammatory fat

Breakfast
Red Pepper Tofu Scramble*
½ cup grilled baby potatoes (slice thinly,
    boil potatoes for 5-6 minutes, brush
    with olive oil and grill)
Classic English Tea with Milk*
Apo E Diet Multivitamins™

Morning Snack
Snack Mix: ½ cup oat bran squares, ¼ cup
    almonds, and ¼ cup dried cranberries
1 oz. soy cheese
Lemon Ginger Green Tea*

Lunch
2 slices whole-grain bread
3 oz. sliced, skinless chicken
Romaine lettuce, fresh tomato, and onions
    (1–2 cups)
1 tbsp. canola mayonnaise†
1–2 peaches, sliced
Sparkling Hibiscus Iced Water*

Afternoon Snack
Vegetable and Bean Tacos* (½ serving)
1 oz. avocado
Ginger Green Tea*

Dinner
4 oz. Grilled or Baked Fish
    (wild black cod)*
½ cup red skin potato
1 cup steamed broccoli
½ cup cooked carrots
Salad: spinach, red pepper, fresh tomatoes,
    and corn (1–2 cups)
Lemon Lime Tea with Wild Mint*
Peach Tea*

Supper (evening snack)
1 cup low-fat soy ice cream
¾ cup fresh sliced strawberries
Chamomile Hibiscus Tea*

Chapter Twenty

RECIPES FOR THE APO E GENE

*"Get people back into the kitchen and combat the trend
toward processed food and fast food."*
— Andrew Weil, M.D.

Here I offer a wide variety of recipes to make your Perfect Gene Diet experience more fun and enjoyable.

For the recipes in this book, use truly organic ingredients whenever possible. When it's not possible, use ingredients free of pesticides, antibiotics, preservatives and genetically modified organisms (GMO). Be sure to reread the general comments about special food items and where to obtain them on page 263.

Apo E Gene Breakfasts

Scottish Oatmeal 338
Scottish Oatmeal with Walnuts 338
Scottish Oatmeal with Dates 339
Scottish Fruit Oatmeal 340
Scottish Spiced Pear Oatmeal 340
Breakfast Bread 341
Raspberry Oat Bread 341
Blueberry Sultana Oat Bread 342
Black Currant Oat Bread 342
Banana Berry Muffins (Jen's) 343
Blueberry Muffins (Jen's) 343
Blueberry Oat Bread or Muffins 344
"Green" Toast 344
Omelet or Burrito 345
Red Pepper Tofu Scramble 346
Banana Almond Shake-to-Go 346
Quick Fresh Fruit Shake-to-Go 347
Lemon Shake-to-Go 347
Orange Shake-to-Go 348
Golf Snack Mix 348

Apo E Gene Soups

Simple Vegetable Broth 349
Creamed Spinach Carrot Soup 349
Miso Pasta Soup 350
Pam's Vegetable Soup 350
Tomato, Carrot, and Butternut Squash Soup 351
Butternut Lemon Soup 351
Sunflower Split Pea Soup 352
Cornish Pea Soup 352
Simple Vegetarian Black Bean Soup 353
Cream Potato Corn Soup 353
Spring and Fall Nettle Soup 354

Apo E Gene Entrées

Pam's Lime Rosemary Baked Chicken. 355
Roast Rosemary Turkey 355
Grilled or Baked Fish 356
Grilled or Baked Salmon with
  Teriyaki Shiitake Mushroom Sauce 357
Grilled Wild Halibut with
Raspberry Honey Ginger Glaze 357
Pacific Rim Fish (or Tofu) and Veggies in a Wok 358
Shrimp Curry. 358
Mevagissey Fish Tacos. 359

Apo E Gene Vegetarian Entrées

Rustic Tuscany Pizza 360
Mevagissey Ratatouille 361
Cornish Chili. 361
Vegetable and Garbanzo Bean Curry 362
Vegetable Spaghetti or Pasta 362
Shiitake Mushroom and Spinach Lasagna 363
Vegetable and Bean Tacos 364
Tofu and Bean Tacos 364
Thai Hazelnuts and Currant Tofu 365

Apo E Gene Pacific Rim Sauces and Salsa

Peanut Sauce. 366
Thai Hazelnut Sauce 367
Teriyaki Sauce 368
Soy Ginger Sauce 368
Fresh Tomato Salsa 368
Hawaiian Mango Salsa 369
Tomato Salsa Cream 369
Mango Salsa Cream 370
Papaya Salsa Cream 370
Nonfat Papaya Salsa Cream 371

Apo E Gene Salads and Salad Dressings

Fish Salad 372
Chicken Salad 372
Tuna or Tofu Salad 372
Wheat Pasta Salad 373
Carrot and Cucumber Yogurt Salad 373
Green Salad 374
Sultana, Carrot, Ginger Coleslaw 374
Daily Veggie Bag 375
Cilantro Soy Ginger Dressing 375
Simple Salad Dressing 376
Fat-Free Salad Dressing 376
Nonfat Spicy Lime Ginger Dressing 376

Apo E Gene Side Dishes

Pam's Baked Potato 377
Olive Oil Potato Wedgewood Fries 377
Original Hummus 378
Guacamole 378
Homemade Corn and Lime Tortilla Chips 379
Tomato-Olive Tapenade 379
Almond Milk 380
Almond Cheese 380
Vegan Cottage Cheese 381
Soy Yogurt 381

Happy Families and a Cornish Tradition—Pasties

Nana Caine and Uncle Brian's Cornish Pasty 386
Pam's Cornish Pasty—the Heart-Healthy Version 388

Apo E Gene Desserts

Very Berry Fruit Salad 389
Pear and Currant Crumble 390
Apple and Peach Crumble 391
Apple and Grape Crumble 391
Apple and Blueberry Crumble 392
Pear and Blueberry Crumble 392
Peach and Blackberry Crumble 392
Black Currant and Rhubarb Crumble 393
Baked Pears or Apples 393
Scottish Fruit Pottage 393
Kelly's Fore Street Dessert 394
English Vanilla Custard 394
Ginger Biscuits (Cookies) 395
Lemon Ginger Biscuits (Cookies) 395
Raspberry Ginger Biscuits (Cookies) 396
Orange Ginger Biscuits (Cookies) 396

Apo E Gene Teas

Simple Teas 397
Rosehip Green Tea 398
The Green and Red Tea 398
Ginger Green Tea 398
Lemon Ginger Green Tea 398
Ginger Cinnamon Tea 399
Ginger and Turmeric Tea 399
Black Currant, Ginger, and Turmeric Tea 399
Hibiscus Elder Tea 399
Chamomile Hibiscus Tea 399
Chamomile Peach Tea 400
Chamomile Tea with Peach 400
White Tea with Cranberries 400
White Mint Tea 400
Classic English Tea with Milk 400

Apo E Gene Waters and Iced Tea/Lemonades

Sparkling Lime Juice Iced Water 401
Sparkling Orange Juice Iced Water 401
Sparkling Lemon Juice Iced Water 401
Sparkling Hibiscus Iced Water 401
Sparkling Vanilla Orange Iced Water 401
Lavender Chamomile Iced Water 402
Cornish Pixie Rose-Lemon Green Tea 402
Lemon Lime Tea with Wild Mint 402

Apo E Gene Breakfasts

Have you every wondered what the word "breakfast" means? Very simply, it means "breaking" the "fast." What this means is that you must refuel your body with the energy that was used while you were sleeping; and also provide new energy for the coming day.

Here are some recipes my patients have enjoyed:

Scottish Oatmeal

Ingredients
¼ cup Scottish oatmeal   1 tsp. ground flaxseed
4 oz. vanilla soymilk or nonfat milk   ½ tsp. honey
These additional toppings can be added if desired: ginger, cinnamon,
    banana, or nuts.

Directions
Cook oatmeal in a pan with milk or soymilk. When the oats are soft and creamy, add a yummy topping; try banana topped with organic honey and nuts. Serve in your favorite cereal bowl.

1 serving.

Nutritional serving information:　carbohydrate—grain/starch 1
　　　　　　　　　　　　　　　　　protein ½
　　　　　　　　　　　　　　　　　fat 1

Scottish Oatmeal with Walnuts

Ingredients
¼ cup Scottish oatmeal[1]   4 oz. soymilk or nonfat milk
½ banana   1 tsp. chopped walnuts
1 tsp. freshly ground flaxseed

Directions
Cook oatmeal in a pan with milk and flaxseed. When the oats are soft and creamy, add a yummy topping; in this case, banana topped with honey and nuts. Serve in your favorite cereal bowl.

1 serving.

Nutritional serving information:　carbohydrate—grain/starch 1
　　　　　　　　　　　　　　　　　protein ½
　　　　　　　　　　　　　　　　　fat 1

1　See organic Scottish oatmeal at **www.bobsredmill.com**, or use organic quick oats.

History of Scottish Oatmeal

Oatmeal comes from the grain we call oats (Avena sativa), which is actually the seed of the plant. Also known as porridge, oatmeal has been eaten in Scotland and England for centuries, although in England, oats were mainly fed to horses. Oats is truly a native food in the British Isles, directly related to the climate being better suited to growing oats more effectively than wheat.

In Scotland, oatmeal is used in a variety of recipes ranging from the delicious, simple morning oatmeal with fruit, to the outright yucky in my book—although some people love these cultural foods. One example is "Marag geal" from the Outer Hebrides. This is a white pudding made with oatmeal and vegetables that are boiled in a sheep's bladder. Another recipe is the traditional Scottish Highland Black Pudding—far from a pudding in my book—which includes oatmeal mixed with sheep's blood and an assortment of varying spices, and sometimes meat and fat are added to make an old traditional Scottish highland sausage. Personally, I prefer the traditional Scottish oatmeal in its simplest form. Unprocessed Scottish oatmeal offers a highly nutritional, heart-healthy food.

Scottish Oatmeal with Dates

Ingredients

¼ cup Scottish oatmeal[1]
4 oz. soymilk or nonfat milk
1 tbsp. currants
½ tsp. honey

1 tsp. ground flaxseed
1 small cooked apple
2 dates, chopped[2]

Directions

Combine all ingredients except dates and honey in a pan. Bring to boil and simmer for 4–6 minutes. Add dates and honey. Serve in favorite breakfast cereal bowl.
1 serving.

Nutritional serving information: carbohydrate—fruit 1
carbohydrate—grain/starch 1
protein ½
fat 1

---

1   See organic Scottish oatmeal at **www.bobsredmill.com**, or use organic quick oats.

2   Dates are known for a high tannin level and are used to help with intestinal conditions. Dates have also been known to help with fever, sore throat, colds, and bronchial conditions.

Scottish Fruit Oatmeal

Ingredients

¼ cup Scottish oatmeal[1]
4 oz. vanilla soymilk or nonfat milk
1 tbsp. sultanas
¼ tsp. honey

½ tsp. ground flaxseed
1 small diced and cooked apple
1 tbsp. cranberries
Ground cinnamon to taste

Directions

Combine all ingredients in a pan. Bring to boil and simmer for 4–6 minutes. Serve in favorite breakfast cereal bowl.

1 serving.

Nutritional serving information: carbohydrate—fruit 1
carbohydrate—grain/starch 1
protein ½
fat 1

Scottish Spiced Pear Oatmeal

Ingredients

¼ cup Scottish oatmeal[1]
4 oz. soymilk or nonfat milk
Sprinkle of clove spice to taste
½ tsp. ginger spice
Ground cinnamon to taste

½ tsp. ground flaxseed
1 small baked pear
¼ tsp. honey
1 tsp. currants and/or 1 tsp. sultanas

Directions

Heat oatmeal and milk. Add honey and spices as desired. Bring ingredients to a low boil and simmer for 2–3 minutes. Add currants or sultanas, pear, and flaxseed. Serve in your favorite china bowl. Mine is a beautiful English bone china.

1 serving.

Nutritional serving information: carbohydrate—fruit 1
carbohydrate—grain/starch 1
protein ½
fat 1

---

1   See organic Scottish oatmeal at **www.bobsredmill.com**, or use organic quick oats.

Breakfast Bread

Ingredients

2 cups blueberries
2 cups whole-grain wheat flour
2 cups oat bran
1 tsp. baking soda
2 egg whites
¼ cup honey

¼ cup hazelnuts or walnuts
⅛ cup canola oil
⅛ cup peanut oil (double canola oil if
   you don't wish to use peanut oil)
2 cups low-fat soymilk

Directions

Preheat oven to 375°F. Set blueberries and nuts aside. In a medium-size bowl, combine all other dry ingredients. In a large bowl, mix all liquid ingredients. Add dry ingredients to liquid mixture and mix well. Carefully fold in nuts and blueberries. Pour batter into a bread or cake pan. Bake for about 30 minutes. Test with a toothpick to see if fully baked. Remove from pan and allow to cool before slicing.

8 servings.

Nutritional serving information: carbohydrate—fruit ½
carbohydrate—grain/starch 2
protein ½
fat 2

Raspberry Oat Bread

Ingredients

1¾ cups whole-grain flour
2¼ cups oat bran
1 tsp. baking powder
2 egg whites
¼ cup canola oil

1 tsp. orange rind
2 tsp. fresh orange juice
¼ cup honey
2 cups soymilk
2 cups fresh or frozen raspberries

Directions

Preheat oven to 350°F. Set raspberries aside. Mix all dry ingredients. In a separate bowl, mix all wet ingredients until they are completely blended. Gradually add dry ingredients to your blended mixture and stir well. Gently fold in the berries. Pour mixture into a bread pan. Bake for 40–50 minutes or until cooked.

8 servings.

Nutritional serving information: carbohydrate—fruit ½
carbohydrate—grain/starch 2
protein 1
fat 1

Blueberry Sultana Oat Bread

Ingredients

1¾ cups whole-grain flour
2¼ cups oat bran
1 tsp. baking powder
2 egg whites
2 cups soymilk
¼ cup canola oil

2 tsp. fresh orange juice
1 tsp. orange rind
¼ cup honey
1½ cup fresh or frozen blueberries
¼ cup sultanas

Directions

Preheat oven to 350°F. Set blueberries and sultanas aside. In a mixing bowl, combine flour, bran, and baking powder. In a separate bowl, stir all wet ingredients until fully blended. Gradually add dry ingredients to your blended wet mixture and stir well. Gently fold in berries and sultanas. Pour mixture into a bread pan. Bake for 40–50 minutes or until bread is brown on top.

8 servings.

Nutritional serving information: carbohydrate—fruit ½
carbohydrate—grain/starch 2
protein 1
fat 1

Black Currant Oat Bread

Ingredients

1¾ cups whole-grain flour
2¼ cups oat bran
1 tsp. baking powder
2 cups soymilk
¼ cup canola oil

1 tsp. orange rind
¼ cup honey
2 tsp. fresh orange juice
2 egg whites
2 cups fresh or frozen black currants

Directions

Preheat oven to 350°F. Set black currants aside. In a mixing bowl, combine all dry ingredients. In a separate bowl, mix all wet ingredients until thoroughly blended. Gradually add dry ingredients to your blended mixture and stir well. Gently fold in the currants. Pour mixture into a bread pan. Bake for 40–50 minutes or until cooked.

8 servings.

Nutritional information/serving: carbohydrate—fruit ½
carbohydrate—grain/starch 2
protein 1
fat 1

Banana Berry Muffins (Jen's)

Ingredients

2 very ripe bananas, mashed
3 tbsp. honey
2 tbsp. canola oil
1 tsp. vanilla
½ cup unsweetened applesauce
2 cups coarsely chopped mixed
    berries (blackberries, blueberries,
    raspberries, or currants)

1 cup whole-wheat pastry flour
½ cup whole-grain flour
1½ tsp. baking soda
¾ cup chopped walnuts
¼ tsp. salt

Directions

Preheat oven to 350°F. Combine bananas, honey, oil, vanilla, and applesauce. In a separate bowl, stir together flours, baking soda, salt, and walnuts. Add dry ingredients to liquid mixture and blend together until just combined. Add berries and stir gently. Spoon batter into muffin pan or paper-lined cups in pan. Bake for 16 minutes and check to see if fully baked. Remove from pan and allow to cool completely on rack.

12 servings.

Nutritional information/serving: carbohydrate—fruit ½
    carbohydrate—grain/starch 2
    protein ½
    fat 1

Blueberry Muffins (Jen's)

Ingredients

3 tbsp. honey
2 tbsp. canola oil
1 tsp. vanilla
½ cup unsweetened applesauce
1 cup whole-wheat pastry flour

½ cup whole-grain flour
1½ tsp. baking soda
¼ tsp. salt
¾ cup chopped walnuts
2 cups coarsely chopped mixed berries
    (blackberries, blueberries, raspberries,
    or black currants)

Directions

Preheat oven to 350°F. Mix honey, oil, vanilla, and applesauce. In a separate bowl, stir together flours, baking soda, salt, and walnuts. Add dry ingredients to liquid mixture and blend together until just combined. Add berries and stir gently. Spoon batter into bread pan or paper-lined cups in muffin pan. Bake for 16 minutes for muffins, or 25 minutes for bread. Check to see if fully baked. Remove from pan and allow to cool completely on rack.

12 servings.

Nutritional information/serving: carbohydrate—fruit ½
    carbohydrate—grain/starch 2
    protein ½
    fat 1

Blueberry Oat Bread or Muffins

Ingredients

3 tbsp. honey

2 tbsp. canola oil

1 tsp. vanilla

½ cup unsweetened applesauce

1 cup whole-wheat pastry flour

½ cup whole-grain flour

½ cup Scottish oatmeal[1]

1½ tsp. baking soda

¼ tsp. salt

¾ cup chopped walnuts

2 cups coarsely chopped mixed berries (black berries, blueberries, raspberries, or black currants)

Directions

Preheat oven to 350°F. Mix honey, oil, vanilla, and applesauce. In a separate bowl, stir together flours, ¼ cup oatmeal, baking soda, salt, and walnuts. Add dry ingredients to liquid mixture and blend together until just combined. Add berries and stir gently. Spoon batter into bread pan or paper-lined cups in muffin pan. Sprinkle remaining oatmeal on top of muffins. Bake for 16 minutes for muffins, or 25 minutes for bread. Check to see if fully baked. Remove from pan and allow to cool completely on rack.

12 servings.

Nutritional information/serving: carbohydrate—grain/starch 2
protein ½
fat 1

"Green" Toast

Pam's "Green Toast" is a fun breakfast for children. Try it!

Ingredients

1 slice of whole-grain oat bread or bran flax bread.

1 serving of avocado

Directions

Toast the bread to your liking. Top with avocado (the green stuff). Cut into green fingers and enjoy. Mmm, good!

1 serving.

Nutritional information/serving: carbohydrate—grain/starch 1
fat 1

---

1   See organic Scottish oatmeal at **www.bobsredmill.com**, or use organic quick oats.

Omelet or Burrito

Ingredients
Extra-virgin olive oil (spray bottle)
2 egg whites
1 small chopped shallot
2 tbsp. diced red bell pepper

½ tsp. curry mix with turmeric
1 tomato, sliced
⅛ avocado

For burrito:
1 whole-wheat or corn tortilla (fat-free or made with olive oil). When purchasing tortillas, make sure they do not contain trans fat, a common ingredient in commercial tortillas.

Note: you may wish to add some low-fat soy cheese if it is included in your dietary plan.

Directions for omelet:
Mix egg whites, shallot, bell pepper, and curry mix in a bowl. Lightly spray frying pan with olive oil. Place over medium heat. Pour the egg mixture into the pan and swish around so that a fine layer of egg sticks to the side of the pan. Leave the egg mixture alone for a few minutes to allow it to "set." You will know the egg has cooked enough to proceed when the egg whites have actually turned white. When the egg is about 70% cooked solid, it is time for the second swish. Whatever liquid mixture is left in the skillet, swirl it around the edges again to make the crispy edge layer thicker.

Place the avocado and tomato in the center of the omelet and fold it in half. Cook for an additional minute before serving.

For burrito:
Heat the tortilla. Place cooked eggs and all your toppings on top of it. Roll up and enjoy. I have to say this is one of my favorite breakfasts!

1 serving.

Nutritional information/serving: carbohydrate—vegetable 1
carbohydrate—grain/starch 1
protein 2
fat 1

Red Pepper Tofu Scramble

Ingredients

4 oz. firm tofu or 2 egg whites
Extra-virgin olive oil (spray bottle)
1 small shallot, chopped
2 oz. shiitake mushrooms
1 tortilla or oat flax toast (optional)
2 tbsp. diced red bell pepper

1 vine-ripened tomato, chopped
½ tsp. curry mix with turmeric
⅛ of an avocado
1 tbsp. salsa (optional)
Salt and pepper to taste

You may wish to add some low-fat soy cheese if this is included in your
recommended dietary plan.

Directions

If using tofu, break it into small pieces. Spray pan with olive oil and place over
medium heat. Add the shallot, mushrooms, tomato, and pepper and stir until
lightly browned. Add the tofu or eggs, then the curry/turmeric mixture, salt,
and pepper. Cook for 2–3 minutes, stirring constantly. Serve with salsa, sliced
avocado, and warm whole-wheat tortillas or toast.

1 serving.

Nutritional information/serving: carbohydrate—vegetable ½
carbohydrate—grain/starch 1
protein 1
fat 1

Shakes-to-Go

A shake is an excellent way to include fresh fruit in your diet. Here are four
shakes-to-go. This can also be a snack selection.

Banana Almond Shake-to-Go

Ingredients

½ banana
1⅓ tbsp. natural almond butter
1 tbsp. honey
1 tbsp. ground flaxseed

¼ cup fresh or frozen mixed berries
2 tbsp. Scottish oatmeal[1]
8 oz. vanilla Vitasoy[2]

Directions

Put all ingredients in blender and blend until smooth. Serve in a cup to go. Or, if
serving at home, serve in a glass dessert dish.

1 serving.

Nutritional information/serving: carbohydrate—fruit 1½
carbohydrate—grain/starch ½
protein 2
fat 2

---

1   See organic Scottish oatmeal at **www.bobsredmill.com**, or use organic quick oats.
2   **www.vitasoy-usa.com**

Quick Fresh Fruit Shake-to-Go

Ingredients

4 strawberries
1 tbsp. raspberries
1 cup fresh pineapple, crushed or sliced
2 tbsp. Scottish oatmeal[1]
1 cup plain soy yogurt or
    vanilla nonfat yogurt

1 tbsp. blueberries
½ tbsp. ground flaxseed
1 medium banana
4 ice cubes

Directions

Place all ingredients in a blender and blend until smooth. Serve in a cup to go. Or if serving at home, serve in a glass dessert dish.

1 serving.

Nutritional information/serving: carbohydrate—fruit 5
carbohydrate—grain/starch ½
protein 1
fat ½

Lemon Shake-to-Go

Ingredients

1 small peach
½ medium banana
Juice of 1 lemon
1 cup plain soy yogurt or
    vanilla nonfat yogurt

2 tbsp. Scottish oatmeal[1]
1 tsp. vanilla extract
4 ice cubes

Directions

Place all ingredients in a blender and blend until smooth. Serve in a cup to go. Or if serving at home, serve in a glass dessert dish.

1 serving.

Nutritional information/serving: carbohydrate—fruit 2
carbohydrate—grain/starch ¼
protein 1

---

1   See organic Scottish oatmeal at **www.bobsredmill.com**, or use organic quick oats.

Orange Shake-to-Go

Ingredients

1 medium orange
2 tbsp. Scottish oatmeal[1]
½ medium banana
4 ice cubes

1 small peach
1 tbsp. ground flaxseed
1 tsp. vanilla extract
1 cup plain soy yogurt or vanilla
    nonfat yogurt

Directions

Place all ingredients in a blender and blend until smooth. Serve in a cup to go. Or, if serving at home, serve in a glass dessert dish.

1 serving.

Nutritional information/serving: carbohydrate—fruit 2
                                      carbohydrate—grain/starch ½
                                      protein 1
                                      fat 1

Golf Snack Mix

A lot of my patients are avid golfers. The big question is: "Pam, you don't want me to have a hot dog on the course. So what do I do for my morning snack?" Yep, you guessed it! Golf Snack Mix slips, oh so nicely, into that golf bag. The serving amount is based on your individual diet. By the way, this can be great for kids, too, morning or afternoon. It fits nicely into a backpack.

Tip for moms and dads—this is a great activity to do with your children. Get them measuring and mixing all the ingredients in a big bag, then dance around the kitchen with a big baggie of Golf Snack Mix. See who can do the best shake dance. Dads usually do the silliest dances, and children think this is really funny. Then use a measuring cup to dole out serving sizes into individual baggies.

Mix ½ cup of any of the following nuts or seeds: pumpkin seeds, almonds, walnuts, along with ½ cup of any of the following: dried blueberries; diced, dried apricots; sultanas; currants; or dried cranberries.

Add 1 cup oat bran cereal flakes or whole oat bran biscuit pieces. Mix all ingredients in a bowl and pop into paper or wax snack bags for a morning or afternoon snack. Do the big shake. Make a big batch of this snack mix on Sunday evenings to last (maybe) through the whole week.

4 servings.

Nutritional information/serving: carbohydrate—fruit 1
                                      carbohydrate—grain/starch ½
                                      protein ½
                                      fat 1

---

1   See organic Scottish oatmeal at **www.bobsredmill.com**, or use organic quick oats.

Apo E Gene Soups

Simple Vegetable Broth

Ingredients

3 cups carrots, sliced	2 tbsp. extra-virgin olive oil
8 cups water	1 cup chopped shallots
1 cup chopped turnip	1 cup chopped onion
2 crushed garlic cloves	1 cup fresh parsley
1 cup chopped celery	½ cup fresh thyme
1 bay leaf	1 tsp. white pepper
3 sticks astragalus root	Salt to taste

Directions

Combine all ingredients, except water, in a large saucepan. Cover the vegetables with water. Bring to a boil and then reduce heat and simmer for 45 minutes. Liquidize in blender and strain for broth.

4 servings.

Nutritional information/serving: carbohydrate—vegetable 1½
fat 1

Creamed Spinach Carrot Soup

Ingredients

2 tbsp. extra-virgin olive oil	2 tbsp. whole-wheat flour
2 shallots, chopped	1 tsp. flaxseed
1 cup chopped leeks	¼ tsp. ginger
2 sticks astragalus root	4 cups vegetable broth
4 cloves of garlic, crushed	4 cups spinach
1½ cups lentils	2 cups soymilk
1 large potato, chopped	1 sprig cilantro or parsley
3 cups chopped carrots	white pepper to taste

Additional ½ cup vegetable broth or water if needed

Directions

Heat olive oil in a medium-size skillet. Add shallots, leeks, astragalus root, and garlic. Add lentils, potato, and carrots and cook for 5–7 minutes until they begin to soften. Gradually add the wheat flour, flaxseed, and ginger; and stir well. Gradually add 1 cup of vegetable stock. Transfer all ingredients to a larger saucepan for further cooking. Allow to cook for another 5 minutes. Add the remaining 3 cups of stock, then add the spinach. Bring soup to a boil, then lower heat to simmer for 20–30 minutes. Add the soymilk and any additional water (if needed). Simmer 7–10 minutes. Liquidize in a blender for 1 minute. Serve hot in a china bowl, with cilantro or parsley to garnish. Add white pepper to taste.

8 servings.

Nutritional information/serving: carbohydrate—vegetable 1½
carbohydrate—grain/starch ½
protein 1
fat 1

Miso Pasta Soup

Ingredients

2 tbsp. extra-virgin olive oil
1 cup chopped shiitake mushrooms
2 cups chopped shallots
4 cups chopped carrots
2 cups sliced celery

6 cups water
1 cup whole-wheat noodles
2 cups spinach
2 tbsp. fresh miso
Green onion for garnish (optional)

Directions

In a medium skillet, heat olive oil. Add mushrooms, shallots, carrots, and celery and stir until brown, 2–3 minutes. Bring water to the boil in a large saucepan, add vegetables and pasta. Simmer for 7–10 minutes. Add the spinach. Dissolve miso in a bowl of warm water. Add this to the pasta and vegetables. Serve in a Japanese-type bowl. Top with chopped green onion if desired.

8 servings.

Nutritional information/serving: carbohydrate—vegetable 2
carbohydrate—grain/starch 1
fat 1

Pam's Vegetable Soup

Ingredients

3 tbsp. extra-virgin olive oil
2 cups chopped shallots
2 cloves crushed garlic
4 cups chopped carrots
1 cup sliced celery
8 cups chopped potato
2 cups chopped zucchini
1 cup whole-wheat pasta shells
8 cups vegetable broth
4 cups additional broth if needed

2 cups black beans
1 cup pearl barley
2 cups chopped yellow squash
2 sticks astragalus root
2 cups chopped fresh tomatoes
1 cup lentils
2 cups spinach
White pepper and salt to taste
1 avocado

Directions

In a very large saucepan, heat olive oil. Add shallots and garlic, cook for 2–3 minutes; then add carrots, celery, and potato. Cook for an additional 5 minutes. Add remaining ingredients except for salt, white pepper, and avocado. Bring to a boil. Boil slowly for 5 minutes. Reduce heat to a simmer. Simmer for 45–60 minutes or until done. Serve in a rustic bowl, topped with chunks of avocado. (This soup freezes well.)

8 servings.

Nutritional information/serving: carbohydrate—vegetable 2
carbohydrate—grain/starch ½
protein ½
fat ½

Tomato, Carrot, and Butternut Squash Soup

Ingredients

1 tbsp. extra-virgin olive oil
1 cup chopped shallots
4 garlic cloves, crushed
1 cup cooked white navy beans
3 cups chopped carrots
2 sticks astragalus root
2 cups butternut squash

¼ tsp. ground ginger
¼ tsp. cumin
2 cups tomato soup
2 cups vegetable broth
½ cup soymilk
Salt and white pepper to taste
Parsley

Directions

Heat olive oil in a skillet. Add shallots and garlic. Then add beans, carrots, astragalus, squash, ginger, and cumin. Stir well. Add vegetable broth and tomato soup and bring to a boil. Simmer and cook for about 20–30 minutes until the beans and carrots are soft. Add salt and white pepper. Liquidize in blender with soymilk. Serve in a china bowl. Add parsley to garnish.

8 servings.

Nutritional information/serving: carbohydrate—vegetable 2
protein ½
fat 1

Butternut Lemon Soup

Ingredients

2 tbsp. extra-virgin olive oil
1 cup chopped shallots
4 cloves crushed garlic
2 cups butternut squash
4 cups vegetable broth
Juice from ½ lemon

½ cup soymilk
¼ tsp. cinnamon
¼ tsp. nutmeg (if desired)
Salt and white pepper to taste
⅛ avocado (cut into chunks)
Grated lemon rind

Directions

Heat olive oil in a skillet. Add shallots and garlic. Brown lightly. Add squash, vegetable broth, and lemon juice; and bring to a boil. Turn heat to a simmer and cook for 20–25 minutes. Add soymilk. Add seasonings, and liquidize in a blender. Serve in a china bowl. Top with avocado chunks and grated lemon rind.

4 servings.

Nutritional information/serving: carbohydrate—vegetable 1½
fat 1

Sunflower Split Pea Soup

Ingredients

2 cups split peas
2 tsp. extra-virgin olive oil
1 cup chopped shallots
2 cloves crushed garlic
4 cups chopped carrots

1 cup chopped celery
1 cup chopped potato
8 cups vegetable broth
½ cup soymilk
Salt and pepper to taste
½ tsp. toasted sunflower seeds

Directions

Soak split peas in warm water for 4 hours or overnight. In a medium saucepan, warm olive oil. Add shallots, garlic, carrots, celery, and potato—cook for 3–5 minutes. Add vegetable broth, then bring to a boil. Reduce heat and simmer for 45–50 minutes or until the peas are cooked. Add salt and pepper to taste and soymilk. Liquidize in a blender. Serve in a white china bowl. Top with toasted sunflower seeds.

8 servings.

Nutritional information/serving: carbohydrate—vegetable 1½
carbohydrate—grain/starch ½
protein 1
fat 1

Cornish Pea Soup

Ingredients

1 cup split peas
4 cups cold water
¼ cup fresh thyme
1 medium leek, chopped
¼ cup fresh parsley
1 cup sliced celery
1 cup chopped potato

1 cup carrots
1 tbsp. extra-virgin olive oil
¼ cup shallots
Salt and pepper
2 cups soymilk
Croutons (optional)
Mint (optional garnish)

Directions

Soak peas in warm water for 4 hours or overnight. Rinse and place peas in a large saucepan with 4 cups of cold water. Add remaining ingredients, leaving out the soymilk and croutons. Bring soup to a boil, then turn heat to low and simmer for 2 hours. Add soymilk and return to the boil. Simmer for 10 minutes. Serve in your china soup bowl. Add the croutons and chopped mint as a garnish if desired.

6 servings.

Nutritional information/serving: carbohydrate—vegetable 1
carbohydrate—grain/starch 1
protein 1
fat 1

Simple Vegetarian Black Bean Soup

Ingredients

1 tbsp. extra-virgin olive oil
2 shallots, chopped
1 cup carrots coarsely chopped
1 cup chopped red pepper
3 cups vegetable broth
1 tsp. cumin
1 tsp. turmeric

2 stalks of astragalus root
1 cup tomato puree
1 can black beans[3]
1 cup chopped tomatoes
¼ cup fresh parsley
¼ cup fresh ginger root slices
Ground pepper to taste

Directions

Heat olive oil in a heavy pot for 30 seconds. Add shallots, carrots, and red pepper. Cook for 3–5 minutes. Then add vegetable broth, spices, astragalus root, tomato puree, beans, and tomatoes. Cook for about 25 minutes. Serve in your favorite bowl. Add parsley and sliced fresh ginger root to the top. Add ground pepper to taste.

4 servings.

Nutritional information/serving: carbohydrate—vegetable 2
carbohydrate—grain/starch 1
protein 1
fat ½

Cream Potato Corn Soup

Ingredients

2 tbsp. extra-virgin olive oil
1 cup chopped shallots
2 cloves crushed garlic
4 cups chopped carrots
4 cups chopped celery
8 cups chopped potatoes

3 cups vegetable broth
2 cups white beans
1 cup chopped onion
1 cup soymilk
white pepper and salt as seasoning
2 cups fresh cut white corn to garnish

Directions

Heat olive oil in a large saucepan. Add shallots and garlic. Cook for 2–3 minutes. Then add carrots, celery, and potato. Cook for an additional 5 minutes. Add remaining ingredients. Bring to a boil. Boil for 5 minutes and then reduce heat to a simmer. Simmer for 45–50 minutes or until done. Mash soup with a potato masher immediately after cooking. Serve in a china bowl, topped with a spoonful of white corn.

10 servings.

Nutritional information/serving: carbohydrate—vegetable 2
carbohydrate—grain/starch 1
protein 1
fat 1

---

3   Amy's brand: www.amys.com

Spring and Fall Nettle Soup

Yes, this is the stinging nettle that may have stung you as a young child. However, nettles have been found to be helpful with prostate disorders, joint disorders, allergies, and certain respiratory disorders. Now I'm sure you're wondering whether the nettles keep their sting—well, they don't. When you cook stinging nettle, the sting goes away.

Ingredients

2 tbsp. extra-virgin olive oil

2 cups shallots

2 cloves crushed garlic

2 sticks astragalus root

4 cups small leaf stinging nettles
(caution with fresh nettle handling!)

2 tbsp. whole-wheat flour

2 cups vegetable broth

1 cup soymilk

Salt and pepper to taste

Mint leaf and lemon rind (garnish)

Directions

Heat olive oil in a saucepan, then add shallots, garlic, and astragalus. Cook for 2–3 minutes, then add nettle. Cook for an additional 5 minutes. Add whole-wheat flour, stir through, then gradually add vegetable stock and soymilk. Bring to a boil, boil slowly for 5 minutes, and then reduce to simmer for 30 minutes or until done. Liquidize in a blender immediately. Serve in a china bowl, topped with a mint leaf and grated lemon rind.

6 servings.

Nutritional information/serving: carbohydrate—vegetable 1½
fat 1

Apo E Gene Entrées

Pam's Lime Rosemary Baked Chicken

My sister Heather made this chicken dish while I was visiting her in England. The herbs and juices from the chicken roasting made her English Tudor kitchen smell divine. As she made the chicken, we reviewed her recipe and together came up with ingredients to add even further flavor and health benefits to it. Here you have it all!

Ingredients

1 large chicken (6–7 lbs.), free range　　4 whole garlic cloves, crushed
1 fresh lime　　　　　　　　　　　　　2 sprigs each: sage, lavender, and rosemary
1 tbsp. extra-virgin olive oil　　　　　　¼ tsp. fresh ground pepper

Directions

Preheat oven to 350°F. Place chicken in a large roasting pan. Cut and squeeze lime over the chicken, and then place it inside the chicken. Rub oil and garlic over the chicken. Place 1 of the sage, lavender, and rosemary sprigs inside and 1 on the outside of the chicken. Sprinkle with the pepper. Cook for 60–90 minutes, basting occasionally. Cut breast meat off the bone. Serve in 3–5 oz. portions.

15 servings.

Nutritional information/serving:　　protein 4

Roast Rosemary Turkey

Ingredients

1 large turkey, organic, free-range　　4 garlic cloves, crushed
2 sprigs each: thyme and rosemary　　1 tbsp. extra-virgin olive oil
1 pinch fresh ground pepper　　　　　1 lime

Directions

Preheat oven to 350°F. Place turkey in a large roasting pan. Cut and squeeze lime over turkey and then place inside, along with 1 of the thyme and rosemary sprigs, and half of the garlic. Rub oil and remaining garlic over the turkey, sprinkle with pepper. Place remaining sprigs of thyme and rosemary on the turkey. Cooking time depends on size of turkey, approximately 15–20 minutes per pound. Baste occasionally. Cut breast meat off the bone. Serve in 3–5 oz. portions.

1 serving.

Nutritional information/serving:　　protein 3

Grilled or Baked Fish

Here's a tip I learned from my Nana, Bertha McDonald, as a young girl: "You want to know the secret of good eating, my love? Eat the best fish you can find and eat it often."

The fishermen of Cornwall are on their fishing boats, catching fish for your dinner tonight. For centuries the Cornish fishing industry has made Cornwall what it is today. An abundance of fresh fish, including pilchards, mackerel, and cod, was hauled into the famous harbors of Polperro, Mevagissey, Fowey, and Charlestown. The Cornish pilchards were so fresh and delicious, they were shipped far and wide, even to Italy as far back as the mid-1700s.

Make sure your fish is fresh, wild, and not farm raised. Farm-raised fish has been shown to contain food color, environmental toxins, PCBs, heavy metals such as mercury and lead, and other toxic contaminants, as well as residues of antibiotics and other drugs. Wild salmon is only available between April and October. Two reliable sources of wild fish I have found are Whole Foods Market and an Internet site called Vital Choice (**www.vitalchoice.com**).

Ingredients
You can use these types of fish: mackerel, shrimp, scallops, black cod, sea bass, herring, salmon, ahi tuna, halibut, tuna, sardines, and pilchards.

Consider herbs and flavors for fish: lemons, limes, garlic, shallots, lavender, thyme, rosemary, cilantro, parsley, teriyaki, Thai peanut, and soy ginger.

Directions
Preheat oven to 350°F. Place raw fish on a favorite baking sheet that has been brushed with a little olive oil. Brush fish with a little olive oil. Squeeze fresh lime over the fish. Add fresh herbs: rosemary, cilantro, thyme, lavender, etc. Bake for 12–15 minutes. As an alternative, you can use your grill.

Fish serving size—average 3–5 oz.—as per your individual dietary recommendation. Consume the recommended amount of fish per your suggested protein allowance.

1 serving.

Nutritional information/serving: protein 3

Grilled or Baked Salmon with
Teriyaki Shiitake Mushroom Sauce

Ingredients

5 oz. fresh wild salmon

Sliced shiitake mushrooms

1 clove fresh garlic, crushed

Teriyaki Sauce*

1 shallot, chopped finely

Juice of ½ lime

Directions

Marinate the fish in the sauce for 20–30 minutes. Sprinkle with lime juice, garlic, and shallot. Bake or grill with mushrooms until done to your liking.

1 serving.

Nutritional information/serving: protein 3

Grilled Wild Halibut with
Raspberry Honey Ginger Glaze

Ingredients

5 oz. fresh wild halibut

¼ cup fresh raspberries

1 clove fresh garlic, crushed

¼ cup Soy Ginger Sauce*

1 shallot, chopped finely

Juice of ½ lime

Directions

Marinate by covering the fish with all the ingredients for about 30–40 minutes. Grill or bake until cooked to your liking.

1 serving.

Nutritional information/serving: protein 4

Pacific Rim Fish (or Tofu) and Veggies in a Wok

You may add any of the Pacific Rim Sauces to this dish (see page 366). When choosing your Pacific Rim Sauce, keep in mind your available daily servings of fat, based on your individual Apo E genotype and calories allowed.

Ingredients
Olive oil in pump spray bottle
½ tsp. extra-virgin olive oil
¼ cup green onion
⅛ cup shallots
¼ cup water chestnuts
¼ cup grated carrots
¼ cup young English pea pods
¼ cup vegetable stock
¼ cup red bell pepper
3 oz. tofu or fish

Directions
Lightly spray the wok with olive oil, then add and heat ½ tsp. of extra-virgin olive oil. Cook the onion and shallots lightly. Add all other vegetables and cook for 2–3 minutes more, adding stock slowly to keep vegetables from going dry. Then add tofu or fish and cook until lightly browned. Add the Pacific Rim Sauce of your choosing. Cook for an additional 2–3 minutes, or until the sauce is warm.

1 serving.

Nutritional information/serving: carbohydrate—vegetable 2
protein 1
fat ½

Shrimp Curry

Ingredients
4 oz. cooked, peeled, deveined shrimp
⅛ tsp. cayenne
2 small cooked, diced potatoes
1 tsp. tomato paste
½ tsp. honey mustard
1 tbsp. lime juice
1 tsp. cumin powder
⅛ tsp. paprika
¼ tsp red pepper
¼ tsp. whole-wheat flour
¼ tsp. dried lavender
2 tbsp. low-fat soy yogurt

Directions
Mix all ingredients in bowl; chill for at least 1–2 hours before serving.

1 serving.

Nutritional information/serving: carbohydrate—grain/starch 2
protein 4

Mevagissey Fish Tacos

Ingredients

2 six-inch corn tortillas
¼ cup romaine lettuce
5 oz. fresh wild white fish, cooked
⅛ avocado
½ cup grilled vegetables
(red onion, red peppers, zucchini)

¼ cup diced tomato
¼ cup nonfat soy cheese
¼ cup Hawaiian Mango Salsa* or
Fresh Tomato Salsa*
Fresh sliced ginger (garnish)

Directions

In the center of each tortilla place half of each ingredient: lettuce, fish, avocado, grilled vegetables, tomato, and soy cheese. Top with mango or tomato salsa. A ginger garnish adds a sparkle to your taco and a tingle to your tongue.

2 servings.

Nutritional information/serving: carbohydrate—vegetable 1
carbohydrate—grain/starch 1
protein 2½
fat 1½

Apo E Gene Vegetarian Entrées

Rustic Tuscany Pizza

Ingredients

1¼ cups lukewarm water
1 tbsp. honey
1 packet yeast
1 cup white flour
½ cup whole-wheat flour
Salt
1 tsp. extra-virgin olive oil
½ cup fresh tomato sauce
1 tbsp. fresh sweet basil
1 tbsp. each fresh cilantro and parsley

1 tsp. fresh sage
1 tbsp. fresh marjoram
1 tsp. fresh rosemary
4 oz. soy cheese, shredded
1 thinly sliced tomato
1 small roasted garlic clove
1 cup chopped red bell pepper
¼ cup shiitake mushrooms
¼ cup kalamata olives

Directions

Step One: Make pizza dough. Pour water into a large bowl. Stir honey through the water. Whisk the yeast through, and set the mixture aside until a "sponge" forms on top of the mixture. This usually takes 5–10 minutes. Meanwhile, mix flours and salt together, and make a "well" in the center. Put the yeast mixture into the "well," and work the flour in gradually until a ball of soft dough is formed. Rub the inside of a large, clean bowl with olive oil, and place the dough in the bowl. Cover the dough with a clean, damp cloth; and let it rise in a warm place until it has doubled in size, approximately 30 minutes. After dough has risen, knead again and roll out on a clean, dry, floured surface. Divide into two equal portions and roll each piece into a ball. Place the dough, covered, in the refrigerator to rest for 1 hour. Bring the dough to room temperature before preparing to use.

Preheat oven to 450°F.

Step Two: Coat pizza pan with a little olive oil. Roll dough portions to fit pizza pan, and place in the pan to form the pizza crust. Combine tomato sauce and herbs, spread over the dough, and add soy cheese evenly over the surface. Top with vegetables, spreading them evenly over the cheese. Bake for 10–14 minutes or until crust is cooked to a light brown.

4 servings.

Nutritional information/serving:　carbohydrate—vegetable ½
carbohydrate—grain/starch 3
protein 1
fat ¼

Mevagissey Ratatouille

I first had this dish in a little bistro in Mevagissey, Cornwall, when I was about 15 or 16. It was so delicious. The flavors from this dish were extremely memorable. What a clever way to eat vegetables, I thought to myself, and to make them taste great!

Ingredients

2 tsp. extra-virgin olive oil
1 sweet red onion, roughly cut
1 red bell pepper, roughly cut
1 cup eggplant and zucchini, roughly cut
4 shallots, roughly chopped
½ cup water

1 clove garlic, crushed
1 bunch spinach, rinsed, torn into pieces
1 cup cooked corn
2–4 large tomatoes, roughly cut
⅛ tsp. lavender

Directions

Preheat oven to 350°F. Heat olive oil in pan over low to medium-high heat. Add onion, pepper, eggplant and zucchini, shallots, and garlic to the pan. When lightly browned, add spinach with ½ cup of water. When greens are wilted, add corn and tomatoes and cook for another 5–7 minutes. Pour all ingredients into an oval ceramic baking dish. Bake for 30–40 minutes. Garnish with lavender before serving.

12 servings.

Nutritional information/serving: carbohydrate—vegetable 2

Cornish Chili

Ingredients

16 oz. chili beans (black)
8 oz. tomatoes, chopped
2 medium sweet onions (Maui, if available), coarsely chopped
1 chopped red bell pepper
2 tbsp. jalapeño peppers (if desired)

½ cup water
1 tbsp. scallions, chopped
8 oz. firm tofu, cubed
1 tsp. turmeric and chili spices (to taste)
1 tsp. extra-virgin olive oil

Directions

Combine all ingredients in medium saucepan. Bring to boil, cover, and simmer over a low heat for 20–30 minutes.

4 servings.

Nutritional information/serving: carbohydrate—vegetable 1
carbohydrate—grain/starch 1
protein 3

Vegetable and Garbanzo Bean Curry

Ingredients

1 large red potato
1 cup carrots
2 shallots, chopped
1 tbsp. extra-virgin olive oil
1 tbsp. tomato paste
1 tbsp. whole-grain flour
2 garlic cloves, crushed

3 tsp. freshly grated ginger
½ cup vegetable broth
1 tbsp. curry powder
1 cup green peas
1½ cups garbanzo beans
1 cup low fat soymilk
2 tsp. lemon juice

Optional herbs and seasonings include any or all of these: freshly ground coriander seeds, turmeric, fenugreek, black pepper, dried chilies, cardamoms, and cinnamon.

Directions

Cut potato and carrot into bite-size pieces. Heat oil in a pan. Add shallots, potato, carrots, tomato paste, flour, garlic, and ginger. Add stock slowly, and cook for a few minutes. Add curry. Cook, stirring, for 1–2 minutes. Add peas, garbanzo beans, and soymilk. Cook until vegetables are soft. Stir in lemon juice.

4 servings.

Nutritional information/serving: carbohydrate—vegetable 2
carbohydrate—grain/starch ½
protein 1
fat 1

Vegetable Spaghetti or Pasta

Ingredients

2 tbsp. extra-virgin olive oil
16 oz. tofu
1 large shallot, chopped
2 garlic cloves, crushed
1 cup shiitake mushrooms
1 cup zucchini, chopped
4 baby eggplants, quartered
⅛ cup fresh grated ginger

2½ cups coarsely cut tomatoes, sieved
2 tbsp. tomato paste
2 tsp. honey
½ cup kalamata olives
½ cup basil sprigs
Salt and pepper
16 oz. whole-wheat spaghetti or pasta
1 tbsp. lemon juice

Directions

Heat 1 tbsp. of the oil in a large, heavy skillet. Add the tofu, shallot, garlic, mushrooms, zucchini, lemon juice, eggplants, and ginger. Cook over low heat, stirring occasionally, for 4–5 minutes or until lightly browned. Pour in the sieved tomatoes, season with salt and pepper, and stir in the honey and tomato paste. Bring to a boil, reduce the heat, and simmer gently for 25 minutes. While vegetables are simmering, bring a large pan of lightly salted water to a boil. Add the pasta, return to a boil, and cook for 8–10 minutes or until tender but firm to the bite. Drain, and toss in the remaining oil. Serve with tomato veggie sauce. Sprinkle with olives and basil.

6 servings.

Nutritional information/serving: carbohydrate—vegetable 4
carbohydrate—grain/starch 2
protein 2
fat 1

Shiitake Mushroom and Spinach Lasagna

Ingredients

1 tbsp. extra-virgin olive oil
1 cup chopped shallots
1 tsp. crushed garlic
2 cups shiitake mushrooms, roughly cut
1 cup sliced zucchini
10 oz. fresh spinach, torn

½ lb. whole-wheat lasagna
3 cups nonfat marinara sauce
½ tsp. salt to taste
1 cup high-quality tofu
2–4 oz. low-fat soy cheese (optional)
Basil for garnish

Directions

Preheat oven 450°F. In frying pan, heat olive oil; then add shallots, garlic, shiitake mushrooms, and zucchini. Cook until all reach a soft consistency, about 5–7 minutes. Add spinach and slowly cook throughout, about 7 minutes. Do not drain. Move these vegetables to a large bowl. Boil lasagna in a large pot of boiling water until slightly soft. Do not cook completely. Drain. Alternate layers of noodles, sauce, tofu, and vegetables until the pan is filled, ending with noodles and cheese to cover the top of the lasagna. Bake covered for the first 20 minutes. Remove lid and cook for an additional 10–15 minutes. End with a 2- to 3-minute broil to brown the cheese on top of the dish. Garnish with basil. Let sit 10 minutes before serving.

6 servings.

Nutritional information/serving: carbohydrate—vegetable 3
carbohydrate—grain/starch 1
protein 1
fat 1

Vegetable and Bean Tacos

Ingredients

2 six-inch corn tortillas

½ cup diced red pepper

½ cup grilled vegetables (red onion, eggplant, zucchini)

¼ cup fresh vine-ripened tomatoes, chopped

¼ cup romaine lettuce

½ cup pinto beans

2 tsp. extra-virgin olive oil

⅛ avocado

¼ cup low-fat soy cheese

¼ cup salsa with garlic

Cilantro

Directions

In the center of each corn tortilla place half of each ingredient: red pepper, grilled vegetables, tomatoes, beans, avocado, soy cheese, lettuce. Top with salsa and cilantro.

2 servings.

Nutritional information/serving: carbohydrate—vegetable 1½
carbohydrate—grain/starch 1½
fat 1½

Tofu and Bean Tacos

Ingredients

1 tsp. extra-virgin olive oil

4 oz. firm tofu

2 cloves garlic, if desired

½ cup cooked pinto or black beans

¼ cup vine-ripened tomatoes

1 oz. grated cheese

¼ cup chopped romaine lettuce

⅛ cup finely chopped red cabbage

½ cup sweet white onion, chopped (mild Maui onion, if available)

⅛ avocado

2 six-inch white corn tortillas

Directions

Chop tofu into bite-size pieces; finely chop garlic. Brown garlic and tofu in a lightly seasoned skillet over medium heat until golden brown. Heat beans in a saucepan over medium heat. Mix beans, tofu, and grated cheese together. Set aside. Warm tortillas in lightly seasoned pan with olive oil; place tofu and bean mixture on one half of the tortilla; fold other half over the tofu mixture; and add desired toppings: lettuce, cabbage, onions, tomatoes, and avocado.

1 serving

Nutritional information/serving: carbohydrate—vegetable 1½
carbohydrate—grain/starch 1
protein 2
fat 1½

Thai Hazelnuts and Currant Tofu

Ingredients

Extra-virgin olive oil (spray bottle)
3 oz. tofu
½ cup chopped red pepper
⅓ cup currants

½ cup chopped mango
Thai Hazelnut Sauce(see page 367)
Honey
1 cup young English pea pods

Directions

Spray pan with oil. Heat, and brown tofu. Add red pepper, currants, and mango. Stir through sauce and honey. Cook for 7–12 minutes. Add pea pods and simmer for an additional 5–7 minutes.

1 serving.

Nutritional information/serving: carbohydrate—vegetable 5
protein 1
fat ½

Apo E Gene Pacific Rim Sauces and Salsa

The sauces can be used on fish, beans, tofu, lentils, and chicken. If you don't have the time to make a sauce yourself, you may be able to locate a premade sauce similar to this recipe at a local store. Choose one with the best possible ingredients in it. Look for a product made with natural flavorings and a monounsaturated or polyunsaturated oil, such as olive oil or canola oil. Choose a product that does not have artificial flavorings or preservatives. Stay with natural whole foods as much as possible.

The Ancient Chinese Wok

The wok has been used in Chinese cooking for approximately 2,000 years. Usually made out of metal, the wok has a distinct wide, deep bowl shape and can be used for either slow or rapid cooking. The versatility of this cooking tool is one of the main reasons why it has remained a major part of Asian cooking and is now used by cooks around the world. In addition, it requires little fuel, making it economical to use.

Peanut Sauce

This all-around delicious sauce can be stirred into rice, noodles, or vegetables, as well as served on beans, fish, tofu, etc.

Ingredients

1 tbsp. extra-virgin olive oil
1 small onion or scallion
3 tsp. fresh crushed garlic
1 tsp. freshly grated ginger
1 tsp. turmeric
¼ cup nonfat soymilk
1 tbsp. freshly ground peanut butter

¼ cup fresh cilantro
1 tbsp. honey
1 tbsp. lime juice
1 tbsp. lemon juice
1 tsp. tomato paste
2 tbsp. tamari sauce
¼ cup water

Directions

Heat the olive oil in a pan over moderate heat. Cook the onion, garlic, and ginger until the onion is transparent. Cook for 1 minute while mixing in turmeric. Add soymilk, peanut butter, cilantro, honey, lime and lemon juices, tomato paste, tamari, and water. Bring the sauce to a gentle boil, then simmer for 12–15 minutes.

4 servings.

Nutritional information/serving: fat 2

History and Benefits of Soy Sauce

Soy sauce dates back centuries. Initially used as a means of preserving food, soy sauce became a valuable flavor enhancer and was used in many ways in cooking. Several cultures use soy sauce in this way today; Japan and China especially come to mind when we think of soy sauce. Whether it was first developed by the Japanese or the Chinese has been much debated. Regardless, the English have used soy sauce for hundreds of years and it is thought to have been introduced in the mid-1600s by English philosopher John Locke. I definitely enjoyed soy sauce while growing up in England. In our family it was used in many sauces and gravies to produce a richer flavor.

Some people view soy sauce like a fine wine or sherry, and it is said to contain more antioxidants than red wine. This high level of antioxidants boasts protection for the cardiovascular system.

Note

Not all soy sauces are created equal. Many brands of soy sauces available in our supermarkets are artificially hydrolyzed and contain isolated soy protein along with preservatives and flavor enhancers such as MSG. These types of soy sauces create health risks.

A high-quality soy sauce should be made from organic soy and brewed from a natural bacterial and fungal culture.

Thai Hazelnut Sauce

Ingredients

2½ tsp. tamari	2 tsp. freshly grated ginger
¼ cup honey	1 tsp. low sodium soy sauce
1½ tsp. vinegar	¼ tsp. cayenne
¼ tsp. paprika	½ cup miso
¼ cup sweet vinegar	1 cup freshly ground hazelnut butter
2 chopped garlic cloves	

Directions

Blend all ingredients, either by hand or in a blender. Let sit for 1 hour in refrigerator to allow the flavors to mingle together.

4 servings.

Nutritional information/serving: fat 2

Teriyaki Sauce

Ingredients

1 tsp. sesame oil
1 clove garlic, finely chopped
1 tbsp. honey
¼ cup apple cider
2 tsp. shallots, finely chopped

¼ cup low-sodium soy sauce
1 tsp. freshly grated ginger
¼ cup of water
¼ cup vinegar
1 tbsp. lime juice

Directions

Heat oil in a skillet. Add garlic and cook for 2 minutes. Gradually stir in all other ingredients. Then cook for another 5–7 minutes on medium heat.

8 servings.

Nutritional information/serving: fat 1

Soy Ginger Sauce

Ingredients

1 tbsp. extra-virgin olive oil
2 tsp. freshly crushed garlic
1 tsp. freshly grated ginger
¼ tsp. turmeric
¼ cup water

1 tbsp. lime juice
1 tbsp. lemon juice
¼ cup low-sodium soy sauce
1 tbsp. honey
¼ cup chardonnay vinegar

Directions

Heat oil in skillet on low heat. Add garlic and cook for 2 minutes. Add all other ingredients slowly, stirring as you add each ingredient. Then cook for another 5–7 minutes on medium heat.

4 servings.

Nutritional information/serving: fat ½

Fresh Tomato Salsa

Ingredients

2 jalapeño peppers (optional)
5 large tomatoes
¼ lemon
2 oz. fresh ginger, peeled and grated
4 cloves garlic

1 red chili pepper (optional)
1 red onion, quartered
2 tbsp. expeller-pressed olive oil
1 cup fresh cilantro
Salt and pepper to taste

Directions

If using jalapeño peppers, grill on both sides until well browned or blackened. This will give your salsa a smoky flavor. After browning, cool for 10 minutes. Place jalapeños and all other ingredients, except the cilantro, into a blender.

Pulse-blend your salsa to the consistency you like, less blending for chunky salsa. Children love to do this. Allow them to press the button on the blender while mom or dad keeps a hand on the lid. Coarsely chop the cilantro and fold into the blended salsa. Place salsa into a glass or ceramic bowl and chill for at least 30 minutes.

4 servings.

Nutritional information/serving: carbohydrate—fruit 1
fat ¼

Hawaiian Mango Salsa

Ingredients

½ cup chopped red pepper
1 cup chopped cucumber
Juice of two fresh limes
1½ cups ripe mango fruit—
chopped into small pieces

1 mild jalapeño pepper, finely diced
½ cup chopped cilantro
1 avocado, chopped
1 cup Maui sweet onion—
chopped into small pieces

Directions

Mix all ingredients in a bowl.

4 servings.

Nutritional information/serving: carbohydrate—vegetable 1
carbohydrate—fruit 1
fat ½

Tomato Salsa Cream

Ingredients

1 cup Fresh Tomato Salsa*
1 tsp. lemon juice

1 cup soy yogurt
1 tsp. freshly grated ginger

Directions

Combine all ingredients. Chill for 1 hour before serving.

2 servings.

Nutritional information/serving: carbohydrate—fruit 1
protein ½
fat ½

Mango Salsa Cream

Ingredients

1 cup mango salsa
1 tsp. lemon juice
1 tsp. fresh ginger

1 cup soy yogurt
⅓ cup chopped cilantro

Directions

Mix ingredients together. Chill for 1 hour before serving.

2 servings.

Nutritional information/serving: carbohydrate—fruit 1
protein ½
fat ½

Papaya Salsa Cream

This is one of my favorite salsa creams. When our family goes to Maui for a vacation, we often lease a home and invite our friends along. One great thing about staying in a home in Hawaii instead of a hotel is cooking your own meals. We love to prepare food and grill together—our friend Rick Sharkey is an excellent griller. Our favorite foods include fresh Hawaiian fish (heads removed), fresh vegetables, and salads. We love potatoes baked in olive oil and topped with this fresh Papaya Salsa cream. Life doesn't get any better—great place, great friends, and fantastic food. My dear friend Rick inspired this recipe, since we share a real love for fresh ingredients, fresh vine-ripened tomatoes, basil, extra-virgin olive oil, and our Papaya Salsa Cream. (Rick should have been a chef.)

Ingredients

1 cup freshly chopped papaya
1 tsp. lime
½ cup sweet onion (Maui)

1 cup soy yogurt
1 tsp. fresh grated ginger
⅓ cup chopped cilantro

Directions

Mix ingredients together. Chill for 1 hour before serving.

4 servings.

Nutritional information/serving: carbohydrate—fruit 1
protein ¼

Nonfat Papaya Salsa Cream

Ingredients

1 cup freshly chopped papaya

1 tsp. lemon

½ cup sweet (Maui) onion

1 cup nonfat soy yogurt

1 tsp. fresh grated ginger

⅓ cup chopped cilantro

Directions

Mix ingredients together. Chill for 1 hour before serving.

4 servings.

Nutritional information/serving: carbohydrate—fruit 1
protein ½
fat ½

Apo E Gene Salads and Salad Dressings

Fish Salad

Ingredients

1 tsp. lemon juice
1 tsp. mustard—optional
2 tsp. chopped avocado
1 tbsp. diced tomato
3–5 oz. shrimp, black cod, or
 tuna, cooked

1 tsp. vinegar
4 finely chopped almonds
2 tsp. chopped sweet onions
2 tbsp. chopped red pepper
1 tsp. olive oil mayonnaise

Directions
Mix together in bowl.

1 serving.

Nutritional information/serving: carbohydrate—vegetable 1
protein 3
fat 3

Chicken Salad

Ingredients

3–5 oz. chicken, cooked
2 tbsp. chopped red pepper
1 tsp. lemon juice
2 tsp. cilantro

2 tbsp. chopped sweet onions
1 tsp. olive oil mayonnaise
1 tsp. vinegar
1 tsp. chardonnay mustard

Directions
Mix all ingredients together in bowl.

1 serving.

Nutritional information/serving: carbohydrate—vegetable 4
protein 1
fat 1

Tuna or Tofu Salad

Ingredients:

4 oz. tuna or tofu
2 cups fresh spinach
1 cup broccoli tips
1 cup shiitake mushrooms
1 cup sweet onion
1 cup vine-ripened tomatoes
3 tsp. extra-virgin olive oil

1 tsp. turmeric
1 cup grated carrot
1 cup cabbage
1 cup red bell pepper
1 cup asparagus
2 tbsp. chopped walnuts
1 tbsp. balsamic vinegar

Directions

Chop vegetables, and mix all ingredients in salad bowl.

4 servings.

Nutritional information/serving:　　carbohydrate—vegetable 4
　　　　　　　　　　　　　　　　　　　protein 1
　　　　　　　　　　　　　　　　　　　fat 1

Wheat Pasta Salad

Ingredients

1 lb. whole-wheat noodles

1 cup asparagus

1 tsp. extra-virgin olive oil

1 small tomato, chopped

¼ cup cooked sweet potato

⅛ cup fresh grated ginger

1 cup garbanzo beans

10 kalamata olives

1 red bell pepper

4 oz. soy cheese

¼ cup fresh basil

¼ cup Shiitake & Sesame Vinaigrette salad dressing[4]

Directions

Cook pasta and asparagus in separate saucepans. Combine with all other ingredients.

6 servings.

Nutritional information/serving:　　carbohydrate—vegetable 1
　　　　　　　　　　　　　　　　　　　carbohydrate—grain/starch 2
　　　　　　　　　　　　　　　　　　　protein 2
　　　　　　　　　　　　　　　　　　　fat 1

Carrot and Cucumber Yogurt Salad

Ingredients

⅛ cup freshly grated ginger

1½ peeled, grated cucumbers

½ tsp. freshly ground cumin seeds

½ tsp. fresh cilantro

1 tsp. fresh-squeezed lemon juice

2 carrots, grated

⅛ tsp. lavender

1 tbsp. chardonnay vinegar

3 cups nonfat plain soy yogurt

Directions

Combine all ingredients. Chill for at least 1 hour.

4 servings.

Nutritional information/serving:　　carbohydrate—vegetable ½
　　　　　　　　　　　　　　　　　　　carbohydrate—fruit ½
　　　　　　　　　　　　　　　　　　　protein ½

4　www.anniesnaturals.com/organic_dressings

Green Salad

Ingredients

2 cups romaine lettuce, leaves torn
2 cups spinach leaves
½ cup cilantro
3 vine-ripened, chopped tomatoes
¼ tsp. fresh ground white pepper

¼ cup vinaigrette dressing
½ cup chopped red pepper
½ cup peeled and chopped cucumber
1 tbsp. shredded soy cheese

Directions

Combine lettuce, spinach, cilantro, cucumber, tomatoes, red pepper, and ¼ cup vinaigrette. Toss. Sprinkle each serving with soy cheese. Add fresh ground pepper.

4 servings.

Nutritional information/serving: carbohydrate—vegetable 3
fat 2

Sultana, Carrot, Ginger Coleslaw

Ingredients

⅛ cup fresh grated ginger
½ cup sultanas
½ cup nonfat plain soy yogurt

1½ cups grated carrot
¼ cup almonds
1 tsp. fresh-squeezed lime juice

Directions

Combine all ingredients. Chill for at least 1 hour.

2 servings.

Nutritional information/serving: carbohydrate—vegetable 1
carbohydrate—fruit 1
protein—½
fat 1

Daily Veggie Bag

One way of getting servings of veggies into your day is to prepare a bag or container of fresh-cut, raw veggies—these can be eaten at work, in the car, or placed in the refrigerator at home to snack on between household chores. Your bag should contain two cups of veggies, with three or four different types of veggies in each.

Ingredients
Can include any of the following: carrots, red or green bell pepper, cherry tomatoes, broccoli spears, asparagus, cauliflower, green beans, celery, squash, zucchini, snap peas, or English pea pods. Remember to choose organic vegetables whenever possible.

Directions
Slice vegetables into manageable-size pieces. Place into a portable container or refrigerate to enjoy at home. These veggies can be enjoyed with a serving of nut butter or hummus, as suggested in your own individual Apo E food menu.

If you would like to take these veggie snacks to work or school, you can use a wax paper bag or a reuseable muslin bag.

2 servings.

Nutritional information/serving: carbohydrate—vegetable 2

Cilantro Soy Ginger Dressing

Ingredients
¼ cup extra-virgin olive oil   1 roasted garlic clove, crushed
¼ cup fresh chopped cilantro   ¼ cup balsamic vinegar
1 tsp. low sodium soy sauce   1 tsp. freshly grated ginger
¼ tsp. white pepper

Directions
Place all ingredients in a glass salad dressing container; mix well. For best results, let stand in the refrigerator for 8–24 hours.

4 servings.

Nutritional information/serving: fat 3

Simple Salad Dressing

Ingredients

¼ cup extra-virgin olive oil
Juice of 1 lime
1 tsp. freshly grated ginger

¼ cup chardonnay vinegar
1 tsp. low-sodium soy sauce
¼ tsp. white pepper

Directions

Place all ingredients in a glass salad dressing container; mix well. For best results, let stand in the refrigerator for 8–24 hours.

4 servings.

Nutritional information/serving: fat 3

Fat-Free Salad Dressing

Ingredients

¼ cup finely chopped fresh cilantro
2 tbsp. chopped chives
¼ cup chardonnay vinegar
¼ tsp. finely grated fresh lime rind

1 tsp. low-sodium soy sauce
1 tsp. freshly grated ginger
¼ tsp. white pepper
¼ tsp. of mustard

Directions

Place all ingredients in a glass salad dressing container; mix well. For best results, let stand in the refrigerator for 8–24 hours.

4 servings.

Nutritional information/serving: carbohydrate—vegetable ¼

Nonfat Spicy Lime Ginger Dressing

Ingredients

¼ cup fish sauce or
   vegetable broth
   (vegetarian alternative)
½ cup rice vinegar
1 tsp. minced cilantro

2 cloves finely minced garlic
2 tsp. crushed chili pepper flakes
2 tsp. minced, pressed ginger
Juice of 2 medium limes
1 tsp. honey

Directions

Mix all ingredients together in a blender. Chill for two hours before serving.

4 servings.

Nutritional information/serving: carbohydrate—vegetable ¼

Apo E Gene Side Dishes

Pam's Baked Potato

Ingredients

1 medium potato, 3 oz.   ½ tsp. extra-virgin olive oil
Salt

Directions

Preheat oven to 350°F. Wash potato well under warm water and pat dry. Cover with the olive oil. Add a pinch of salt on the potato and a pinch of salt over your shoulder for good luck. Bake your potato 45–60 minutes.

1 serving.

Nutritional information/serving: carbohydrate—grain/starch 1

Olive Oil Potato Wedgewood Fries

I call these "Wedgewood" fries because they are big wedges and look like wood.

Ingredients

3 russet potatoes   Salt and pepper
1 tbsp. extra-virgin olive oil
   (in spray bottle)

Directions

Preheat oven to 450°F.

Cut potatoes into ½" wedges. Place potatoes in boiling water—use just enough water to cover the wedges. Boil for 5 minutes. Drain and place on a cookie sheet that has been lightly sprayed with olive oil. Lightly spray potato wedges with olive oil. Bake for 25 minutes or until golden brown.

6 servings.

Nutritional information/serving: carbohydrate—grain/starch 1
                                         fat 1

Original Hummus

Ingredients

1 cup sesame seeds
1 oz. pine nuts
30 oz. cooked chickpeas
⅛ cup expeller-pressed olive oil
½ cup water

½ lemon
1 oz. ginger, freshly grated
2 cloves garlic, finely chopped
½ bunch cilantro or 1 small
    red pepper

Directions

Lightly stir sesame seeds and pine nuts in cast-iron pan until well toasted. Allow to cool. Grind to a smooth consistency in a coffee grinder or blender. Chill for a few minutes. Place seeds, nuts, and all remaining ingredients, except ¼ cup of water, in a food processor. Blend, gradually adding remaining water until hummus reaches the desired consistency. Place in a glass container and chill for a minimum of 1 hour.

This is also something children love to make and love to eat. My daughter Alison, who is in her first year of high school, loves to eat it with fresh-cut carrots and red peppers.

Alison highly recommends enjoying a serving of hummus with fresh vegetables such as carrots, radishes, English pea pods, asparagus, red and yellow peppers, small baby tomatoes, and organic whole-grain crackers or flax crackers.[5]

8 servings.

Nutritional information/serving: carbohydrate—vegetable 1
                                          carbohydrate—grain/starch 1

Guacamole

I just love the natural goodness of avocado. Until I moved to the United States in 1981, I had never eaten an avocado. Since I arrived, I have eaten them often for their healthful qualities—and flavor! Don't forget, avocado contains large amounts of good fat and plant stanols. Plant stanols may reduce cholesterol and are a promising addition to interventions aimed at lowering heart-disease risk. One serving of avocado has 137 mg. of plant stanol and no partially hydrogenated fats. Compare this to the leading margarine/butter substitute spread that has 2–7 mg. of plant stanols per serving. Yep, I choose to put fresh avocado in my food.

Ingredients

1 medium soft avocado
2 ripe tomatoes
½ cup chopped mild sweet onion
½ green pepper

2 medium garlic cloves, finely chopped
2 tbsp. lime juice
1 jalapeño

5   **www.gluten-free-crackers.com/index.html**

Directions

Place all ingredients in blender, and blend until smooth.

Or for a fun game your children will love, place all ingredients into a ziplock bag and squish to your heart's content until all the ingredients are blended. Cut off one corner of the ziplock bag and squeeze into a bowl.

4 servings.

Nutritional information/serving: carbohydrate—vegetable 1
                                         fat 2

Homemade Corn and Lime Tortilla Chips

Ingredients

1 packet (8) six-inch corn tortillas   1 fresh lime
1 tsp. canola oil

Directions

Cut each tortilla into 8 slices, and place on a slightly oiled baking sheet. Put a squeeze of lime over each tortilla. Place slices under a broiler for 2 minutes. Turn over to broil the other side for 2 minutes. Place on a decorative plate with your fresh salsa and you have a refreshing and tasty healthy snack.

8 servings.

Nutritional information/serving: Carbohydrate—grain/starch 1

Tomato-Olive Tapenade

Ingredients

1 tsp. canola oil   ½ cup fresh basil
1 cup sun-dried tomatoes   ¼ lemon
16 kalamata olives   1 oz. avocado
2 garlic cloves   2 tsp. expeller-pressed olive oil
¾ cup water

Directions

Soak sun-dried tomatoes in hot water for 10 minutes. Drain tomatoes and save liquid. Place all the ingredients, except water and oil, into a food processor. Slowly add water and oil, blending until you have a smooth consistency. Place tapenade into a glass bowl and chill for 4 hours. Serve with whole-grain crackers or whole-grain bread.

4 servings.

Nutritional information/serving: carbohydrate— vegetable 1¼
                                         fat 1¼

Almond Milk

Ingredients

2 cups almonds   2 cups water
Cheesecloth

Directions

Soak almonds overnight. They may begin to sprout. Bring a pot of water to boil, and blanch the almonds by dipping them in the boiling water for 5–10 seconds. Remove the skin by transferring them immediately into ice-cold water. Blend almonds with 2 cups of water until liquid. Squeeze through cheesecloth to remove the almond pulp. Refrigerate.

2 servings.

Nutritional information/serving: protein 1
                                        fat 1

Almond Cheese

Ingredients

2 cups almonds   2 cups water
Herbs: can include basil, rosemary,   Cucumber or sun-dried tomatoes
   chives, spicy red cayenne peppers,   (optional)
   finely chopped chili peppers   Cheesecloth

Directions

Soak almonds overnight. They may begin to sprout. Bring a pot of water to boil, and blanch the almonds by dipping them in the boiling water for 5–10 seconds. Remove the skin by transferring them immediately into ice-cold water. Blend almonds with 2 cups of water until liquid. Do not remove the almond pulp. Place the blended almond mixture in a clean glass bowl. Cover the mixture with a clean, dry cloth or cheesecloth; and leave it at a cool temperature for 12 hours to allow it to ferment. Place mixture into a cheesecloth bag, and allow it to drain for an additional 8 hours at room temperature. This cheese can now be left plain; or spices and herbs, cucumber, or sun-dried tomatoes can also be added. The cheese is best left to sit again for 3–4 days after adding herbs and seasoning to absorb the flavor of the herbs. Store in a glass container only.

8 servings.

Nutritional information/serving: protein 1
                                        fat ½

Vegan Cottage Cheese

Ingredients

1 lb. tofu

1 tsp. lemon juice

Pinch of salt

2–3 drops of honey (optional)

Directions

Mash ingredients together until the mixture has the curd appearance of cottage cheese. Refrigerate for at least 6 hours.

4 servings.

Nutritional information/serving: protein 1

fat 2

Soy Yogurt

Ingredients

1 qt. soymilk   1 package yogurt starter

Directions

Heat milk to 180°F. Allow milk to cool. Add yogurt starter to the milk, and pour into glass container. Refrigerate for at least 8 hours.

8 servings.

Nutritional information/serving: protein ½

fat 1

Food for Thought

At the second nutrition conference Dr. Andrew Weil held in Tucson, Arizona, a physician from Norway spoke about a group of older ladies who used to get together and have tea, sandwiches, and cake while they socialized and shared the traditional recipes for an afternoon tea. Eventually, two of these ladies were told by their doctors that they had to change their diet and stop eating the foods they loved. Soon after they quit attending the daily gatherings, they become much sicker, depressed, and lonely.

Based on this situation, the Norwegian physician learned that these daily gatherings served as much more than a meal. They were also a cultural experience and welcome social occasion. What the women needed was a little recipe modification and nutritional help—not orders to disband a cherished get-together. It was this doctor's nurse who actually said, "No, all you need to do is make some changes, not break up the party."

Food has long been a big part of humans communicating love for their family and friends. Along with sustaining the physical body and satisfying basic physiological needs, food also fills emotional, mental, and spiritual needs. It is only recently that we began looking at food from a health-preserving and disease-preventing perspective in such detail.

Having begun to examine the benefits of good whole food, we need to look at some of the foods our families may have eaten in the past, which we may today call "comfort foods." While we don't necessarily need to remove these comforting foods from our diet, we may need to rework old family recipes. In order to maintain a healthy nutritional regimen, good food must include traditional, local, cultural, and high-quality ingredients. Take some time to look over some of your family recipes and see how you can modify the contents to make them healthier. And it can be fun to share with your family the memories you associate with these recipes.

I want to share with you some of my family traditions and recipes from Scotland and England. These are not foods I eat every day or even every week, yet they are traditional foods of my English-Scottish heritage that I prepare occasionally for my family and friends. While it is important to eat a healthy diet for your Apo E genotype most of the time, it is important not to leave behind those wonderful foods that brought you so much joy. Keep such foods close to your heart and use them to generate good feelings whenever you need them in your life.

Happy Families and a Cornish Tradition—Pasties

Pasties are a cultural food for me and an example of how traditional foods can be enjoyed once in a while so as not to lose the traditional cultural aspect of one's upbringing. I include below the following recipe for Cornish pasties, one I have enjoyed since childhood, in memory of my Nana, Peggy Caine, who died just before this book was published, and my Uncle Brian. Nana Caine lived in Bodmin, Cornwall, all her life, and, believe me, she was a master Cornish pasty maker. I loved her very much. Her very presence emanated love, comfort, and joy. I was not able to share much time with her over the past few years, since she lived in the south of England and I live in California, but she taught me the importance of the family dinner table in keeping the family together. Research today shows us that this is true, and I imagine she would be delighted to know that. So always make sure you and your children share at least one meal together each day, and if possible, make that meal dinner. It's such a good way to end the day. I assure you, the end result is a happy family.

Nana had a very specific way of making her pasties (pronounced "pass-tees"), and I am going to share the recipe she taught to me from about the age of 10.

But first I would like to tell you a little history of the Cornish pasty. Pasties are said to be the original handheld convenience food, with a lineage that dates back to the Middle Ages, although no one knows for certain when they showed up on our ancestors' lunch plates—possibly as far back as the 1100s or 1300s, or maybe centuries afterward in the late 1700s or early 1800s. A common story told in Cornish inns, fishing villages, misty moorlands, and coastlines is that the history of the Cornish Pasty stretches back to the time of King Arthur—they may have come from Tintagel, his birthplace. Stories of King Arthur's Cornwall, with the legends of Camelot, are without question the best known and most fascinating of all Cornish folklore.

But no matter when they were first created, we have no doubt that Cornish pasties came from Cornwall. This dish grew out of a basic need to take hot, satisfying, high-calorie food into the cold Cornish tin mines. Served at lunchtime, pasties were meant to provide the miners with the fuel to get them through the rest of the day. The classic tin-mine pasty contained meat and root vegetables in one end and fruit, such as apples, plums, or fruit preserves, in the other. It was also common to see a person's initials on one side of the pasty casing, in order to avoid mix-up at lunchtime. Nana carried on this time-bound tradition by putting our initials on the pasties so we didn't get someone else's, which was good because I would never want a pasty that was made for my sister. She never liked turnips, and turnips were my favorite part.

One very distinct feature of the Cornish pasty is the way it is put together. To close the pasty, you need to perform a special seal technique called crimping, which makes the wavelike seal that holds the pasty together. It is a little tricky to learn, but once you get the crimping down, it becomes a most enjoyable part of the whole pasty-making process. Essentially, to "crimp," you hold the two sides of the dough together, and by making little twists and folds, you seal the dough on the top. A never-ending debate about the Cornish pasty is whether the sealing crimp should be on the side or on top. My vote is to crimp on the side, because that makes the pasty easier to eat.

1

2

3

4

As you can see, there is a lot of history and debate surrounding the Cornish pasty, which nourishes the tummy as well as the heart and soul. Luckily, one thing that all true traditional pasty makers can agree upon is the quality of the ingredients: The food should be the highest quality. If meat is used, it should be the leanest, best cuts available, and it should be cut into bite-size pieces, rendering true flavor. The vegetables should always be neatly sliced and diced, and the ingredients must never be cooked before they are wrapped inside the pasty. All of the ingredients are to be raw and cooked all at once inside the pasty in the oven.

Cornish pasty–making is an art, as my Uncle Brian would say. This is the "culture of our land," and if you want to experience a Cornish pasty you need to make it with the spirit of the past. As a child, when I delivered dairy products for Uncle Brian's dairy delivery company to authentic pasty shops and kitchens, I saw how the cooks followed the old rules of making pasties. A prime requirement was having the intention of delivering healthy food for good, hard-working people: use garden-fresh, wholesome ingredients such as turnips, onions, potatoes, and parsley, and this will feed your body and soul for hours. (Remember to cut parsley with scissors, not a knife.)

The goodness and love wrapped neatly in this little packet we call a Cornish pasty helps me imagine the tin miners taking a break to enjoy theirs. Before you make your pasty, take a minute to set your own mind to good intention—to provide a tasty meal for today made with love and devotion to the delicious details of the Cornish tradition from hundreds of years ago.

Nana Caine's recipe for Cornish pasties has meat in it. If you do not eat meat, you can leave it out. You may want to substitute the traditional lean beef with chicken, fish, tofu, beans, lentils, salmon, lamprey eels, or carrots (even though some say putting carrot in a pasty is a sin, I love carrot in mine, so I put it in, transgression or not). Even though these ingredients are not in the traditional recipe, I have tried them all, and they are delicious. Tales from the past tell us that some miners actually ate only the filling and discarded the buttery crust. So if you wanted to do that, you could.

"Betho whye lowenack!" (Cornish for "Happiness to you!")

Nana Caine and Uncle Brian's Cornish Pasty

Pasty Crust

Ingredients

3 cups unbleached flour

Traditional recipe: 1½ sticks butter (never use margarine)

1½ tsp. salt

Heart-healthy recipe: 1½ cups canola oil

6 tbsp. water

Directions

In a large bowl, combine flour, butter or oil, and salt. Add water, one tablespoon at a time, mixing well until combined to form a ball of dough. Knead dough with heel of the hand to distribute oil or butter evenly. Lightly dust the dough with a little flour, cover with wax paper. Place the dough, covered, in the refrigerator to rest for 30 minutes. Bring the dough to room temperature before preparing to use.

Pasty Filling

Ingredients

1 lb. round steak, very coarsely ground

2 potatoes, peeled and chopped

2 tsp. salt

½ tsp. pepper

2 large onions, chopped

½ cup turnip or rutabaga, chopped

1 egg, beaten

Tiny pieces of butter

Directions

Preheat oven to 350°F. Combine all filling ingredients (except for the salt, pepper, egg, and butter) in a large bowl, then set aside. Next, divide the dough into 6 pieces and roll one of the pieces into a 10-inch round on a lightly floured surface. Put 1½ cups of filling in the middle of the pastry round, add salt and pepper to taste, and top with your tiny piece of butter. Moisten the edges of the pastry with a little water, and fold the edges together to enclose the filling. Pinch the edges together to seal them, and crimp (see directions on page 384). Place pasty onto a lightly greased baking sheet and draw your initials in the top of your pasty. Also, use a knife to make a slit in the top. Brush the top of the pasty with beaten egg to help seal the crimping and give it a beautiful glazed finish. Bake in preheated oven for 60 minutes. Remove from oven, cover with a tea towel, and cool for 15 minutes. Mmm, mmm—I can hear Nana tell me it is time for my pasty right now.

6 servings.

Nutritional information/serving: carbohydrate—grain/starch 3
protein 3
fat 10

The Magic Ingredient for Cornish Pasties

One winter afternoon around 4 o'clock, I was making Cornish pasties in our kitchen when my daughter Paige, who was 5 years old, dragged her little wooden stool next to me so she could help me and also hear the stories of the Cornish pixies and fairies, Blue Bell Woods, the Cornish castles, and King Arthur. (Victoria and Alison, my older daughters, used to cook with me, too, but they are 11 and 20 years of age now, and while they don't quite believe in my fairy stories anymore, they believe in my pasties.)

Paige said, "So, Mum, do fairies and pixies from Blue Bell Woods like Cornish Pasties, too?"

"Of course they do," I replied. "Cornish fairies love vegetables and fruit, and Cornish pastics have lots of those. Cornish fairies are a big part of making pasties. Who do you think collects all those herbs for the green grocer to sell to all the mummies to bake our pasties? Parsley is the magic ingredient of pasties. That magic comes from the fairies."

"Oh, that's right, Mum, I forgot. How silly of me!" Then she paused, thinking about the information I had just given her. "So, Mum, how do they carry so many herbs, when fairies are so small?"

"They have a magic herb pouch," I said, "just like the pixie and fairy dust pouch that they carry with them wherever they fly."

"They do? Fairies must be very strong. No, I think they have help, Mum."

Oh boy, these 5-year-olds keep you thinking! However, at dinnertime, Paige told the whole family about how the fairies collected the magic herbs for the green grocer so Mummy could make the pasties.

Keep your children dreaming and cooking with you. And always allow them to sprinkle the magical ingredients into the dish you are making.

Pam's Cornish Pasty—the Heart-Healthy Version

Pasty short-crust ingredients

1 cup white flour, regular or
   gluten free
1½ cups whole-wheat flour
Pinch of salt

¾ cup extra-virgin olive oil
3 tbsp. water

Pasty filling ingredients

Note: all filling ingredients are to be kept separate. All kinds of vegetables and herbs can be placed inside a pasty—potatoes being one main ingredient. Additional possibilities include fish, spinach, shallots, leeks, carrots, parsnips, onion, parsley, turnip, or watercress.

For this recipe, I am going to use: fish, potatoes, carrots, onion, and the magic ingredient—parsley.

Glaze: egg white and soymilk

Directions

Make your short-crust following directions for pastry crust in Nana Caine's Cornish Pasty recipe on page 386. Allow to cool in the refrigerator. Bring out your short-crust and roll it out on a floured kitchen counter to the size of a dinner plate. In the middle of the short-crust, ingredient by ingredient, layer the vegetables and fish filling, ending with the fish and a magic sprinkle of parsley. Dampen the edge of the pastry with water. Then take one edge of the circle of short-crust and fold it over to meet the other edge, and press the edges of the dough together to make a half-moon shape. Then crimp (see directions on page 384) the edges of the pasty. Make a small hole with a knife to let out steam while cooking. Brush with an egg white and soymilk glaze. Place your pasty on a lightly greased metal baking sheet; bake for 1 hour at 450°F. Allow to cool and serve on your best English china plate with a fresh, mixed-garden salad.

3 servings.

Nutritional information/serving: carbohydrate—vegetable ½
carbohydrate—grain/starch 3
protein 2
fat 9

Apo E Gene Desserts

Very Berry Fruit Salad

Ingredients

1 cup black currants

1 cup blackberries

1 cup blueberries

1 cup strawberries, cut in quarters

1 cup raspberries

Directions

Wash fruit well. Place in a chilled bowl. Serve with your favorite frozen yogurt.

Alternative Directions

Freeze fresh berries in individual baggies in ¾-cup portions. When you are ready to serve a dessert, remove berries from the freezer, place on your favorite china dessert plates, and cover with warm English Vanilla Custard. This makes a delicious after-dinner or nighttime snack.

10 servings.

Nutritional information/serving: carbohydrate—fruit 1
   If served with custard, add: protein 1

Fruit Crumbles

Here are some examples of fresh fruit crumble recipes. These are a well-known English dessert, which I grew up eating at dinner. Our crumble usually consisted of apple, blackberry, raspberry, gooseberry, and rhubarb—the fruits my grandmother had in our garden. Of course, the crumbles I ate were made a little differently back then and usually were smothered with either Cornish clotted cream (a delicious decadent cream with 60 g. of saturated fat per serving) or Kelly's Cornish Ice Cream. Very delicious memories! Today my focus is on modifying this delicious food to a healthy alternative. I hope you enjoy these recipes. The love from my grandmothers, Nana McDonald and Nana Caine, is in every one.

Consider Black Currants

In World War II England, fresh citrus fruit was difficult to get from 1940 on, so black currant became a very popular fruit for its vitamin C, and the British government encouraged people to cultivate it. The taste became so popular that a black currant cordial was given out free to all British children, including me. Even Rowntrees, one of the largest candy makers in England, produced a candy called Fruit Gums, and the best flavor in my book is black currant. Ask any British Fruit Gum lover and they will tell you the black currant Fruit Gums are one of the best candies. Whether black currant is eaten fresh off the bushes in the garden or in popular candies, or whether it's turned into juice, the flavor is very good. Why should you consider eating black currant? In addition to vitamin C, black currants contain a very important source of essential fatty acid called gamma-linolenic acid (GLA).

Pear and Currant Crumble

Ingredients

2 pears, peeled, cored, and sliced
1 cup black currants
1½ cups Scottish oatmeal[1]
¼ tsp. vanilla extract

²/3 cup apple juice
1 tsp. arrowroot
½ tsp. cinnamon
¹/3 cup honey

Directions

Preheat oven to 350°F. Layer sliced pears and currants in a baking dish. Mix the remaining ingredients in a bowl. Spread over fruit. Bake for 40 minutes. Delicious alone, or serve with your recommended accompaniment such as nonfat ice cream or low-fat soy yogurt.

4 servings.

Nutritional information/serving: carbohydrate—fruit 1½
carbohydrate—grain/starch 2

---

1   See organic Scottish oatmeal at **www.bobsredmill.com**, or use organic quick oats.

Apple and Peach Crumble

Ingredients

2 fresh peaches, peeled and sliced
1 russet apple, peeled and sliced
1 cup sultanas
½ tsp. cinnamon
⅛ tsp. vanilla extract

⅔ cup apple juice
1 tsp. arrowroot
1½ cups Scottish oatmeal[1]
1 sprinkle of lavender, if desired
⅓ tsp. honey

Directions

Preheat oven to 350°F. Layer sliced peaches and apple in a baking dish. Mix the remaining ingredients in a bowl. Spread over fruit. Bake for 40 minutes. Delicious alone or serve with your recommended accompaniment such as nonfat ice cream or soy yogurt.

4 servings.

Nutritional information/serving: carbohydrate—fruit 1½
carbohydrate—grain/starch 2

Apple and Grape Crumble

Ingredients

2 fresh apples, peeled and sliced
1 cup concord red grapes
½ tsp. cinnamon
⅓ tsp. honey
1 tsp. arrowroot

¾ cup low-fat granola
¾ cup Scottish oatmeal[1]
⅛ tsp. vanilla extract
⅔ cup red grape juice

Directions

Preheat oven to 350°F. Layer apples and grapes in a baking dish. Mix the remaining ingredients in a bowl. Spread over fruit. Bake for 40 minutes. Delicious alone or serve with your favored accompaniment—nonfat ice cream or soy yogurt.

4 servings.

Nutritional information/serving: carbohydrate—fruit 1½
carbohydrate—grain/starch 2

---

1   See organic Scottish oatmeal at **www.bobsredmill.com**, or use organic quick oats.

Apple and Blueberry Crumble

Ingredients

2 large apples, peeled and sliced

1 cup fresh or frozen blueberries

⅔ cup blueberry juice

1 tsp. arrowroot

1 ½ cups Scottish oatmeal[1]

½ tsp. cinnamon

¹⁄₁₆ tsp. nutmeg

⅛ tsp. vanilla extract

⅓ tsp. honey

Pear and Blueberry Crumble

Ingredients

2 pears, peeled and sliced

1 cup fresh or frozen blueberries

1½ cups Scottish oatmeal[1]

⅛ tsp. vanilla extract

⅔ cup blueberry juice

1 tsp. arrowroot

½ tsp. cinnamon

⅓ honey

Directions

Preheat oven to 350°F. Layer pears and blueberries in a baking dish. Mix the remaining ingredients in a bowl. Spread over fruit. Bake for 40 minutes. Delicious alone or serve with your recommended accompaniment—nonfat soy ice cream or low-fat soy yogurt.

4 servings.

Nutritional information/serving: carbohydrate—fruit 2
carbohydrate—grain/starch 1
protein ½

Peach and Blackberry Crumble

Ingredients

2 peaches, peeled and sliced

1 cup fresh or frozen blackberries

1½ cups Scottish oatmeal[1]

⅓ tsp. honey

1 tsp. arrowroot

½ cup black currant or blackberry juice

⅛ tsp. vanilla extract

Directions

Preheat oven to 350°F. Layer peaches and blackberries in a baking dish. Mix the remaining ingredients in a bowl. Spread over fruit. Bake for 40 minutes. Delicious alone, or serve with your recommended accompaniment—nonfat soy ice cream or soy yogurt.

4 servings.

Nutritional information/serving: carbohydrate—fruit 1½
carbohydrate—grain/starch 2

Black Currant and Rhubarb Crumble

Ingredients

2 stalks fresh rhubarb, peeled and sliced
1 cup fresh or frozen black currants
1½ cups Scottish oatmeal[1]
⅓ tsp. honey

1 tsp. arrowroot
½ cup black currant juice
⅛ tsp. vanilla extract

Directions

Preheat oven to 350°F. Layer sliced rhubarb in a baking dish, add black currants. Mix the remaining ingredients in a bowl. Spread over fruit. Bake for 40 minutes. Delicious alone, or serve with your recommended accompaniment—nonfat soy ice cream or soy yogurt.

4 servings.

Nutritional information/serving: carbohydrate—fruit 1½
carbohydrate—grain/starch 2

Baked Pears or Apples

Ingredients

4 pears or apples
½ cup of sultanas
¼ cup black currant juice
¼ cup honey
1 tsp. lemon juice

¼ tsp. fresh ground cinnamon
1½ cups of water
2 tsp. fresh whole cloves
¼ cup slivered almonds
fresh mint

Directions

Preheat oven to 350°F. Core and peel pears, leaving the stems on for decoration. Stir sultanas, black currant juice, honey, and lemon juice together in a saucepan. Bring mixture to a boil, and remove to cool. Sprinkle cinnamon over pears. Place pears and water with cloves in a heavy dish. Bake until pears are tender, approximately 20–30 minutes. Remove pears and put each on individual decorative plates. Drizzle some of the warm fruit sauce over each pear. Top with slivered almonds and fresh mint. This recipe can be made with apples instead of pears.

4 servings.

Nutritional information/serving: carbohydrate—fruit 1½

Scottish Fruit Pottage

Ingredients

2½ cups fresh mixed berries, *mix and match:* loganberries, gooseberries, blueberries, bilberries, huckleberries, blackberries, raspberries, currants, cranberries, grapes, strawberries

2 tsp. grated lemon rind   2 tsp. honey
⅛ tsp. lavender (optional)

Directions
Puree berries in blender. Blend in lemon rind and honey. Use as a topping for desserts. 1 serving is ¾ cup.

4 servings.

Nutritional information/serving: carbohydrate—fruit 1

Kelly's Fore Street Dessert

I literally made this dessert hundreds, if not thousands, of times as a young waitress. It was a Kelly's Cornish ice cream favorite. People came from all over England to have one of these. I have modified the recipe to be heart-healthy.

Ingredients
1 banana   ¼ cup Scottish Fruit Pottage*
6 oz. vanilla soy frozen yogurt   ½ cup berries
2 tbsp. dark chocolate (70%), melted   2 tbsp. chopped almonds

Directions
Slice banana in half lengthwise. Place in glass dessert dish, with one half on either side of dish. Place vanilla frozen yogurt in between the banana halves. Top with melted chocolate and Scottish Fruit Pottage, and then berries and nuts.

2 servings.

Nutritional information/serving: carbohydrate—fruit 2
                                         protein ½
                                         fat 1

English Vanilla Custard

This is the modified English custard, also known as the classic traditional British dessert sauce.

Ingredients
1 cup nonfat milk or soymilk   1 tbsp. arrowroot
1 tsp. vanilla extract   2 oz. honey
1 cup egg substitute

Directions
Heat milk and vanilla in a saucepan, over low heat, to just below boiling point. While the milk is heating, whisk the egg substitute, arrowroot, and honey together in a medium bowl, using a balloon whisk. Then, while whisking the egg mixture with one hand, slowly pour the hot milk into the bowl. Immediately

return all the ingredients to the saucepan, then place on a low, gentle heat and continue stirring until the custard is thick and creamy.

4 servings.

Nutritional information/serving: protein 1

Ginger Biscuits (Cookies)

Ingredients

1 cup unbleached whole-wheat flour	¾ cup canola oil
1 cup unbleached white flour	½ cup brown sugar
2 tsp. baking soda	¾ tsp. freshly grated ginger
Pinch of salt	½ cup applesauce, unsweetened
1 tsp. cinnamon	2 egg whites
1 pinch of clove spice	¼ tsp. vanilla

Directions

Preheat oven to 350°F. Sift flours, soda and spices together. In another bowl mix canola oil and sugar; add the ginger. Add all the wet ingredients to the canola mixture, and mix well. Gradually add the dry ingredients. Roll mixture into 1-inch balls and place on a cookie sheet. Bake 12–14 minutes, until lightly browned. Allow to cool before removing from cookie sheet.

24 servings.

Nutritional information/serving: carbohydrate—grain/starch ½
fat ½

Lemon Ginger Biscuits (Cookies)

Ingredients

1 cup unbleached whole-wheat flour	¾ cup canola oil
1 cup unbleached white flour	½ cup brown sugar
2 tsp. baking soda	¾ tsp. freshly grated ginger
1 tsp. cinnamon	2 egg whites
Pinch of salt	½ cup applesauce
¼ tsp. pure vanilla bean extract	¾ tsp. grated lemon rind

Directions

Preheat oven to 350°F. Sift flours, spices, lemon rind, and soda together. In another bowl mix canola oil and sugar; add the ginger. Then add all the wet ingredients to the oil and sugar mix, and mix well. Gradually add the dry ingredients. Shape into 1-inch balls and place on a cookie sheet. Bake 12–14 minutes or until done. Allow to cool on a cooling sheet.

24 servings.

Nutritional information/serving: carbohydrate—grain/starch ½
fat ½

Raspberry Ginger Biscuits (Cookies)

Ingredients

1 cup unbleached whole-wheat flour	½ cup brown sugar
1 cup unbleached white flour	¾ cup canola oil
2 tsp. baking soda	¾ tsp. freshly grated ginger
Pinch of salt	½ cup applesauce
1 tsp. cinnamon	½ cup raspberries
2 egg whites	¼ tsp. pure vanilla bean extract

Directions

Preheat oven to 350°F. Sift flours, soda and spices together. In another bowl, mix canola oil and sugar; add the ginger. Then add all the wet ingredients to the oil and sugar mix, and mix well. Gradually add the dry ingredients. Mix well. Shape into 1-inch round balls, and place on a cookie sheet. Bake 12–14 minutes, or until done. Allow to cool on a cooling sheet.

24 servings.

Nutritional information/serving: carbohydrate—grain/starch ½
fat ½

Orange Ginger Biscuits (Cookies)

Ingredients

1 cup unbleached whole-wheat flour	½ cup brown sugar
1 cup unbleached white flour	¾ tsp freshly grated ginger
2 tsp. baking soda	¼ cup applesauce, unsweetened
1 tsp. cinnamon	¼ tsp. vanilla extract
Pinch of salt	2 egg whites
¾ cup canola oil	⅛ cup orange juice
¼ tsp. grated orange rind	

Directions

Preheat oven to 350°F. Sift flours, spices, and soda together. In another bowl mix canola oil and sugar; add the ginger. Then add all the wet ingredients to the oil and sugar mix, and mix well. Gradually add the dry ingredients. Form mixture into 1-inch round balls, and place on a cookie sheet. Bake 12–14 minutes, or until done. Allow to cool on a cooling sheet.

24 servings.

Nutritional information/serving: carbohydrate—grain/starch ½
fat ½

Apo E Gene Teas

What to drink? As we have learned, pure water is one the best beverages for the human body, but what we put into our water can be either beneficial or harmful. Drinking only water all the time can be boring for many people—a fact that drives our beverage industry. However, adding flavors in the form of teas can do a body good. I have added some interesting options here for you to try. I enjoy these flavors, and so do my patients.

We have been using plants and foods as medicines for thousands of years, ever since humans learned to draw medicinals from a plant by extracting substances through steeping leaves in hot or cold water. From these ancient practices come some of our foundational beverage traditions, such as the tradition of steeping tea and coffee. However, other plants and beans have been used for beverages for hundreds of years. Today, we are exploring various steeped beverages for their health benefits, such as tea.

A famous evening tea I know well from my childhood is chamomile tea, known for its gentle, calming effects. And, of course, I think the best variety of chamomile is English (Chamaemelum nobile). Growing up in England, we were all told the stories of our little furry friend Peter Rabbit. As the story goes, Peter Rabbit's mother used chamomile tea to help calm him down and send him off to sleep after his adventures in Mr. McGregor's garden.

A note about sweeteners in teas: While many people like to add them to their teas, sweeteners are not included in the nutritional calculations here (and artificial ones are basically toxic chemicals). If you're in the habit of adding them, I strongly recommend you to wean yourself from any sweetener you've been using by gradually reducing the amount until you can enjoy the tea for its own unique flavor.

Dried rosehips are loaded with vitamin C. Add two hips per cup to the pot while brewing. You can buy them at your local health-food store.

My patients ask me all the time: "What do you drink if you don't drink soda or coffee? Water is boring." Here are a few delicious substitutes.

Simple Teas

Choose your favorite tea bag or loose tea (with or without caffeine), for example: White Tea, Peach Tea, Mint Tea, Peach Herbal Tea, Green Tea, Lemon Tea, or Chamomile Tea.

Ingredients
1 bag of tea or 1 tsp. of loose tea

Directions
To a warmed, dry teapot add a bag of tea or your favorite loose tea and any additional flavors or herbs you might like, such as a squeeze of orange or lemon, a slice of peach, or ginger. Add boiling water. Wait 2–5 minutes for the tea and added flavors to infuse. Serve in your favorite teacup. Take a moment to rest and sip your delicious tea.

Rosehip Green Tea

Ingredients

1 bag of green tea   4 slices of fresh orange peel
2 rosehip buds (dried)

Directions
To a warmed, dry teapot, add a bag of your favorite green tea, rosehips, and orange peel. Add boiling water. Wait a few minutes for the tea to infuse. Serve in your favorite teacup. Take a moment to rest and sip your delicious tea.

Dried rosehips can be found in health-food stores, add a delicious flavor to your tea, and are loaded with vitamin C.

The Green and Red Tea (This is a pretty drink)

Ingredients

1 bag of green tea   1 bag of hibiscus tea
1 slice of lemon

Ginger Green Tea

Ingredients

1 bag of green tea   1 bag of ginger tea

Lemon Ginger Green Tea

Ingredients

1 bag of green tea   Squeeze of fresh lemon
Slice of fresh ginger

Directions
To a warmed, dry teapot, add a bag of green tea, a squeeze of lemon, and a slice of ginger. Add boiling water. Wait 2–5 minutes for the green tea, ginger, and lemon to infuse. Serve in your favorite teacup. Take a moment to rest, and sip your delicious tea.

Ginger Cinnamon Tea

Ingredients

6 white tea bags (or equivalent leaves)
½ cup of sliced fresh ginger
3 tbsp. agave nectar

6 cups boiled water
6 cinnamon sticks
1 slice of lemon

Directions

In your teapot add white tea, fresh ginger, cinnamon sticks—allow tea ingredients to sit and steep for 5 minutes. Add agave nectar and lemon slice to taste.

Ginger and Turmeric Tea

Ginger and turmeric have been found to be beneficial for reducing inflammation in the body. Adding these delicious herbs as an anti-inflammatory drink to your daily diet may be very helpful in reducing your risk of inflammatory diseases.

Ingredients

1 cup boiling water
½ tsp. turmeric powder
1 tbsp. honey

½ tsp. ginger powder
¼ tsp. cloves
Juice of ½ lime or lemon

Directions

In your teapot, place ginger, cloves, and turmeric. Add boiling water and steep for 5 minutes. Add honey and lemon to taste. Best drunk immediately.

Black Currant, Ginger, and Turmeric Tea

Ingredients

1 cup boiling water
½ tsp. ginger powder
¼ tsp. cloves

2 tsp. black currant juice
½ tsp. turmeric powder
1 tbsp. honey

Directions

In your teapot, place ginger, cloves, and turmeric. Add boiling water and steep for 5 minutes. Add honey and black currant juice. Best drunk immediately.

Hibiscus Elder Tea

Ingredients

1 bag of hibiscus elder tea

1 serving of natural honey if desired

Chamomile Hibiscus Tea

Ingredients

1 oz. dried chamomile flowers
    or 3 bags of chamomile tea

1 bag of hibiscus tea

Chamomile Peach Tea

Ingredients

1 bag of chamomile tea   1 bag of peach tea

Chamomile Tea with Peach

Ingredients

1 bag of chamomile tea   Slice of peach

White Tea with Cranberries

Ingredients

1 bag of white tea   1 bag of cranberry tea
A few fresh cranberries

Directions

In a warmed, dry teapot, add your tea bags, and cranberries. Add boiling water. Wait 2–5 minutes for the tea to infuse. Serve in your favorite teacup. Take a moment to rest, and sip your delicious tea. Then reflect on your day.

White Mint Tea

Ingredients

1 oz. of your favorite loose-leaf   1 bag of mint tea
   white tea or white tea bag   1 sprig of fresh mint

Directions

To a warmed, dry teapot, add teas and a sprig of fresh mint. Add boiling water. Wait a few minutes for the tea to infuse. Serve in your favorite teacup. Take a moment to rest and sip your delicious tea.

Classic English Tea with Milk

(A classic afternoon tea-break drink)

English people believe in taking a break in the afternoon—try adding a little British into your day, and take a rest. It doesn't have to be long, even 5 or 10 minutes. You will be surprised how much better you feel after your break.

Ingredients

English China teapot—warmed   English China teacup
Loose-leaf tea or tea bags   Nonfat milk or soymilk, if desired

Directions

To your teapot add 1 serving per person of either loose-leaf tea or traditional tea bags—1 tsp. or bag per person and 1 for the pot. Add freshly boiled water to the pot, then brew for 3–5 minutes. Not longer or shorter—shorter doesn't give you all the flavor, longer can make it bitter. Pour your piping hot tea into your English china teacup. If you prefer milk in your tea, pour a little milk in the bottom of the teacup before you pour the tea. Sip your tea and dream of your perfect day.

Apo E Gene Waters and Iced Tea/Lemonades

Earlier in the book I encouraged you to drink fresh, pure water. However, water can be a wonderful beverage if fresh fruit juices, berries, and herbs are added. Consider the following combinations for a refreshing change to your water; and for even more variety, try sparkling water.

Sparkling Lime Juice Iced Water

Ingredients
Crushed ice
Lime slices

Sparkling water
Juice of 1½ limes

Sparkling Orange Juice Iced Water

Ingredients
Crushed ice
Orange slices

Sparkling water
Juice of 1½ oranges

Sparkling Lemon Juice Iced Water

Ingredients
Crushed ice
Lemon slices

Sparkling water
Juice of 1½ lemons

Sparkling Hibiscus Iced Water

Ingredients
Crushed ice
Lemon slices

Sparkling water
1 cup hibiscus tea

Sparkling Vanilla Orange Iced Water

Ingredients
Crushed ice
Juice of 1½ oranges
½ tsp. vanilla extract

Sparkling water
Orange slices

Lavender Chamomile Iced Water

Ingredients

1 bag chamomile tea

Crushed ice

(available in health-food stores)

Hot water

1 tbsp culinary lavender buds

Directions

Pour 1 cup of hot water over lavender buds and chamomile tea.
Allow tea to steep and pour over ice. Very refreshing.

Cornish Pixie Rose-Lemon Green Tea

Ingredients

1 bag green tea

Juice of 1 lemon

Baby rose petals

1 bag hibiscus tea

Slices of lemon

Crushed ice

Directions

Add boiling water to tea and allow to cool. Steep for 5 minutes, remove teabags
or loose tea, and then let cool. Mix tea and lemon juice together and pour over
crushed ice. Drop sliced lemons and baby rose petals on the top of your drink
and glasses. Listen for the whispers of the fairies and pixies. For the moms of
the world, this is a very good drink to sip with little girls while you share a story
about fairies.

Lemon Lime Tea with Wild Mint

Ingredients

1 bag green tea

Juice of 1 lemon and 1 lime

1 bag wild mint tea (or fresh mint)

Lemon and lime slices

Directions

Place tea bags in teapot. Add boiling water. Steep for 5 minutes and then remove
teabags or loose tea. Leave to cool. Mix tea and juice together and pour over
freshly crushed ice. Add sliced lemons and limes to the top of your drink.

Apo E Gene Herbs for Cooking and Health

TURMERIC (CURCUMA LONGA):

A yellow spice generally used in Asian and Indian food, turmeric is akin to the ginger family and has been shown to reduce inflammation. Some research states this herb can reduce the development of beta amyloids in the brains of patients who are prone to, or have, Alzheimer's disease. Turmeric has also been shown to provide some anti-cancer benefits with melanoma, colorectal cancer, and breast cancer.

GINGER (ZINGIBER OFFICINALE):

This spice is a root or underground stem with a highly pungent spiced bite to it. It also has anti-inflammatory properties.

CHAMOMILE (ANTHEMIS NOBILIS):

Chamomile is a plant found throughout Europe. As a child in England, I saw it growing wild as a common weed. This plant is used mainly as an infusion that can help with intestinal colic, fever, and mild acid indigestion. Chamomile is commonly used for restlessness.

PEPPERMINT (MENTHA PIPERITA):

A flavor historically used in candy, gum, toothpaste, tea, and ice cream. Medicinal benefits include reducing gastric upset and helping to the body to relax.

CAYENNE (CAPSICUM BACCATUM):

Cayenne is a spice of the nightshade family. This is a hot spice. It also has some anti-inflammatory properties.

GARLIC (ALLIUM SATIVUM):

Garlic is part of the family Alliaceae and genus Allium, and it is connected to leeks, shallots, and the onion families. Garlic has a very strong flavor and odor, and it has some benefits for cardiovascular health and diabetes.

PARSLEY (PETROSELINUM CRISPUM):

Parsley is a pretty leafy green herb with a mild flavor. Commonly used as a garnish for food, parsley has been known to help with high blood pressure and enhancing the immune system.

CHIVES (ALLIUM SCHOENOPRASUM):

Connected to the onion family Alliaceae, chives grow in clusters and have very pretty purple flowers. Chives have been known to relieve pain.

TARRAGON (ARTEMISIA DRACUNCULUS):

Tarragon is an herb with a smooth, spicy flavor. National Institutes of Health Botanical Research Center is carrying out a research project investigating the actions of Russian tarragon on insulin in the human body.

THYME (THYMUS):

You may be familiar with many varieties of this herb. Garden thyme (T. vulgaris), citrus thyme (T. citriodorus), and wild thyme (Thymus serpyllum) are a few of the most common varieties. Thyme has been said to aid with inflammation in the body.

BASIL (OCIMUM BASILICUM):

Basil is an herb traditionally found in Asia. It has a unique flavor and has been said to have antibacterial and antifungal benefits.

ROSEMARY (ROSMARINUS OFFICINALIS):

Rosemary's translated Latin name is "dew of the sea." It is a multicolored, flowering herb plant and a distant relation of the mint family. Thanks to its unique flavor, rosemary can be used in many ways from fish and poultry to lemonade. It has the potential to aid with memory.

SAGE (SALVIA OFFICINALIS):

Sage grows as a beautiful light-purple flower. It was first cultivated in the southern parts of Europe. Sage is a common herb often used at Christmas and Thanksgiving as a poultry seasoning. Sage can help settle the digestive system and calm the mood.

DILL (ANETHUM GRAVEOLENS):

This herb has a rugged white and yellow flower. Dill was originally found in Asia, but now has a strong British connection, and the word "dill" has a British meaning of soothing or calming. Dill has some pain-relieving properties.

Appendix A

OPTIMAL NUTRITION FOR BABIES AND YOUNG CHILDREN

My first advanced clinical education was in a women's health-care nurse-practitioner program. Prior to this advanced course, I had worked in a labor-and-delivery unit at a local hospital for eight years. At this hospital I worked with not only uncomplicated births, but also high-risk deliveries, C-sections, and highly technological IVF (*in vitro* fertilization) surgeries.

All these medical situations had the same end result—a brand new baby. Once a baby is on the way, the parents need to make a host of decisions. By the time of the birth, some have already been made, but others are still pending. I was most surprised to observe the decision-making process new mothers went through in deciding what to feed their new little person. It puzzled me that they were given very little information about feeding their babies. They seemed ill prepared, confused, and often did not make the decision as to whether to breast-or bottle-feed until 30 minutes to an hour after the baby was born.

Many times their feeding decisions were made with no nutritional considerations whatsoever. With regard to breast-feeding, I heard mothers say many negative things, ranging from it being too messy or too much work to her wanting to quickly get back into prepregnancy clothes, to get back to work, or take a prearranged trip, without having to worry about breast-feeding.

Whether to use breast or bottle is up to the new mother. However, there is often a vacuum in which the new mother makes such decisions, because the medical system often does not provide adequate guidance. Cultural factors may also influence her decision. In the U.S., bottle-feeding is the norm, but some cultures don't consider it to be an option. Unfortunately, mothers who emigrate to the U.S. from breast-feeding cultures and who give birth in a hospital often buy into the our misguided norms of bottle-feeding, much to their children's detriment. If we look at the history of infant feeding, we can see that, like other products from the processed-food industry, infant formulas make a good profit. In the early 1920s, the dairy industry improved its sanitation practices, and milk storage was facilitated by the invention of the home refrigerator. These two improvements allowed the public to increase their use of milk and milk products—including processed infant formula. As a result, breast-feeding rates declined from the late 1920s through the early 1970s. Instead, cow's milk and strained solid foods, called "baby food," were given to babies at increasingly earlier ages. This led to various nutritional problems, including iron-deficiency anemia.[1] In response, "iron fortified" formulas were introduced.

By 1970, the World Health Organization (WHO) and UNICEF were becoming extremely concerned about the decline in breast-feeding. In the United States, thanks to a small but vocal group, La Leche League International, breast-feeding rates began to increase. In 1990, the WHO Innocenti Declaration recommended breast-feeding for two or more years. U.S. recommendations, of only one year, have yet to match this. And, distressingly, in large part, the U.S. medical system is not even promoting this minimal period.

Historically, the medical field has moved at a slow-as-molasses pace; and by the time new information reaches the consumer, it can be several years, or even decades, afterward. We need to act now with respect to the children. One major factor that can help with our obesity epidemic in very young children is deciding how to feed our babies. The sooner we learn about human genomics, our internal genetic instructions, and how nutrition affects our health, the sooner we will be guided in making the decisions that nature intended us to make where nutrition is concerned.

Which is best? Feeding your baby processed food products or human milk? My answer is: nature's way is best. Give your baby what nature intended—breast milk. Deciding how and what to feed your baby should be based on what is best for your baby—not on what is most convenient for you. Furthermore,

---

1   Committee on Nutrition. Iron Fortification of Infant Formulas. *J Am Acad Pediatr.* 1999;104(1):119-123. **pediatrics.aappublications.org/cgi/content/full/104/1/119.**

your diet during pregnancy and the breast-feeding period is extremely important for a baby's health. There is no longer any question about this; it is a fact.

Breast Milk and the Apo E Gene

Our body's innate intelligence has guided us through millions of years to nourish our offspring with human milk. It is odd to think that baby-food companies could provide a better food than nature. The American Academy of Pediatrics (AAP) has issued clear guidelines emphasizing that breast milk is the foundation of good infant nutrition. As parents and health-care providers, we need to be guided by this recommendation.

In my own practice, I am finding that breast milk provides a perfect diet for babies based on the mother and baby's Apo E genotype. For example, women who have the Apo E 4 gene have between 50 to 75 percent less total fat in their breast milk than an Apo E genotype mother, so they need to nurse their babies more often.

We also know that the correct proportions of the fatty acid DHA and the omega-3 and omega-6 ratios for each Apo E genotype is critical for the baby's brain development and eye health. Breast milk is perfect in this respect, too. A substantial body of research shows that conditions such as anxiety disorders, mood disorders, hyperactivity disorders, learning disabilities, and even autism relate to the fat content of an infant's diet and the mother's genetics. All these diseases could be greatly reduced by feeding babies breast milk rather than processed formula.

Recommendations of the American Academy of Pediatrics

The AAP recommends that infants be fed *exclusively* breast milk (no water, formula, or other liquids) for at least the first six months after birth, and that they continue to be breast-fed for *at least* the next six months while solid foods are introduced. Infants weaned before 12 months should not be given cow's milk, but an iron-fortified infant formula. Science reveals the extreme benefits of breast-feeding, both to mother and infant, for at least one year, and ideally as long as mother and baby desire. Sadly, while 71 percent of American mothers presently attempt to breast-feed their children, only 46 percent of these babies are being breast-fed *exclusively* at three months. That number drops to 13 percent by six months. Once solid foods are introduced in the second half of the first year, the numbers drop further. By a year, only 16 percent of infants receive *any* breast milk at all, and even fewer get the two or more years of breast-feeding recommended by the World Health Organization.

Nutritional Value of Breast Milk

Breast milk contains all the ingredients that a baby needs to thrive. Formulas based on cow's milk provide only 60 of the 200 nutrients found in breast milk. Formula makers simply cannot duplicate breast milk. Why? Because our bodies are as individual as our fingerprints, and each mother's body knows exactly what nutrients to produce for her baby's optimal health. Breast milk includes antibodies and other immune-system enhancing nutrients, as well as hormones and other substances that help your baby grow and develop at the optimal rate for your baby. One exception is vitamin D. Over the past few years, vitamin D research revealed a large percentage of the population has a vitamin D deficiency, including pregnant and lactating mothers. The commercial response to this information has been to recommend supplementation, but adequate vitamin D is created in the skin with only 10–15 minutes of exposure to sunlight a day.

This vitamin D deficiency is due to our spending too much time inside, plus an overconcern about skin cancer that results in using sunblocks that interfere with vitamin D synthesis. If you are exposed to strong sunlight more than the 10–15 minutes you need each day for adequate amounts of vitamin D, apply sunscreen after those 10–15 minutes. On the other hand, if you live in northern latitudes, the sun is too weak to adequate exposure in the winter months so supplementing will be necessary.

I believe infants and small children need sunlight as much as older folks, and should get their 10–15 minutes a day in the sun, but similarly, those living in northern latitudes need to be supplemented with vitamin D in the winter months. The current AAP recommendation for vitamin D for children is 400 IU per day (the amount contained in supplement drops or a liter of fortified formula).

Nutritional Concerns about Formula

Besides the many studies that have shown the superiority of breast milk, with its numerous components that cannot be synthesized and put in formula, there is also no long-term data on the consequences of adding artificial vitamins and fat supplements to humanmade formula. Therefore, the risk of any consequences must be weighed against the possible benefits when any additives are included. Do we know that this type of supplementation does not cause inflammation? When it comes to the baby's Apo E genotype, it is likely that any formula we pick will contain serious mismatches and not promote the health of the baby as well as breast milk would have done. Research confirms that babies' serum cholesterol is elevated as a result of being fed formula and other processed foods.[2]

From this we can conclude that they experience early inflammatory conditions, whether from additives or just the foreign protein from cows. Along with elevated cholesterol, I have noticed these common conditions in my practice:

- allergies
- behavioral disorders—poor concentration, inattention, anger, sleep disorders
- ear infections
- obesity
- anxiety
- tooth decay
- blood-pressure abnormalities
- stomach or intestinal conditions such as diarrhea or constipation
- skin diseases such as eczema, psoriasis, atopic dermatitis

It is only logical to stay with what nature intended and choose breast milk over formula.

Physical and Psychological Benefits to Baby and Mother

In addition to perfect nutrition, there are a host of other benefits, both physical and psychological, to both mother and baby. Breast-feeding is about more than giving milk. It is an entire neurodevelopmental system that encourages optimal physical and emotional well-being. Extensive cross-cultural and clinical research led The Alliance for Transforming the Lives of Children to state: "Breastfeeding, continual physical contact, and being carried on the body are necessary for optimal brain and immune system development and to promote the long-term health of the baby *and* mother. Spontaneous breastfeeding for a minimum of two years supports optimal bonding, immunity, and nutrition. Carrying infants in-arms or wearing them in slings throughout the day provides the near-constant movement that optimizes brain development as well as the touch, safety, and comfort essential to secure bonding."

---

2   Kallio, M. J. T., Salmenpera, L., Shes, M. A., Perheentupa, J., Gylling, H., and Miettinen, T. A. Apoprotein E phenotype determines serum cholesterol in infants during both high cholesterol breastfeeding and low-cholesterol formula feeding. *J. Lipid Res.* 1997;38:759–764.

While the breast-feeding baby feels nurtured and secure snuggled into the warmth of mother's breast, the breast-feeding mother produces prolactin, oxytocin, and other hormones that deepen their physiological bond.

Mothers benefit physically and emotionally from breast-feeding. A baby's breast-feeding contracts the mother's womb, and helps her entire body return to its prebirth condition. The breast-feeding mother's body naturally produces hormones that calm her. And these mothers experience lower breast-cancer rates (rates drop proportionately with the length of time the mother breast-feeds), and less osteoporosis in later life. Breast-feeding generally lengthens the time before menstrual periods begin.

Which is easier, breast or bottle? Surely, anything that enhances the immediate and long-term emotional and physical well-being of our children is going to make life easier. Here, indisputably, breast is better. On top of this, breast-feeding mothers don't need to stress out about which formula is best for baby. They don't need to shop and prepare bottles. Outings with breast-feeding babies don't require bottles and nipples. And with experience, breast-feeding in public is discreet and comfortable.

Studies show that breast-feeding can be one of the best things a working mother can do for herself and her baby. Working mothers find that they feel more connected to their babies when they know their baby is being nurtured by the milk they have left for them. After several hours apart, nursing virtually guarantees a loving reunion. And working mothers who nurse are better employees: breast-fed babies are sick less often—a healthy baby is important to a working mom.

Formulas can't begin to match the natural balance of the nutrients in breast milk and all the other positive factors associated with the process of breast-feeding. Not only is breast milk nutritionally perfect, it is ready to drink at anytime, day or night.

I encourage parents to ask lots of questions! Learn about baby nutrition from a reputable source, such as the La Leche League International, that is not promoting a particular product. Talk with a medical provider who has been trained in pediatric medicine and nutrition.

I have cared for hundreds and hundreds of moms and new babies. Most parents want what is best for their baby, no matter whether it is their first or their seventh. With more evidence-based nutritional education, we will see an entirely new level of health appearing in our children and much less chronic disease in adults. Pediatric medicine has taken care of most of the infectious illnesses that once plagued children, so we can now begin preventing early chronic illnesses by choosing the best nutrition for our babies and children.

Infant Nutrition and the Apo E Gene

The following table lists the nutritional requirements of infants from birth to 12 months. After two years, the caloric requirement needs to be adjusted based on the individual child's caloric needs, related to their Apo E genotype, lean mass, and activity level.

Nutritional Recommendations by Age and Genotype

0–6 Months (all genotypes)
100% breast milk

Introducing Solid Foods

The slow introduction of solid, plant-based, whole foods can begin at six months to a year, although some children do not take to solids as quickly as others. There's no rush to introduce them if breast milk is still their preference. Give a combination of foods and ensure that they are appropriately prepared so that your baby can comfortably swallow them.

- Breast milk
- Rice cereal (consider iron-fortified)
- Rice
- Small amounts of noncitrus, organic whole fruit
- Yellow vegetables
- Green vegetables
- Non-inflammatory fats such as avocado, olives, olive oil, and nut butters
- Small amounts of plant protein such as lentils, beans, legumes, or soy

Suggested Schedules for Introducing Solid Foods

6–12 Months

Breast milk should remain the main source of nutrition while your baby is slowly introduced to solid foods at a pace she chooses.

rice cereal	carrots	yams	sweet potatoes
squash	apricots	apples	blackberries
blueberries	bananas	cherries	grapes
prunes	pears	peaches	cauliflower
broccoli	beets	split peas	millet
oats & oatmeal	lima beans	basmati rice	green string beans
peas	papaya	nectarines	soybeans

Age 1–2 Years

Although few Americans realize it, the World Health Organization recommends breast-feeding through the second year or beyond, so if your child prefers nursing, and you are willing to continue, breast milk can remain a major source of nutrition.

pearl barley	other green leafy vegetables	asparagus
acorn squash	avocado	brown rice
honey	eggplant	garlic
shallots	cabbage	turnips & turnip greens
rye	lettuce	fish
buckwheat	egg whites	corn
ground nuts:	citrus fruits:	peanuts
almonds, walnuts,	lemons, limes,	sunflower seeds
cashews	oranges, pineapples	shellfish
wheat foods with yeast	lentils	

The Apo E 3/3, 2/3, and 2/2 child may have meats such as chicken, Cornish game hen, turkey, or wild meats in small amounts, preferably from an organic source and not more than once every 24–48 hours.

After 2 years

Once breastfeeding has ended, it is important to follow carbohydrate, fat, and protein percentages more closely. Use caloric recommendations based on the American Heart Association—see Table A.2 on page 415.

A.1 Summary of Recommended Nutrients by Age			
Age	0-6 months	6-10 months	10-12 months
Carbohydrates	Breast milk	Breast milk Begin baby cereal if desired. Begin 2–4 oz. soft fruit and vege-tables—mashed; slowly adding soft pieces or cooked fruit and vegetables.	Breast milk Continue baby cereal. Begin bread, 4 servings per day (1 serving bread = ¼ slice). Fruits and vegeta-bles, 4 servings per day (one serving = 2–8 tbsp).
Fat	Breast milk	Breast milk	Breast milk
Protein	Breast milk	Breast milk Gradually introduce yogurt and puréed plant protein—len-tils, beans, legumes, soy.	Nut butters, 2–3½ oz. servings per day.

Nutrient Recommendations for Apo E Genotypes

Apo E 4/4
Carbohydrate: 55% of total calories
Protein: 25% of total calories
Fat: 20% of total calories

Apo E 4/3
Carbohydrate: 55% of total calories
Protein: 25% of total calories
Fat: 20% of total calories

Apo E 4/2
Carbohydrate: 55% of total calories
Protein: 20% of total calories
Fat: 25% of total calories

Apo E 3/3
Carbohydrate: 55% of total calories
Protein: 20% of total calories
Fat: 25% of total calories

Apo E 2/3
Carbohydrate: 50% of total calories
Protein: 20% of total calories
Fat: 30% of total calories

Apo E 2/2
Carbohydrate: 50% of total calories
Protein: 15% of total calories
Fat: 35% of total calories

A.2 Daily Caloric Intake Guidelines and Recommended Foods by Category, Age, and Gender[a]

	1 Yr.	2–3* Yrs.	4–8 Yrs.	9–13 Yrs.	14–18 Yrs.
Calories					
Female	900 kcal	1,000 kcal	1,200 kcal	1,600 kcal	1,800 kcal
Male	900 kcal	1,000 kcal	1,400 kcal	1,800 kcal	2,000 kcal
Fat (% of calories)	30–40%	30–35%	25–35%	25–35%	25–35%
Milk/Dairy[b] Lean Meat/ Beans					
Female	1.5 oz.	2 oz.	3 oz.	4 oz.	5 oz.
Male	1.5 oz.	2 oz.	4 oz.	5 oz.	6 oz.
Fruits[c]					
Female	1 cup	1 cup	1½ cups	1½ cups	1½ cups
Male	1 cup	1 cup	1½ cups	1½ cups	2 cups
Vegetables[d]					
Female	¾ cup	1 cup	1 cup	2 cups	2½ cups
Male	¾ cup	1 cup	1½ cups	2½ cups	3 cups
Grains					
Female	2 oz.	3 oz.	4 oz.	5 oz.	6 oz.
Male	2 oz.	3 oz.	5 oz.	6 oz.	7 oz.

*For children older than 2 years, consider following Apo E fat percentage guidelines for genotypes shown above.

a. Adapted from **americanheart.org/presenter.jhtml?identifier=3033999**

b. Milk listed is fat-free (except for children under the age 2). If 1%, 2%, or whole milk is substituted, this will utilize, for each cup, 19, 39, or 63 kcal of discretionary calories and add 2.6, 5.1, or 9.0 g. of total fat, of which 1.3, 2.6, or 4.6 g. are saturated fat. See: **americanheart.org/presenter.jhtml?identifier=3033999**

c. For 1-year-old children, calculations are based on 2% milk. If 2 cups of whole milk are substituted, 48 kcal of discretionary calories will be utilized. The American Academy of Pediatrics recommends that low-fat/reduced-fat milk not be started before 2 years of age. Adapted from the Executive Office of the President of the AAP and the Department of Health and Human Services. See: **americanheart.org/presenter.jhtml?identifier=3033999**

d. Serving sizes are ¼ cup for 1 year, ⅓ cup for 2 to 3 years, and ½ cup for 4 years. A variety of vegetables should be selected from each subgroup over the week. All grains should be whole grains.

Appendix B

APO E GENE
ADDITIONAL CALORIE LEVELS

The following calorie levels have been provided in addition to those found in Chapter 19. These are based on broader recommendations and allow more freedom to choose various food options in your new eating pattern. All calorie-level tables take into consideration your specific Apo E genotype.

Apo E 2/2: 1,200–3,600-Calorie Serving Sizes

S E R V I N G S   P E R   D A Y

Calories	Carbohydrates	Fruits/Vegetables	Protein	Fat
1,200	4	8	3	8.5
1,400	5	8	4	9.5
1,600	5.5	9.5	4	9
1,800	6.5	9.5	6.5	6
2,000	8	10.5	9	7.5
2,200	10	10	7	15
2,400	8	11	9.5	8
2,600	12	12	8	18
2,800	13	12	9	19
3,000	14	12	9.5	20
3,400	17	14	10.5	22
3,600	18	14	11	23

Apo E 2/3: 1,200–3,600-Calorie Serving Sizes

S E R V I N G S   P E R   D A Y

Calories	Carbohydrates	Fruits/Vegetables	Protein	Fat
1,200	5	8	3.5	7
1,400	6	8.5	5	8
1,600	4.5	7.5	8.5	6
1,800	5.5	9	9	5
2,000	8	6.5	10	7.5
2,200	9.5	12.5	7	12.5
2,400	8.5	11.5	14	5.5
2,600	11	16	9	15
2,800	11.5	16	9.5	15.5
3,000	12	17	9.5	17
3,400	14	21	8	19.5
3,600	15.5	22	12	19.5

Apo E 3/3: 1,200–3,600-Calorie Serving Sizes

SERVINGS PER DAY

Calories	Carbohydrates	Fruits/Vegetables	Protein	Fat
1,200	5	8.5	5.5	5
1,400	5.5	10	6.5	6
1,600	6.5	10	8.5	3
1,800	7.5	11.5	7	5
2,000	10	11	9	5
2,200	10	12	10	9.5
2,400	11	8.5	14	8
2,600	13	12	12.5	10.5
2,800	14	13	13.5	11.5
3,000	15	14	14	12
3,400	18	15	16	14
3,600	19	17	17	15

Apo E 4/2: 1,200–3,600-Calorie Serving Sizes

SERVINGS PER DAY

Calories	Carbohydrates	Fruits/Vegetables	Protein	Fat
1,200	4.5	9	5	5.5
1,400	5.5	10	6.5	6
1,600	6	13.5	7	5
1,800	7.5	11.5	7	5
2,000	6	7	7	5
2,200	9	13	10.5	9.5
2,400	10	11.5	12.5	6
2,600	11	16	11.5	11
2,800	12	16	10	11.5
3,000	13	17	13	12.5
3,400	15	19	15	14
3,600	16	21	16	15

Apo E 4/3 and 4/4: 1,200–3,600-Calorie Serving Sizes				
SERVINGS PER DAY				
Calories	Carbohydrates	Fruits/Vegetables	Protein	Fat
1,200	6	5	7	3
1,400	7	6	9	4
1,600	6	10.5	8	4
1,800	11.5	5.5	10	2.5
2,000	5.5	9	10	5
2,200	11	9	12	6.5
2,400	6.5	9.5	14.5	2.5
2,600	16	13	11	8
2,800	16	14	12	9
3,000	18	17	13	9
3,400	19	19	15	10
3,600	20	21	16	10

Appendix C

AUTISM DIAGNOSES, NUTRITION, AND WINDOWS OF OPPORTUNITY

It was August of 2008 and I had been invited to speak to a group of parents of special-needs children in my local area. I was told that considering nutrition as an option in managing autism was a very intriguing topic to this group of moms and dads, and we would more than likely have a large group attending the lecture that evening.

The day came, and I arrived ahead of the crowd to set up for my presentation. The four staff members I had brought with me set up a table of handouts with relevant nutritional research and books for parents to review in the back of the room.

The moms and dads began to arrive, and it was immediately apparent that these parents were hungry for nutritional information regarding any type of special-needs child—children with autism, Asperger's, ADD, ADHD, Tourette's, anger disorder, depression . . . and the list goes on.

In no time, every seat in the large meeting room was taken, and people were standing. I began by briefly introducing myself—an integrative, medically trained, primary-care nurse-practitioner—and what that meant. I introduced them to integrative medicine and the differences between allopathic and alternative medicine, and what this meant for the patient. I then talked about the role of nutrition in health, and how most of us get our nutritional information.

I presented some relevant scientific research, and discussed its application to children with special needs. I followed this with case studies illustrating the practical application of nutrition, i.e., choosing what to eat and what not to eat, as applied to your Apo E genes.

After about 45 minutes I took questions. I immediately got some excellent ones and found that the parents were very happy with the answers I gave. After the first three or four questions, a woman in the back row stood up with her laptop computer in hand. She gave an elaborate introduction about who she was—the head of this and that committee, and on the board of this and that organization, in what seemed like a hundred different parts of the country.

I had noticed this lady earlier when she walked into the event—partly because she was very loud, and it was obvious that she thought she was in charge as she gave people what I would like to say were directions, but they seemed more like orders. In addition, her weight was in excess of 300 pounds. I also noticed her computer was open the entire time she was giving orders to her staff. Now, having so eloquently introduced herself, she spoke directly to me.

"Let me tell you, Pamela McDonald, that what you have presented over the last 45 minutes is completely misleading, it has no validity at all, and there is zero research showing that nutrition is beneficial for special-needs children. I have been sitting on my computer the entire time, and I have not found one bit of information telling me that nutrition works. And if it does work so well, why are doctors not recommending it? Medication is the only way to go for these children."

I immediately thanked her for her comment but respectfully disagreed with her opinion. I shared with her that nutrition is not widely prescribed by physicians because it is not taught in medical school. If physicians have no training in it, they will not prescribe it—especially when a $10 pill will get a quicker result. But a $10 pill will only treat the symptom, not the problem.

Where special-needs children are concerned, the problem is much deeper than the presenting symptoms. What we are seeing in the medical treatment of special-needs children are multiple system failures at multiple levels. Nutritional medicine, especially integrative medicine coupled with genetic testing, while still in its infancy, offers real solutions, not just Band-Aids. We need to look at all the options for our special-needs children, and this is where integrative medicine comes in.

I had hardly finished my sentence when a mother on the other side of the room stood up and introduced herself as a registered dietitian. She said that with her two special-needs children, if she did not follow some of the recommendations that I had just presented, their health gets worse and her life becomes "a living hell." She ended by saying, "Good nutrition is important and I live by it every day."

Not two seconds after her passionate statement, a woman sitting in front of the 300-pound lady stood up and said, "Pam, I want to thank from my heart for what you have just presented. What you have just shared with us is the future. We all should be so happy that this type of information is now coming to light. So I want to thank you again for being here this evening." The room broke out in applause. The questions kept coming. But what had just happened was amazing: we had moms and dads passionately discussing and debating nutrition and integrative medicine.

This was exciting for me and gives hope that we can be passionate about our children's health and really talk together about this subject. The next day at my office the phone rang and rang—moms and dads wanting to make appointments to talk further about how nutrition could be applied to special-needs children.

It was just over three and half weeks after this lecture that a little bright beam of sunshine walked into my office. I was walking down the hall when a lady came into the waiting room, waving her arms and shouting my name. "Pam! Hi Pam, I am here! I can't believe I am finally here!" In tow was a very cute little 18-month-old boy who immediately got up onto the bench in my waiting room office and said, "Oh, hot, mama, hot!" Mom immediately exclaimed, "Look, did you hear that? He said two words together. I have to talk to you." One of my staff took her back to the exam room where I sat with her. What I was about to hear was something that would warm any mom or dad's heart. It certainly did mine, being a mother of three children myself.

This mom began to tell me her story of the past three-and-a-half weeks. She had been invited to my lecture at the last minute and decided that, because her second son had been given a diagnosis of autism two months earlier, she would gather any information that could possibly make her life and her child's life better. So she attended the lecture.

She admitted that she had no idea that nutrition could be a helpful option for treating an autistic child, but she was open-minded enough to look at the possibility. She told me how excited she had been after my lecture, as it made so much sense. She went home that night and cleaned out her kitchen, getting rid of all the processed food and deciding not to give her son any dairy, processed food, or meat for a trial period.

Once the house was cleaned out, she put him on whole foods only—fresh fruit and vegetables—organic whenever possible—plant protein and fresh wild fish—no processed anything. Within a short period, he had stopped being so aggressive, began to sleep, stopped rocking, had a much better attention span, and had begun to say words, where before he had said nothing, just grunting every now and then. She was so excited she could hardly get the words out fast enough. She pointed to her son and said, "I don't know what to tell you, but this has changed our lives, and I think his health, forever."

She went on to say that she wanted to get tested because she was sure they had an abnormal Apo E gene. She wanted me to test the entire family because they wanted to know why their son has autism. She especially needed to know if the health of her four-year-old son, which has been bad, was because of the food she had been feeding him. We talked at length about her options, and it was clear that this was a possible next step.

The testing was completed and the results came back—Mom: Apo E 4/4; Dad: Apo E 4/3; four-year-old son: Apo E 4/4; and autistic son: Apo E 4/3. With these results the autism possibly had a connection with the Apo E 4 gene and a diet that was not matching its requirements. But I was puzzled—why did the boy's health and behavior change so rapidly after such a short time on the new diet?

Reviewing the diet history with the mom revealed that this boy's diet had included excessive amounts of highly processed foods, fast foods, and multiple exposures of animal protein each day, with the resulting excessive calories from saturated fat, as well as trans fats. In addition, he was getting high glycemic load carbohydrates and excessive preservatives and food dyes. Also, from whole milk, he was getting rBGH (an artificial growth hormone) and high levels of IGF-1 (insulin-like growth factor 1), produced when artificial growth hormones are given to cows. After learning about the reversal of this child's symptoms, I immediately began to analyze the situation.

Clearly what had changed was the nutritional environment—this child was now getting a much better diet. What the mother had described earlier was clearly a highly processed, inflammatory diet—large quantities of chips and candy bars laden with inflammatory trans fats, plus food loaded with antibiotics; high-fructose corn syrup; exogenous sex hormones from dairy products; as well as synthetic hormones, pesticides, and herbicides.

What we did not know prior to testing was this family's inability to clear out the toxic chemistry coming from processed foods, fast foods, food dyes, and high amounts of animal protein (with a 50% saturated fat content from whole cow's milk that the boy consumed three to four times a day). Could this child's nutritional environment have been a contributing factor to his diagnosis of autism?

When his diet became void of all items that were toxic to his Apo E 4/3 biochemistry, we witnessed an immediate shift in his behavior—he began to talk, stopped the aggressive behavior, slept normally, and ceased having chronic diarrhea.

Why would we get such a huge change in such a short time after shifting his diet to only whole foods with organic fruits and vegetables along with omega-3 and essential-fatty-acid supplements? Learning that he was an Apo E 4/3 with its genetic inability to clear the toxic chemistry that resulted from the diet he was being fed, it appeared his neurological system could not develop well enough to express normal speech, behavior, and sleep patterns; and interact appropriately with his parents, siblings, or playmates.

Like many mothers, this mom had little knowledge of nutrition and how to apply it to her young children's health. The American Dietetic Association has completed multiple nutritional-trend surveys and found that most people don't even know that nutrition is connected to health. If we don't even know this, how can we begin to use the nutrition as a tool for health and healing?

I believe that as more patients choose integrative medicine, we will begin to see changes for the better, with more practitioners prescribing nutritional plans that relate to a child's Apo E genetic expression.

Research says that the Apo E gene and autism are not connected. However, what I have learned from knowledgeable colleagues in the field of genetics and nutrition, specifically Ron Krauss, M.D., director of atherosclerosis research at Children's Hospital Oakland Research Institute, and Carl Cotman, Ph.D., professor of neurology and neurobiology, University of California, Irvine, is that the field of human nutrition research is fraught with difficulties and challenges, making it difficult to obtain reliable outcomes, so I remain convinced nutrition is connected to autism-spectrum disorders. Good, sound nutrition and exercise programs may be our best tool for healing and prevention—prevention has yet to be proven *not* to be the best solution.

Appendix D

APO E GENE RESEARCH

Arbonés-Mainar JM, et al. (2006). Trans-10, cis-12- and cis-9, trans-11-conjugated linoleic acid isomers selectively modify hdl-apolipoprotein composition in apolipoprotein E knockout mice. *Journal of Nutrition,* 136:353–359.

Beilby JP, Hunt CC, Palmer LJ, et al. (2003) Apolipoprotein E gene polymorphisms are associated with carotid plaque formation but not with intima media wall thickening: results from the Perth Carotid Ultrasound Disease Assessment Study (CUDAS). *Stroke,* 34(4):869–74.

Berenson GS, et al. (1996). Influence of apolipoprotein E polymorphism on the tracking of childhood levels of serum lipids and apolipoproteins over a 6-year period. The Bogalusa Heart Study. *Atherosclerosis,* Nov 15;127(1):73–79.

Bray MS (2000). Genomics, genes, and environmental interaction: the role of exercise. *Journal of Applied Physiology,* 88:788–792.

Brown AJ and Roberts DC (1991). The effect of fasting triacylglyceride concentration and apolipoprotein E polymorphism on postprandial lipemia. *Arteriosclerosis and Thrombosis,* 11:1737–1744.

Corder EH, Saunders AM, Strittmatter WJ, et al. (1993). Gene dose E type 4 allele and the risk of Alzheimer's disease in late onset families, *Science,* 261:921–923.

de Andrade M, Thandi M, Brown S, Gotto A, Patsch W, and Boerwinkle E, (1995). Relationship of the apolipoprotein E polymorphism with carotid artery atherosclerosis. *American Journal of Human Genetics,* 56:1379–1390.

Djousse L, et al. (2004). Apolipoprotein E polymorphism modifies the alcohol-hdl association observed in the National Heart, Lung, and Blood Institute Family Heart Study. *American Journal of Clinical Nutrition,* 80(6):1639–1644.

Dreon DM, Fernstrom HA, Williams PT and Krauss RM, (2000). Reduced ldl particle size in children consuming a very low-fat diet is related to parental ldl subclass patterns 1,2,3. *American Journal of Clinical Nutrition,* Vol. 71, No. 6, 1611–1616.

Farrer LA, Brin MF, Elsas L, et al. (1995). Statement on use of Apolipoprotein E testing for Alzheimer disease. *JAMA,* 274:1627–1629.

Georgoulias P, Wozniak G, Samara M, et al. (2009). Impact of ACE and ApoE polymorphisms on myocardial perfusion: correlation with myocardial single photon emission computed tomographic imaging. *J Human Genetics,* 54(10):595-602.

Ghebremedhin E, et al. (2005). Relationship of apolipoprotein E and age at onset to Parkinson disease neuropathology. *American Journal of Medical Genetics Part B: Neuropsychiatric Genetics,* 5:136(1):72–74.

Green RC, (2002). Genetic testing for Alzheimer's disease: has the moment arrived? *Alz. Care Quarterly,* 208–214.

Gylling H, Kontula K, Koivisto UM, Miettinen HE, Miettinen TA (1997). Polymorphisms of the gene encoding apoproteins A-I, B, C–III, and E and LDL receptor, and cholesterol and LDL metabolism during increased cholesterol intake. Common alleles of the apoprotein E gene show the greatest regulatory impact. *Arterioscler Thromb Vasc Biol,* 17:38–44.

Heyer EJ, et al. (2005). ApoE-epsilon4 predisposes to cognitive dysfunction following uncomplicated carotid endarterectomy. *Neurology,* 13;65(11):1759–1763.

Huang X, Chen P, Kaufer DI, Troster AI, and Poole CJ (2006). Apolipoprotein E and dementia in Parkinson's disease: a meta-analysis. *Neuropathology Experimental Neurology,* 65(2):116–23.

Kallio MJ, et al. (1997). Apoprotein E phenotype determines serum cholesterol in infants during both high-cholesterol breast feeding and low-cholesterol formula feeding. *Journal of Lipid Research,* 38:759–764,

Lapinleimu H, et al. (2000). Impact of gender, apolipoprotein E phenotypes, and diet on serum lipids and lipoproteins in infancy. *Atherosclerosis,* 152(1):135–141.

Lehtinen S, et al. (1993). Gene dose of apolipoprotein E type 4 allele and the risk of Alzheimer's disease in late onset families. *Science,* 261:921–923.

Leon AS, Togashi K, Rankinen T, et al. (2004). Association of apolipoprotein E polymorphism with blood lipids and maximal oxygen uptake in the sedentary state and after exercise training in the HERITAGE family study. *Metabolism,* 53(1):108–16.

Lim GP, et al. (2005). A diet enriched with the omega-3 fatty acid docosahexaenoic acid reduces amyloid burden in an aged Alzheimer mouse model. *USA Neurology,* 13;65(11):1759–63.

López-Miranda J, et al. (2004). The effect of dietary fat on ldl: Size is influenced by apolipoprotein E genotype in healthy Subjects. *Journal of Nutrition,* 134:2517–2522.

Mahley RW (1988). Apolipoprotein E: cholesterol transport protein with in cell biology. *Science,* 240:622–630.

Mahley RW (1995). Apolipoprotein E polymorphism, serum lipids, myocardial infarction and severity of angiographically verified coronary artery disease in men and women. *Atherosclerosis,* 114:83–91.

Martinez M, et al. (2006). Apolipoprotein E 4 is probably responsible for the chromosome 19 linkage peak for Parkinson disease. *American Journal of Medical Genetics Part B: Neuropsychiatric Genetics,* 37(2):364–370.

Maury CP, Liljestrom M, Tiitinen S, Laiho K, Karela K, and Ehnholm C, (2001). Apolipoprotein E phenotypes in rheumatoid arthritis with or without amyloidosis. *Amyloid,* 8(4):270–273.

McConnell LM, Koenig BA, Greely HT, Raffin TA, and the Alzheimer Disease Working Group of the Stanford Program in Genomics, Ethics, & Society (1998). Genetic testing and Alzheimer disease: has the time come? *Nat Med,* 4:757–759.

Minihane, et al. (2000). Apo E polymorphism and fish oil supplementation in subjects with anatherogenic lipoprotein phenotype. *Arterioscler Thromb Vasc Biol,* 20:1990–1997.

Miura Y, et al. (2001). Tea catechins prevent the development of atherosclerosis in apoprotein E—Deficient mice. *Journal of Nutrition,* 131:27–32.

Moore RJ, Chamberlain RM, and Khuri FR, (2004). Apolipoprotein E and the risk of breast cancer in African-American and non Hispanic white women: A review. *Oncology,* 66:79–93.

Moreno JA, et al. (2005). The apolipoprotein E Gene Promoter (-219G/T) Polymorphism determines insulin sensitivity in response to dietary fat in healthy young adults, *Journal of Nutrition,* 135:2535–2540.

Moysich KB, Freudenheim JL, Baker JA, et al. (2000). Apolipoprotein E genetic polymorphism, serum lipoproteins, and breast cancer risk. *Mol Carcinog,* 27(1):2–9.

Nichol K, Deeny SP, Seif J, Camaclang K, and Cotman CW (2009). Exercise improves cognition and hippocampal plasticity in APOE epsilon4 mice. *Alzheimers Dement,* 5(4):287–94.

Noble JM, Manly JJ, Schupf N, Tang MX, Mayeux R, Luchsinger JA (2010).Association of C-reactive protein with cognitive impairment. *Arch Neurol,* 67(1):87–92.

Obisesan T, Ferrell R, Goldberg A, et al. (2008). APOE genotype affects black-white responses of high-density lipoprotein cholesterol subspecies to aerobic exercise training. *Metabolism,* 57(12):1669-76.

Ordovas JM (2006). Nutrigenetics, plasma lipids, and cardiovascular risk. *J Am Diet Assoc,* 106:1074–81.

Pertovaara M, et al. (2004). Presence of apolipoprotein E epsilon4 allele predisposes to early onset of primary Sjogren's syndrome. *American Journal of Clinical Nutrition,* 80(6):1639–1644.

Roberts JS, Green RC, Relkin N, et al. (2003). How do participants rate the impact of genetic susceptibility testing for Alzheimer's disease? *Neurology,* 60:A453.

Roe CM, Fitzpatrick AL, Xiong C, et al. (2010). Cancer linked to Alzheimer disease but not vascular dementia. *Neurology,* 74(2):106–12.

Roses AD (1997). Genetic testing for Alzheimer disease: practical and ethical issues. *Arch Neurol,* 54:1226–1229.

Roter DL, Stewart M, Putnam S, et al. (1997). Communication patterns of primary care physicians. *JAMA,* 270:350–355.

Sanchez-Muniz FJ, Maki KC, Schaefer EJ, and Ordovas JM (2009). Serum lipid and antioxidant responses in hypercholesterolemic men and women receiving plant sterol esters vary by apolipoprotein e genotype. *J Nutr,* 139(1):13–19.

Sarkkinen E, Korhonen M. Erkkila A, Ebeling T, and Uusitupa M, (1998). Effect of apolipoprotein E polymorphism on serum lipid response to the separate modification of dietary fat and dietary cholesterol. *American Journal of Clinical Nutrition,* 68, 1215–1222.

Simell O, et al. (1997). Impact of gender, apolipoprotein E phenotypes, and diet on serum lipids and lipoproteins in infancy. *J Pediatr,* 131(6):825–32.

Simell O, et al. (2000). Apolipoprotein E4 phenotype increases non-fasting serum triglyceride concentration in infants - the STRIP study. *Atherosclerosis,* 152(1):135–41.

Sisto T, et al. (1995). Apolipoprotein E polymorphism, serum lipids, myocardial infarction and severity of angiographically artery disease in men and women. *Atherosclerosis,* 114:83–91.

Solfrizzi V, Frisardi V, Capurso C, D'Introno A, Colacicco AM, Vendemiale G, Capurso A, Panza F (2009). Dietary fatty acids and predementia syndromes. *Scientific World Journal,* 9:792–810.

Sorlí JV, Corella D, Francés F, Ramírez JB, González JI, Guillén M, Portolés O (2006). The effect of the APOE polymorphism on HDL-C concentrations depends on the cholesterol ester transfer protein gene variation in a Southern European population. *Clin Chim Acta,* 366(1-2):196–203.

Spurway N (2006). Top-down studies of genetic contribution to differences in physical capacity. In *Genetics and Molecular Biology of Muscle Adaptation,* ed. Spurway N & Wackerhage H, pp. 25–59. Churchill Livingstone, Elsevier, London.

Sudlow C, Gonzalez-Martinez NA, Kim J, and Clark C (2006). Does apolipoprotein E genotype influence the risk of ischemic stroke, intracerebral hemorrhage, or subarachnoid hemorrhage. Systematic review and meta-analyses of 31 studies among 5961 cases and 17,965 controls. *Stroke,* 37(2):364–370.

Superko HR, Haskell WL. The effect of apolipoprotein E genotype on postprandial lipoprotein in patients matched for triglycerides, ldlcholesterol, and hdl-cholesterol. *Artery,* 1991:18:315–325.

Taimela S, et al. (1996). The effect of physical activity on serum total and low density lipoprotein cholesterol concentrations varies with apolipoprotein E phenotype in male children and young adults: The Cardiovascular Risk in Young Finns Study. *Metabolism,* 45:797–803.

Tammi A, et al. (1996). Apolipoprotein E 4 phenotype increases non-fasting serum triglyceride concentration in infants—the STRIP study. *Cardiorespiratory Pediatrics,* 98(4 Pt 1):757–62.

Thompson PD, et al. (2006). Angiotensin-converting enzyme genotype and adherence to aerobic exercise training. *Preventive Cardiology,* 9(1):21–24.

Wohlin M, Sundström J, Lannfelt L, et al. (2007). Apolipoprotein E epsilon4 genotype is independently associated with increased intima-media thickness in a recessive pattern. *Lipids,* 42(5):451–6.

Zhongyin Z, Hesheng L, Jun L, and Jihong C. (2006). Association of serum lipids and apolipoprotein E gene polymorphism with the risk of colorectal adenomas. *Saudi Medical Journal,* 27(2):161–164.

Zick CD, Matthews C, Roberts JS, et al. (2005). Genetic susceptibility testing for Alzheimer's disease and its impact on insurance behavior. *Health Aff,* 24(2):483–490.

Appendix E

ANONYMOUS APO E AND ADVANCED CHOLESTEROL TESTING

For those concerned about protecting your privacy with respect to these tests and your medical records, we offer test options so you can get anonymous Apo E gene testing and/or advanced cholesterol testing, along with detailed instructions.

Select the Testing Kit You Want

At **ThePerfectGeneDiet.com**,[1] select the section called "Apo E Gene Testing Options," where a link at the bottom will lead to a description of the three different testing kits that can be ordered:

- **Option 1: The Anywhere Program Test Kit**
  This option provides anonymous testing and telephone support from our specially trained licensed providers to shape an eating plan ideal for your unique gene type.

- **Option 2: The Local Provider Test Kit**
  If you prefer to work with a local medical provider, we offer a testing

---

1   Or call (925) 736-8510, or write to 4165 Blackhawk Plaza Circle, Danville, CA 94506

kit that includes your anonymous identification number. Detailed instructions are included for a local provider to draw and submit the blood sample.

- **Option 3: Advanced Cholesterol Testing Kit**
This test checks 13 different types of cholesterol and other important chemistries that will help you identify critical risk factors.

Apo E Gene Testing Seminars
(check **www.ThePerfectGeneDiet.com** for seminar updates)

Apo E Gene-Testing Seminar 1: This informational seminar provides information about the Apo E gene test and/or advanced cholesterol testing, with an overview of the Perfect Gene Diet program. Please note: The Apo E gene testing is *free* of charge with the Perfect Gene Diet integrative medicine seminar. *This seminar may be covered by your medical insurance plan—individual plans vary.*

Apo E Seminar 2: This seminar is for those who have received Apo E gene test results or advanced cholesterol test results, and provides the Perfect Gene Diet step-by-step approach for accomplishing your goals.

Apo E Gene Testing Companies

23andMe: **www.23andMe.com**

Berkeley HeartLab: **www.bhline.com/clin_test_apoe.php**

Boston Heart Lab: **www.bostonheartlab.com/Patients_ YourProgram.html**

Kimball Genetics: **www.kimballgenetics.com/tests-apo_e.html**

Genova Diagnostics USA: **www.genovadiagnostics.com**

Genova Diagnostics Europe: **www.gdx.uk.net/index.php**

Navigenics: **www.navigenics.com**

Acknowledgments

In completing this project, I am indebted to numerous family members, friends, and colleagues. Expressing my personal gratitude to all who contributed their time, patience, and understanding while I undertook this endeavor cannot be accomplished with a mere "Thank-you." And so I want to offer a personal tribute to the individuals mentioned below. The completion of the manuscript would not have been possible without each and every one of them.

At the top of my list is Robert Superko, M.D. This man had the courage to make it his personal mission to find new ways to prevent heart disease. His drive, passion, and determination inspired me to write this book. Dr. Superko has shared his knowledge with me in many ways. It benefited not only me, but also hundreds of my patients, and particularly my husband, Rick. For that, I will always be grateful. It was my fierce desire and commitment to solving my husband's heart health mystery that led me to Dr. Superko's work. Today, at my integrative-medicine practice in Danville, California, hundreds of patients are being provided answers to many of medicine's mysteries. Dr. Superko made this possible, and I will always be grateful for his knowledge and continued support.

After being blessed with Dr. Superko's knowledge, I was directed to Kona, Hawaii, by a colleague, Andrew Benn, M.D. It was there, at the Integrative

Medicine Cardiology Conference, that I first met Andrew Weil, M.D. Since then, Dr. Weil has given me so much that the words "Thank you" cannot express the depth of my gratitude. It is his knowledge, obtained through my fellowship in the Integrative Medicine Program at the University of Arizona, that helps me facilitate change in myself and in my patients with chronic heart disease and other chronic illnesses.

This fellowship took me on a most amazing journey, one I would encourage any physician or nurse-practitioner to explore. It provided me with a unique and personal education for healing-oriented medicine that takes the whole person into account—body, mind, emotions, and spirit, as well as the surrounding environment—and makes use of all appropriate healing therapies, both conventional and alternative.

Besides Drs. Superko and Weil, I would like to thank John Roberts, M.D.; J. B. Humphrey, M.D.; Claire Humphrey, M.D.; Thomas Gregory Quinn, M.D.; Tieraona Low Dog, M.D.; Victoria Maizes, M.D.; Dan Shapiro, Ph.D.; Randy Horwitz, M.D.; Moira Andre; and Howard Silverman, M.D. These people have taught me about so much more than medicine; they have taught me, through their depth and integrity, to be a better person.

In addition, I offer a personal thank you to Betty and Silvia Johnson; Lynne Schurga; Diane Rozakis; Joanne Moody; Lynn Wiese; Lynn Probert; Walter C. Youngman, Jr.; Nancy Vasko, C.P.A.; Nelson Gwinn, M.D.; Susanne Goeb, P.A.; Julie LaGuardia, N.P.; Rich Cazin, P.A.; Christine Aday, N.P.; Brenda Garrett-Superko, R.N.; Kim Evans, N.P.; Barbara Denison, N.P.; Lynn Chadd, N.P.; Betsy Busilli, Ph.D., N.P.; Patricia Faust, N.P.; Kalama Hochreiter, M.S.W.; Catrina Morefield, M.P.H., R.D., M.S.; Renie Vaharen Tharp, R.D.; Jeannette Kotys, M.S., R.D.; Mary Ann Osborne, D.N.P.; and Molly McCormick, M.S.

I want to extend a very special thank-you to my dear friend and colleague, Carla Enea, whom I have known for almost 20 years. Her unconditional love and support have been nothing short of amazing. She is a true friend and a kind and supportive person who has an exceptional understanding of the human spirit. Without Carla Enea in my life and our company, our mission would not be what it is today.

A special thank-you to Wayne Dyer, Ph.D., an amazing teacher and author whose work has not only resonated and changed my life, but the life and health of thousands of my patients. It is my hope that both my work and the work of Dr. Dyer can continue to come together to help shift the serious diseases in our society.

I also give a thank-you in loving memory of my dear friend Cindy. She, and her husband, Doug, assisted me during the beginning of my private practice. It is one of my hopes that, in some small way, my work will be an extension of the exceptional contributions that Amy Roberts, Ph.D., gave to the field of disease prevention before her death. I dearly miss both Cindy and Amy. A very big thanks to Kirsten Beal, who has supported me and helped so much over the past 15 years that she has become a close member of my family and is one of the nicest, kindest people I could ever have in my life.

It is not an easy task to write a book that promotes healing in a way that all who read it feel included and educated at their personal level of understanding. I was given the gift of being able to work with three amazing people who have helped to craft this message with me—John W. Travis, M.D.; Meryn Callander; and Gayle Vivere, who not only know their art well, they live it. I want to thank them for their contributions to the success of *The Perfect Gene Diet*. I am truly grateful.

Lastly, I deeply appreciate my husband, Rick Cassidy, for supporting me unconditionally for over 25 years in all my hopes and dreams, both professionally and personally, and my children—Victoria, 25; Alison, 15; and Paige, 11—for being so patient.

Health care does not progress through the efforts of professionals alone—patients' feedback is a significant and integral part of each new discovery. So to all those patients, past, present, and future, I express great gratitude to you. Without you, I could not have made this journey.

Pam McDonald
October 10, 2010 (10/10/10)
Walnut Creek, California

About the Author

Pamela McDonald is a board-certified nurse-practitioner, author, and international speaker who has focused her work on the prevention of chronic illness, especially heart disease and Alzheimer's disease. Pam is a graduate of Andrew Weil, M.D.'s, Program in Integrative Medicine at the University of Arizona.

Pam has used her advanced specialty training in surgery, women's health care, adult primary care, pediatrics, pediatric obesity, family practice, cardiovascular- and heart-disease prevention, nutrition, exercise, sports medicine, mind-body medicine, energy medicine, and botanical medicine to develop the groundbreaking diet based on the Apo E Gene.

The foundation of her work utilizes the body's own unique genetic expression in combination with its innate healing system. She brings together leading-edge tools in medical science and technology, as well utilizing today's rigorous scientific research. This enables her to prescribe a unique patient program that honors each person's uniqueness in mind, body, emotion, and spirit, while utilizing resources such as organic whole food, exercise therapies, and powerful effective behavioral changes—all coming together in a powerful healing solution.

Pam was born in Paisley, Scotland, and grew up in the southernmost part of England. Originally trained as a nurse at the Royal Hospital of St. Bartholomew's in London, England, she now lives in Northern California with her husband, Rick, and three children.

Healing Magic

You say you are a healer,
binding up wounds and
applying potions and salves
for a broken humanity.

Tell me, kind healer,
have you found on your journey
a wound deeper
than lovelessness?
A person more broken
than the one who's own heart
was long ago abandoned
in search of what we do not know,
if not for Love itself.

And tell me gentle healer,
how do you bind the wound
of lovelessness?
What potions and salves
do you carry
in your black bag
that can mend a broken heart?

"I'm sorry," you say, "I have nothing,
there is nothing I can do."
And that, dear friend,
is where you are wrong

Put down the bag:
Leave go of the rummaging
for magic other than your own,
open your heart,
pick up a hand,
Gaze into an eye,
Share in
one
true
moment,
and watch healing begin.

Many thanks to Janet Quinn, Ph.D., R.N.
Source: Quinn, Janet, 1996. *Alternative Therapies*

Many thanks to the following people:

Dawson Church, Elite Books, **EliteBooksOnline.com**

Billy Carpenter M.S., R.D.

Carole Dobson, MAN, R.D.

Health Stand Nutrition Consulting Inc., **HealthStandNutrition.com**

Andrea Holwegner, R.D.

Tom Joyce, CreativeWerks, **CreativeWerks.com**

Jessica Keet, Editor, **ProofreadersProofreader.com**

Jeannette Kotrys, R.D.

Deidre Lingenfelter, **ImagesbyDeidre.com**

John MacArthur, Editor

Doug Parks, Spirit 2000, **Spirit2000.com**

Ray Rimmer, Ray Rimmer Studios

Barbara Stahura, Editor, **BarbaraStahura.com**

John W. Travis, M.D., & Meryn Callander, Editors, **TheWellspring.com**

Gayle T. Vivere, The Vivere Design Team, **VivereDesign.com**

Marla Wilson, Printed Page Productions, **PrintedPage.com**

We hope you enjoyed this Hay House book. If you'd like to receive our online catalog featuring additional information on Hay House books and products, or if you'd like to find out more about the Hay Foundation, please contact:

Hay House, Inc.
P.O. Box 5100
Carlsbad, CA 92018-5100

(760) 431-7695 or **(800) 654-5126**
(760) 431-6948 (fax) or **(800) 650-5115 (fax)**
www.hayhouse.com® • **www.hayfoundation.org**

✟✟✟

Published and distributed in Australia by: Hay House Australia Pty. Ltd., 18/36 Ralph St., Alexandria NSW 2015 • *Phone:* 612-9669-4299 • *Fax:* 612-9669-4144 • www.hayhouse.com.au

Published and distributed in the United Kingdom by: Hay House UK, Ltd., 292B Kensal Rd., London W10 5BE • *Phone:* 44-20-8962-1230 • *Fax:* 44-20-8962-1239 • www.hayhouse.co.uk

Published and distributed in the Republic of South Africa by: Hay House SA (Pty), Ltd., P.O. Box 990, Witkoppen 2068 • *Phone/Fax:* 27-11-467-8904 • info@hayhouse.co.za • www.hayhouse.co.za

Published in India by: Hay House Publishers India, Muskaan Complex, Plot No. 3, B-2, Vasant Kunj, New Delhi 110 070 • *Phone:* 91-11-4176-1620 • *Fax:* 91-11-4176-1630 • www.hayhouse.co.in

Distributed in Canada by: Raincoast, 9050 Shaughnessy St., Vancouver, B.C. V6P 6E5 • *Phone:* (604) 323-7100 • *Fax:* (604) 323-2600 • www.raincoast.com

✟✟✟

Take Your Soul on a Vacation

Visit **www.HealYourLife.com®** to regroup, recharge, and reconnect with your own magnificence. Featuring blogs, mind-body-spirit news, and life-changing wisdom from Louise Hay and friends.

Visit **www.HealYourLife.com** today!

Mind Your Body,
Mend Your Spirit

Hay House is the ultimate resource for inspirational and health-conscious books, audio programs, movies, events, e-newsletters, member communities, and much more.

Visit **www.hayhouse.com**® today and nourish your soul.

UPLIFTING EVENTS
Join your favorite authors at live events in a city near you or log on to **www.hayhouse.com** to visit with Hay House authors online during live, interactive Web events.

INSPIRATIONAL RADIO
Daily inspiration while you're at work or at home. Enjoy radio programs featuring your favorite authors, streaming live on the Internet 24/7 at **HayHouseRadio.com**®. Tune in and tune up your spirit!

VIP STATUS
Join the Hay House VIP membership program today and enjoy exclusive discounts on books, CDs, calendars, card decks, and more. You'll also receive 10% off all event reservations (excluding cruises). Visit **www.hayhouse.com/wisdom** to join the Hay House Wisdom Community™.

Visit **www.hayhouse.com** and enter priority code 2723
during checkout for special savings!
(One coupon per customer.)